CLINICS
IN
GASTROENTEROLOGY

CLINICS IN GASTROENTEROLOGY

VOLUME 12/NUMBER 2
MAY 1983

MALABSORPTION AND NUTRITIONAL SUPPORT

Marvin H. Sleisenger, MD, FACP
Guest Editor

W. B. Saunders Company Ltd London · Philadelphia · Toronto

W. B. Saunders Company Ltd: 1 St Anne's Road
Eastbourne, East Sussex BN21 3UN

West Washington Square
Philadelphia, PA 19105, USA

1 Goldthorne Avenue
Toronto, Ontario M8Z 5T9, Canada

Cedro 512
Mexico 4, DF Mexico

9 Waltham Street
Artarmon, NSW 2064, Australia

Ichibancho Central Building, 22-1 Ichibancho
Chiyoda-ku, Tokyo 102, Japan

ISSN 0300-5089

Clinics in Gastroenterology is published three times each year by W. B. Saunders Company Ltd. Subscription price is £21.50 per annum.

The editor of this publication is William Wolvey, W. B. Saunders Company Ltd, 1 St Anne's Road, Eastbourne, East Sussex BN21 3UN.

Printed at The Lavenham Press Ltd, Lavenham, Suffolk, England.

Contributors to This Issue

THEODORE M. BAYLESS, MD, Professor of Medicine, Johns Hopkins University School of Medicine; Physician, Johns Hopkins Hospital, 600 N. Wolfe Street, Baltimore, MD 21205, USA.

DANIEL D. BIKLE, MD, PhD, Assistant Professor of Medicine, University of California, San Francisco; Codirector of Special Diagnostic and Treatment Unit, Veterans Administration Medical Center, 4150 Clement Street (111 N), San Francisco, CA 94121, USA.

LLOYD L. BRANDBORG, MD, Clinical Professor and Lecturer in Pathology, Department of Medicine, University of California, San Francisco; Staff Physician, Veterans Administration Medical Center, 4150 Clement Street, San Francisco, CA 94121, USA.

THOMAS A. BRASITUS, MD, Assistant Professor of Medicine, Department of Medicine, Gastrointestinal Unit, College of Physicians and Surgeons of Columbia University, Black Building 11-1101, 630 West 168th Street, New York, NY 10032, USA; Columbia Presbyterian Medical Center, New York, USA.

JOHN P. CELLO, MD, Associate Professor of Medicine, University of California, San Francisco; Chief, Gastroenterology, San Francisco General Hospital, 339 Building 100, 1001 Portrero Avenue, San Francisco, CA 94110, USA.

WILLIAM F. DOE, MBBS, MSc, MRCP, FRACP, Professor, John Curtin School of Medical Research, Australian National University, Department of Medicine and Clinical Science, 4th Floor, Central Health Laboratory Building, Woden Valley Hospital, Garren, ACT 2606, Australia; Visiting Medical Officer, Royal Canberra Hospital, Canberra; Consultant Medical Physician, Calvary Hospital, Australia.

Z. MYRON FALCHUK, MD, Associate Professor of Medicine, Harvard Medical School, Boston; Investigator, Center for Blood Research, 800 Huntingdon Avenue, Boston, MA 02115, USA; Physician, New England Deaconess Hospital, and Brigham and Women's Hospital, Boston, USA.

HUGH JAMES FREEMAN, MD, CM, FRCP(C), FACP, Associate Professor of Medicine and Head, Division of Gastroenterology, Department of Medicine, University of British Columbia, 2211, Westbrook Mall, Vancouver, British Columbia V6T IW5, Canada; Head, Gastroenterology, University of British Columbia Health Sciences Center Hospital, Vancouver, Canada.

N. D. GALLAGHER, MD, FRACP, Head, A. W. Morrow Department of Gastroenterology, Royal Prince Alfred Hospital, Sydney 2050, Australia.

ROBERT M. GLICKMAN, MD, Samuel Bard Professor of Medicine and Chairman, Division of Gastroenterology, Department of Medicine, Columbia University College of Physicians and Surgeons, 630 West 168th Street, New York, NY 10032, USA; Director of Medical Service, The Presbyterian Hospital of New York City, New York, USA.

PETER H. R. GREEN, MBBS, MD(Sydney), FRACP, Assistant Professor of Clinical Medicine, Division of Gastroenterology, Department of Medicine, Columbia University College of Physicians and Surgeons, 630 West 168th Street, New York, NY 10032, USA; Attending Physician, The Presbyterian Hospital of New York City, USA.

JAMES H. GRENDELL, MD, Assistant Professor of Medicine and Physiology, University of California, San Francisco; Attending Physician, Department of Medicine, 5H-22, San Francisco General Hospital, 1001 Portrero Street, San Francisco, CA 94110, USA.

ANDREW J. HAPEL, MD, Research Fellow, The John Curtin School of Medical Research, Australian National University, PO Box 334, Canberra City, ACT 2601, Australia.

PETER E. T. ISAACS, MD, MRCP, Senior Registrar in Gastroenterology, Gastroenterology Unit, Guy's Hospital, St Thomas Street, London SE1 9RT.

YOUNG S. KIM, MD, FACP, Professor of Medicine, Department of Medicine, University of California, San Francisco; Gastroenterologist, Gastrointestinal Research Laboratory, Veterans Administration Hospital, 4150 Clement Street, San Francisco, CA 94121, USA.

CHARLES E. KING, MD, Associate Professor of Medicine, Division of Gastroenterology and Nutrition, University of Florida College of Medicine, Gainesville; Veterans Administration Medical Center, Gainesville, FL 32610, USA.

JOHN A. MORRIS Jr, MD, Trauma and Burn Research Fellow, University of California at San Francisco General Hospital, 1001 Portrero Avenue, San Francisco, CA 94110, USA.

WARD A. OLSEN, MD, Professor of Medicine, University of Wisconsin, Madison; Chief of Gastroenterology, William S. Middleton Memorial Veterans Hospital, Madison, WI 53705, USA.

ROBERT L. OWEN, MD, Associate Professor, Department of Medicine, University of California, San Francisco; Staff Physician, Cell Biology Service, 151-E, Veterans Administration Medical Center, 4150 Clement Street, San Francisco, CA 94121, USA.

WILLIAM J. RAVICH, MD, Assistant Professor of Medicine, Division of Gastroenterology, The Johns Hopkins University School of Medicine, Baltimore; Attending Physician, The Johns Hopkins Hospital, 600 N. Wolfe Street, Baltimore, MD 21205, USA.

MICHAEL E. RYAN, MD, *formerly* Fellow in Gastroenterology, Department of Medicine, William S. Middleton Memorial Veterans Hospital and University of Wisconsin, Madison, WI 53705, USA; *now* Staff Member, Section of Gastroenterology, Marshfield Clinic, Marshfield, WI 54449, USA.

VAL SELIVANOV, MD, Trauma and Burn Research Felllow, University of California at San Francisco General Hospital, 1001 Portrero Avenue, San Francisco, CA 94110, USA.

GEORGE F. SHELDON, MD, Professor of Surgery, University of California, San Francisco; Chief of Trauma and Hyperalimentation Service, San Francisco General Hospital, 1001 Portrero Avenue, San Francisco, CA 94110, USA.

MARVIN H. SLEISENGER, MD, FACP, Professor of Medicine and Vice-Chairman, Department of Medicine, University of California, San Francisco; Chief, Medical Service, Veterans Administration Medical Center, 4150 Clement Street, San Francisco, CA 94121, USA.

PHILLIP P. TOSKES, MD, Professor of Medicine and Director, Division of Gastroenterology and Nutrition, University of Florida College of Medicine, Florida; Veterans Administration Medical Center, Gainesville, FL 32610, USA.

ELLIOT WESER, MD, Professor of Medicine, Department of Medicine, The University of Texas Health Science Center at San Antonio; Chief, Medical Service, Audie L. Murphy Veterans Hospital, Medical Service (111), 7400 Merton Minter Boulevard, San Antonio, TX 78248, USA.

Table of Contents

RECENT ISSUES

FORTHCOMING ISSUE

Foreword

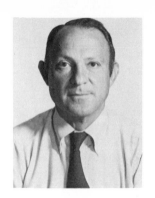

Malabsorption by the small intestine is an identifiable syndrome of nutritional deficiencies, although the spectrum of signs and symptoms is wide. Continuing study of the pathogenesis of disease associated with the syndrome, as well as the pathophysiology underlying its signs and symptoms, has led to significantly greater understanding of normal small bowel function in the past two decades.

The search for clearer understanding of the bases for the spectrum of abnormalities has led to a clearer definition of intestinal transport processes, including fat, carbohydrate and, particularly, protein; of the hormonal role of vitamin D and its metabolites in absorption of calcium; of the contribution of gut microorganisms to homeostasis; of the importance of immunological defence mechanisms which reside in the small gut mucosa; of protein-calorie malnutrition; of the complexity of vitamin B_{12} and folate uptake and metabolism; of factors which stimulate adaptive mechanisms for absorption; and of a logical approach to the clinical detection of malabsorption of fat and carbohydrate, as well as vitamins, folate and minerals.

This issue was planned to present important clinical data regarding the malabsorption syndrome reflecting major pathophysiological sequelae of disease and disorders of the small intestine. Accordingly, chapters are included that deal with disturbances of vitamin D metabolism and of fat absorption, the noxious effects of alcohol, drugs, gluten (and perhaps other food substances) on small gut function, and bacterial contamination of the upper portion of the small bowel, including a review of breath tests. Some aspects of protein digestion and nutrition have been emphasized, namely adaptation following massive bowel resection. Principles of total parenteral nutrition and an overview of nutritional aspects of malabsorption with emphasis on protein malnutrition are included.

On balance, then, we believe that the articles in this *Clinics in Gastroenterology* on malabsorption and nutritional support will review for the reader the important and basic physiological principles of absorption, update the pathophysiological consequences of disturbances of the many mechanisms involved, and offer information on nutritional support.

MARVIN H. SLEISENGER

1

Fat Absorption and Malabsorption

ROBERT M. GLICKMAN

The average western diet contains approximately 100 g of fat. The marked efficiency of the entire process of fat absorption can be judged by the fact that under normal conditions less than 5 per cent of ingested fat is recovered in the stool. A thorough understanding of this process requires an appreciation of the physical chemistry of lipids, the physiology of bile salts, and the formation and metabolism of lipoproteins, all directly influencing the process of fat absorption. Fat absorption is a multistep process involving the coordinated participation of several organs (Figure 1) and can be conveniently considered as being composed of (a) luminal, (b) mucosal, and (c) secretory (lymphatic or portal venous transport) phases.

In the present discussion the major principles of fat absorption will be stressed and correlated with appropriate examples of how this process may become disordered, resulting in steatorrhoea.

INTRALUMINAL DIGESTION

Most dietary fat is ingested in the form of triglycerides containing three long-chain fatty acids on a glycerol backbone. While pancreatic lipolysis is quantitatively more important, hydrolysis of dietary fat begins in the stomach; estimates of the proportion range from 10 to 30 per cent (Hamosh et al, 1973, 1975). Hydrolysis is accomplished by a lingual lipase acting in the stomach, active at gastric pH and not requiring bile salts. Liberation of some fatty acids in the stomach serves to stabilize the surface of the triglyceride emulsion and promotes the binding of pancreatic colipase (see below). In addition, liberated fatty acids also aid in liberating cholecystokinin-pancreozymin (CCK-PZ) from the duodenal mucosa. Lingual lipase may have an important role in fat digestion in situations where pancreatic function is impaired, such as in premature infants and cystic fibrosis (Ross and Sammons, 1955; Hamosh et al, 1981).

Most triglyceride lipolysis occurs in the duodenum secondary to the action of pancreatic lipases. In the duodenum the water-insoluble triglyceride is further emulsified by mechanical factors and mixes with pancreatic secretions, particularly bicarbonate and water, which increase duodenal pH to 6 or 6.5. Pancreatic lipase reversibly hydrolyses triglyceride at the 1,3 positions, leaving β-monoglyceride, diglycerides, and free fatty

Clinics in Gastroenterology — Vol. 12, No. 2, May 1983

0300-5089/83/1202-323 $05.00©1983 W. B. Saunders Company Ltd

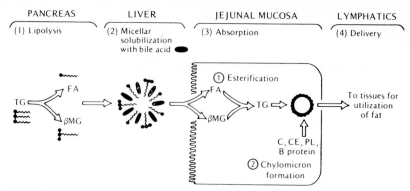

Figure 1. Schematic of intestinal fat absorption showing the participation of pancreas, liver and intestinal mucosal cell in fat absorption. From Wilson and Dietschy (1971), with kind permission of the authors and the editor of *Gastroenterology*.

acid as the products of lipolysis. Recent evidence has shown that for pancreatic lipase to be active in triglyceride hydrolysis an additional pancreatic factor is required. This is a protein of low molecular weight (approximately 10 000), secreted by the pancreas, called colipase (Borgstrom, 1975a). It facilitates lipase action by binding to bile salt-lipid surfaces, facilitating the interaction of lipase with triglyceride and permitting efficient hydrolysis. Isolated colipase deficiency (lipase normal) has recently been described in two brothers with resulting fat malabsorption of 50 per cent (Hildebrand et al, 1982). This is similar to isolated pancreatic lipase deficiency (colipase normal) where steatorrhoea is 50 per cent (Figarella, Negri and Sarles, 1972). Other requirements for effective hydrolysis are bile salts which are necessary for optimum lipase activity (Hofman, 1965). The process of intraluminal triglyceride emulsification and hydrolysis requires the coordination of pancreatic secretion with the presence of lipid in the upper portion of the small intestine. This is accomplished by release of cholecystokinin-pancreozymin (CCK-PZ) from duodenal epithelial cells in response to the presence of lipid and protein in the lumen (Meyer and Jones, 1974). In addition, this hormone causes gall-bladder contraction and simultaneous relaxation of the sphincter of Oddi (Lin, 1975), enabling bile salt secretion to be synchronous with the presence of fat in the upper part of the intestine. In addition, secretin is released from the duodenal mucosa by gastric acid, and this hormone stimulates pancreatic fluid and bicarbonate secretion, an important factor in raising duodenal pH to permit effective lipolysis (Rayford, Miller and Thompson, 1976). Impaired lipolysis due to clinical disorders can now be classified with respect to the aforementioned considerations (Table 1).

Bile salts and their role in intraluminal fat absorption

Bile salts are trihydroxy or dihydroxy bile acids that are conjugated with either taurine or glycine. Eighty per cent of the bile salts released into the bile are primary bile salts, cholic acid and chenodeoxycholic acid, which are

Table 1. *Conditions associated with impaired lipolysis*

Postgastrectomy
  Rapid transit ('dumping')
  Improper emulsification of triglyceride, bicarbonate and lipase, e.g., Billroth II anastomosis

Altered duodenal pH
  Acid hypersecretion — Zollinger-Ellison syndrome

Decreased CCK-PZ release
  Severe intestinal mucosal destruction, e.g., sprue, regional enteritis

Congenital lipase or colipase deficiency

Pancreatic insufficiency
  Loss of lipase and bicarbonate secretion
  Chronic pancreatitis
  Pancreatic duct obstruction

Decreased luminal bile salts
  See Table 2

---

synthesized in the liver. The secondary bile salts, deoxycholic and litho-cholic acids, which contribute 20 per cent of the pool, are formed from the primary bile acids as metabolic products of intestinal bacterial action. Approximately 600-800 mg of bile salts are synthesized each day by the liver, an amount equal to that lost in the stool. Although the total bile salt pool is only 2-4 g, the amount of bile salts actually passing through the intestine each day is 20-30 g. This is the result of enterohepatic circulation whereby bile salts are actively absorbed in the terminal ileum and returned to the liver by the portal venous system. In order to accommodate the needs of lipid absorption, the bile acid pool may be recycled several times during the course of a single meal (Borgstrom, 1975b).

The products of triglyceride lipolysis — monoglyceride, free fatty acids and glycerol — still have only limited solubility in the aqueous environment of the intestinal lumen. This is also true for other lipids such as cholesterol and the fat-soluble vitamins. Efficient absorption depends on micellar formation in which these lipid moieties interact with bile salts in mixed aggregates or micelles. The bile salt molecule, consisting of hydrophobic and hydrophilic portions, can interact with lipids in an aqueous environment and solubilizes these moieties. These multimolecular aggregates of bile salts, monoglyceride, fatty acids and cholesterol are called 'micelles'. The lowest concentration of bile salts at which such aggregates are present in solution is termed the 'critical micellar concentration'.

In a recent report it is suggested that the traditional concept of micellariz-ation and absorption may be subdivided into several coexisting phases. Direct observation of lipolysis by light microscopy reveals an initial crystalline phase of digestion in which calcium and fatty acids are formed, and this is followed by the production of a viscous isotropic phase composed predominantly of monoglycerides and protonated fatty acids. Thus, other phases may coexist with the micellar phase during fat absorption. However, the exact sequence of events and the quantitative importance of these events require further elucidation.

Successful micellarization of lipids within the intestinal lumen permits these lipid products to diffuse to the surface of the intestinal epithelium and to make intimate contact with the microvillus membrane. This is particularly important since it has been shown experimentally that covering the surface of the intestine is an unstirred water layer (Wilson et al, 1971, 1972) which functionally may pose a significant barrier to the diffusion of hydrophobic molecules such as lipids. This relatively immobile aqueous layer is more easily penetrated by the micellar complex, thus increasing the efficiency of lipid uptake into the intestinal mucosal cell. The apparent thickness of this layer is largely unknown, but recent estimates suggest that it may be substantial (600 μm) (Read, Leven and Holdsworth, 1976; Smithson et al, 1981).

Any condition which results in a reduced concentration of bile salts within the intestinal lumen (below the critical micellar concentration) will result in impaired micellar solubilization of lipids (Table 2). A particularly graphic example of impaired micelle formation leading to steatorrhoea is that associated with ileal resection (Austad, Lack and Tyor, 1967; Hofmann and Poley, 1972). With modest degrees of ileal resection (less than 100 cm), increased hepatic synthesis of bile salts can compensate for increased faecal losses, maintaining the micellar concentration of bile salts in the jejunum within normal limits; hence, there is no steatorrhoea. With larger degrees of ileal resection (greater than 100 cm), hepatic synthesis is maximally increased but cannot compensate for these large faecal losses, resulting in reduction of jejunal bile acid concentration and steatorrhoea. In this situation, lipolysis and mucosal epithelial function are normal, and the malabsorption is a 'pure' example of bile salt deficiency. This example also illustrates the obligatory requirement of active ileal bile salt absorption, a function which cannot be assumed by the more proximal small bowel.

Table 2. *Conditions associated with impaired micelle formation*

Decreased hepatic synthesis of bile salts
  Severe parenchymal liver disease

Decreased delivery of bile salts to the intestinal lumen
  Biliary obstruction (stone, tumour, primary biliary cirrhosis)
  Cholestatic liver disease

Decreased effective concentration of conjugated bile acids
  Increased acidity (Zollinger-Ellison) — decreased ionization of bile salts with increased
    proximal absorption
  Drugs affecting micelle formation — neomycin, cholestyramine
  Stasis syndromes with secondary bacterial overgrowth and bile salt deconjugation

Increased intestinal loss of bile salts
  Ileal disease or resection

MUCOSAL PHASE OF FAT ABSORPTION

The uptake of lipids, such as fatty acids and monoglycerides, across the microvillus membrane is a passive process which results from the solubility of the lipid moieties within the lipid-rich surface membrane of the epithelial cell. A low-molecular-weight cytosolic protein, fatty acid binding protein (FABP), has been isolated from the intestine (Ockner and Manning, 1976). Fatty acid binding protein avidly binds fatty acids and appears to function as an intracellular transport protein for long-chain fatty acids; it may serve a transport function within the intestinal epithelium, directing intracellular fatty acids to the smooth endoplasmic reticulum, the site of triglyceride resynthesis. A schematic representation of events within the cell is shown in Figure 2. Triglyceride resynthesis reduces the effective concentration of fatty acids within the cell and maintains an effective concentration gradient for continued passive uptake.

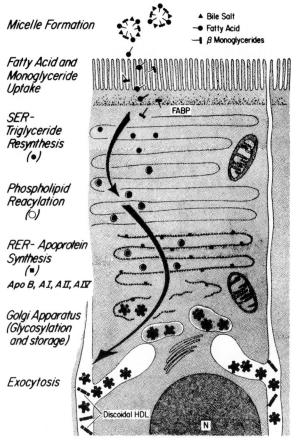

Figure 2. Schematic representation of events within an intestinal epithelial cell during fat absorption.

The enzymes for triglyceride resynthesis have been localized bio-chemically in the smooth endoplasmic reticulum in the apical portion of the intestinal epithelial cell beneath the microvillus membrane. This is corroborated morphologically in that the earliest time triglyceride can be observed within the intestinal epithelial cell is within the profiles of the smooth endoplasmic reticulum (Cardell, Badenhausen and Porter, 1967). With time, one can follow the movement of these triglyceride droplets through the profiles of the endoplasmic reticulum to the Golgi apparatus in the supranuclear portion of the cell. Here, clusters of chylomicrons can be seen within the saccules of the Golgi apparatus. Golgi vesicles then migrate towards the laterobasal membrane where they appear to fuse with the membrane and discharge their contents into the intercellular space by reverse pinocytosis. Experimental evidence suggests that this directed intracellular movement may, in part, depend on intact microtubular function (Glickman, Perrotto and Kirsch, 1976).

CHARACTERISTICS OF INTESTINAL LIPOPROTEINS

Although the morphological events of triglyceride transport have been well defined, less is known concerning the biochemical events of chylomicron formation. Table 3 shows the chemical composition of rat mesenteric lymph chylomicrons (Glickman, 1975) and of chylomicrons obtained from the urine of two patients, studied in our laboratory, with chyluria due to long-standing filarial disease and documented communications between mesenteric and renal lymphatic systems (Green et al, 1979a, b). It can be seen that triglyceride comprises the major portion of chylomicron lipid, which reflects the major physiological role of this particle in fat absorption. Phospholipid, the next most abundant lipid, is important in chylomicron structure; together with free cholesterol and chylomicron protein, it is arranged on the surface of this particle. Although the intestine can synthesize phospholipid de novo for the chylomicron surface, it appears that a variable proportion of chylomicron phospholipid may be derived from luminal sources (i.e., biliary lecithin) after reacylation of absorbed lysolecithin.

Table 3. *Characteristics of rat (Glickman, 1975) and human (Green et al, 1979a) lymph chylomicrons*

Chemical composition	Percentage composition by weight	
	Rat	Human
Triglyceride	84	91
Phospholipid	13	7.5
Cholesterol	2	1.6
Protein	1	1.3

Although quantitatively small (1 per cent of chylomicron mass), chylomicron apoproteins contain a characteristic complement of specific proteins (Glickman and Green, 1977; Imaizumi, Fainaru and Havel, 1978). Figure 3 shows the apoprotein composition of rat and human lymph chylomicrons after delipidation and electrophoresis on sodium dodecyl sulphate polyacrylamide gels. Note the similarity in the protein patterns from these two species. Of particular importance to intestinal lipid transport is apoB.

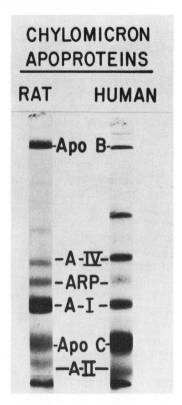

Figure 3. Apoprotein composition of rat (mesenteric lymph) and human chylomicrons (isolated from chyluria). The apoproteins are separated by sodium dodecyl sulphate polyacrylamide gel electrophoresis.

In addition, apoA-I, the major apoprotein of circulating high density lipoprotein in most species, is also an important chylomicron component and comprises 20 per cent of chylomicron protein in man (Green et al, 1979a) and 40 per cent in the rat (Glickman and Kirsch, 1973). This apoprotein is also an activator of lecithin:cholesterol acyltransferase (LCAT), a plasma enzyme responsible for cholesterol esterification. ApoA-IV is a newly described chylomicron apoprotein in man (Weisgraber, Bersot and Mahley, 1978; Green et al, 1979b) and is analogous to a similar apoprotein in the rat (Wu and Windmeller, 1978). Its metabolic importance remains to be determined. A group of apoproteins of low molecular weight, the C apoproteins, are also found on lymph chylomicrons (Imaizumi, Fainaru and Havel, 1978). One of this group, apoC-II, is an activator of lipoprotein lipase and, hence, is of extreme importance in the catabolism of chylomicrons after secretion (Ganesan et al, 1971; Brown and Baginsky, 1972). In a recent report (Breckenridge et al, 1978) a man was described with severe hypertriglyceridaemia and a complete deficiency of this lipoprotein lipase activator, apoC-II, resulting in a marked impairment of chylomicron lipolysis. After partial replacement of apoC-II by transfusion of plasma from a normal subject, the patient's plasma triglyceride levels fell, within one day, from 1000 to 250 mg/dl.

A variety of studies have demonstrated the active synthesis of several chylomicron apoproteins during fat absorption (Glickman and Kirsch, 1973; Weisgraber, Bersot and Mahley, 1978; Wu and Windmeller, 1978; Green et al, 1979b). In many species, including man, apoB, apoA-IV and apoA-I appear to be actively synthesized by the enterocyte. Small amounts of the C proteins may also be synthesized by the intestine (Wu and Windmeller, 1978), but most is acquired by chylomicrons after secretion by the cell.

The presence of apoB in intestinal epithelial cells and its role during fat absorption have been demonstrated using fluorescent antibody techniques (Glickman, Khorana and Kilgore, 1976). A progressive, rapid increase in apoB fluorescence, which gradually fills the entire apex of the cell, has been shown. The distribution of fluorescence in the apical and supranuclear portions of the cell suggests that a pool of the apoprotein is present within the cell and, with active lipid absorption, that there is a progressive increase in apoB fluorescence consistent with the known increase in the synthesis of this apoprotein during chylomicron formation (Windmeller, Herbert and Levy, 1973). Recent work in in our laboratory in the rat has shown a sustained increase in the apoB content of mucosal cells during triglyceride absorption.

Although quantitatively a small proportion of chylomicron mass, apoprotein synthesis appears to be extremely critical for triglyceride transport through the intestinal mucosa. Figure 4 shows an intestinal biopsy specimen from a patient after an 18-hour fast. The mucosa is engorged with large droplets which, on analysis, are triglyceride droplets. Such an appearance in the fasting state is abnormal and suggests an impairment in triglyceride transport. This biopsy specimen was obtained from a patient with abetalipoproteinaemia (Levy, Fredrickson and Laster, 1966), a rare hereditary disorder associated with a total inability to form triglyceride-rich lipoproteins. It has recently been shown that the intestinal mucosa of such patients, despite being engorged with triglyceride, completely lacks immunoreactive apoB (Glickman et al, 1979), and this apoprotein is also absent in the plasma. It appears that other apoproteins are normal. Thus, this rare disease has clearly shown that apoB synthesis is an obligatory step in chylomicron formation and that in its absence there is a total inability to form chylomicrons. Recently, compelling evidence has been presented that organ-specific forms of apoB may be present in man, i.e., intestinal and hepatic apoB (Kane, Hardman and Paulus, 1980). The description of a patient with the inability to secrete apoB from the liver while preserving intestinal apoB and chylomicron secretion is of great interest in this regard (Molloy et al, 1981). It is also probable that disorders will be discovered of impaired intestinal apoB synthesis with hepatic apoB synthesis preserved. Such patients will have intestinal biopsies similar to that in Figure 4 but will retain hepatic lipoprotein secretion. Thus, plasma very low density and low density lipoprotein levels will be largely normal and such patients will not be suspected of having a form of 'abetalipoproteinaemia'. There are no human

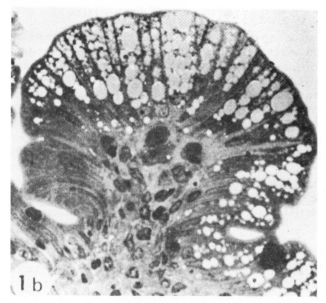

Figure 4. Biopsy specimen of the intestine after an 18-hour fast in a patient with abetalipo-proteinaemia.

disease states associated with an inability to synthesize apoA-I or apoA-IV, and experimental studies in animals suggest that these apoproteins are not absolutely required for chylomicron formation to proceed. Similar biopsy specimens showing engorgement of the mucosa with triglyceride have been seen in human protein calorie malnutrition (Theron, Wittmann and Prinston, 1971) as well as in experimental conditions in animals with impaired protein synthesis (Glickman and Kirsch, 1973). Thus, intact protein synthesis appears to be necessary for chylomicron formation to proceed.

Although studies of chylomicron apoprotein synthesis have not been carried out in various human malabsorptive disorders, it is probable that in mucosal destructive disease (e.g., sprue) or severe protein calorie malnutrition, impaired apoprotein synthesis is a contributing factor in the resulting malabsorption. In addition, it is probable that the complex series of synthetic steps required for chylomicron formation is most fully developed in mature, differentiated villus epithelial cells. While less differentiated cells along the villus contain apoproteins, it is not known whether they can secrete lipoproteins. Disease states, such as sprue and other conditions associated with intestinal repair or regeneration, are characterized by functionally immature (less differentiated) epithelial cells populating the intestinal villus, perhaps with a limited capacity for chylomicron formation.

INTESTINAL HDL SECRETION

While the preceding discussion has focused on triglyceride absorption and chylomicron secretion, there is increasing evidence that the intestine may elaborate lipoproteins in the absence of triglyceride absorption. Specifically, high density lipoproteins have been isolated from rat mesenteric lymph and have been shown to have distinctive chemical and morphological differences from plasma HDL (Green, Tall and Glickman, 1978). In lymph, HDL exist as either discoidal or small spherical particles and contain more phospholipid and apoA-I than plasma HDL. These particles continue to be secreted during experimental biliary diversion (Bearnot et al, 1982) despite markedly reduced lymphatic triglyceride secretion. Such evidence supports the hypothesis that the intestine can elaborate lipoproteins, independent of triglyceride absorption, and may contribute an important class of lipoproteins (HDL) to systemic lipoprotein metabolism.

LIPOPROTEIN SECRETION

Lymphatic transport is required for triglyceride-rich lipoproteins to reach the systemic circulation after secretion from the intestinal cell. With lymphatic obstruction, intestinal fat transport is impaired. This is the case in such diseases associated with lymphatic obstruction as intestinal lymphangiectasia (Dobbins, 1976), Whipples' disase (Trier, 1978) and lymphoma, in which lymphatic obstruction is not uncommon. In such situations the therapeutic use of medium-chain triglycerides is advantageous since fatty acids of less than 12 carbons in length are not incorporated into chylomicrons (Greenberger and Skillman, 1969) but pass directly into the portal blood. Therefore they provide the caloric supplementation of fat without requiring micellarization, chylomicron formation or lymphatic transport.

THE IMPORTANCE OF THE INTESTINE IN SYSTEMIC LIPOPROTEIN METABOLISM

There is mounting evidence that the intestine is a major synthetic source of apoprotein constituents of important plasma lipoproteins. As already noted, apoproteins such as apoB, apoA-I and apoA-IV are actively synthesized by the intestine during triglyceride absorption. As noted above, high density lipoproteins are also secreted (Green, Tall and Glickman, 1978), and constitute an additional source of apoA-I for plasma. Since these lipoproteins of intestinal origin enter the systemic circulation they directly contribute to the levels of these apoproteins in plasma. This is especially true for apoA-I which has been shown to leave the chylomicron surface after secretion and eventuate in plasma high density lipoproteins (Redgrave and Small, 1979; Tall, Green and Glickman, 1979). Estimates in man indicate that as much as 30-50 per cent of the total daily synthesis of this apoprotein may originate in the intestine and thus directly influence plasma high density lipoprotein metabolism (Green et al, 1979a). A detailed review of intestinal lipoprotein metabolism has recently been published (Green and Glickman, 1981). Further research is required to determine factors which modulate the intestinal synthesis of such apoproteins. Sufficient data are already available to indicate that dietary influences and their effect on the quantitative and qualitative aspects of intestinal lipoprotein formation will have important consequences for systemic lipoprotein metabolism.

REFERENCES

Austad, W. I., Lack, L. & Tyor, M. P. (1967) Importance of bile acids and of an intact distal small intestine for fat absorption. *Gastroenterology,* **52,** 638.

Bearnot, H. R., Glickman, R. M., Weinberg, L. et al (1982) Effect of biliary diversion on rat mesenteric lymph apolipoprotein-I and high density lipoprotein. *Journal of Clinical Investigation,* **69,** 210-217.

Borgstrom, B. (1975a) On the interaction between pancreatic lipase and colipase and the substrate, and the importance of bile salts. *Journal of Lipid Research,* **16,** 411.

Borgstrom, B. (1975b) On the importance of bile salts. *Journal of Lipid Research,* **16,** 415.

Breckenridge, W. C., Little, J., Steiner, G. et al (1978) Hypertriglyceridaemia associated with deficiency of apolipoprotein C-II. *New England Journal of Medicine,* **298,** 1265.

Brown, W. V. & Baginsky, M. L. (1972) Inhibition of lipoprotein lipase by an apoprotein of human very low density lipoprotein. *Biochemical and Biophysical Research Communications,* **46,** 375.

Cardell, R. R. Jr, Badenhausen, S. & Porter, K. P. (1967) Intestinal triglyceride absorption in the rat. An electron microscopical study. *Journal of Cell Biology,* **34,** 125.

Dobbins, W. O. III (1976) Electron microscope study of the intestinal mucosa in intestinal lymphangiectasia. *Gastroenterology,* **51,** 1004.

Figarella, C., Negri, G. A. & Sarles, H. (1972) Presence of colipase in cogenital pancreatic lipase deficiency. *Biochimica et Biophysica Acta,* **280,** 205-210.

Ganesan, D., Bradfort, R. H., Alaupovic, P. et al (1971) Differential activation of lipoprotein lipase from human post-heparin plasma, milk and tissue by polypeptides of human serum apolipoproteins. *FEBS Letters,* **15,** 205.

Glickman, R. M. (1975) Chylomicron formation by the intestine. In *Lipid Absorption: Biochemical and Clinical Aspects* (Ed.) Rommel, K. pp. 99-112. Essen, FR Germany: University of Ulm and H. Goebel.

Glickman, R. M. & Green, P. H. R. (1977) The intestine as a source of apolipoprotein A-I. *Proceedings of the National Academy of Sciences of the USA,* **74,** 2569.

Glickman, R. M. & Kirsch, K. (1973) Lymph chylomicron formation during the inhibition of protein synthesis. *Journal of Clinical Investigation,* **52** (11), 2910.

Glickman, R. M., Khorana, J. & Kilgore, A. (1976) Localization of apolipoprotein B in intestinal epithelial cells. *Science,* **193,** 1254.

Glickman, R. M., Perrotto, J. L. & Kirsch, K. (1976) Intestinal lipoprotein formation: effect of colchicine. *Gastroenterology,* **70,** 347.

Glickman, R. M., Green, P. H. R., Lees, R. S. et al (1979) Immunofluorescence studies of apolipoprotein B in intestinal mucosa. Absence in abetalipoproteinaemia. *Gastroenterology,* **76,** 288.

Green, P. H. R. & Glickman, R. M. (1981) Intestinal lipoprotein metabolism. *Journal of Lipid Research,* **22,** 1153-1171.

Green, P. H. R., Tall, A. R. & Glickman, R. M. (1978) Rat intestine secretes discoid nascent high density lipoprotein. *Journal of Clinical Investigation,* **61,** 528.

Green, P. H. R., Glickman, R. M., Saudek, C. D. et al (1979a) Intestinal lipoprotein secretion in chyluric man. *Journal of Clinical Investigation,* **64,** 233.

Green, P. H. R., Glickman, R. M., Riley, J. W. et al (1979b) Human apolipoprotein A-N — intestinal origin. *Journal of Clinical Investigation,* **76,** 1143.

Greenberger, N. J. & Skillman, T. G. (1969) Medium chain triglycerides. Physiological considerations and clinical implications. *New England Journal of Medicine,* **280,** 1045.

Hamosh, M. & Scow, R. O. (1973) Lingual lipase and its role in the digestion of dietary fat. *Journal of Clinical Investigation,* **52,** 88-95.

Hamosh, M., Klaeveman, H. L., Wolf, R. O. & Scow, R. O. (1975) Pharyngeal lipase and digestion of dietary triglyceride in man. *Journal of Clinical Investigation,* **55,** 908-913.

Hamosh, M., Scanlon, J. W., Ganot, D. et al (1981) Fat digestion in the newborn. Characterization of lipase in gastric aspirates of premature and term infants. *Journal of Clinical Investigation,* **67,** 838-846.

Hilderbrand, H., Borgstrom, B., Bekassy, A. et al (1982) Isolated co-lipase deficiency in two brothers. *Gut,* **23,** 243-246.

Hofmann, A. F. (1965) Clinical implictions of physicochemical studies on bile salts. *Gastroenterology,* **48,** 484.

Hofmann, A. F. & Poley, J. R. (1972) Role of bile acid malabsorption in pathogenesis of diarrhea and steatorrhea in patients with ileal resection. I. *Gastroenterology,* **62,** 918.

Imaizumi, I., Fainaru, M. & Havel, R. J. (1978) Composition of proteins of mesenteric lymph chylomicrons in the rat and alterations upon exposure of chylomicrons to blood serum and serum proteins. *Journal of Lipid Research,* **19,** 212.

Kane, J. P., Hardman, D. A. & Paulus, H. E. (1980) Heterogeneity of apolipoprotein B: isolation of a new species from human chylomicrons. *Proceedings of the National Academy of Sciences of the USA,* **77,** 2465-2469.

Levy, R. I., Fredrickson, D. S. & Laster, L. (1966) The lipoproteins and lipid transport in abetalipoproteinemia. *Journal of Clinical Investigation,* **45,** 531.

Lin, T.-M. (1975) Actions of gastrointestinal hormones and related peptides on the motor function of the biliary tract. *Gastroenterology,* **69,** 1006.

Meyer, J. G. & Jones, R. S. (1974) Canine pancreatic responses to intestinally perfused fat and products of fat digestion. *American Journal of Physiology,* **226,** 1178.

Molloy, M. J., Kane, J. P., Hardman, D. A. et al (1981) Normotriglyceridemic abetalipoproteinemia. Absence of the B-100 apolipoprotein. *Journal of Clinical Investigation,* **67,** 1441-1450.

Ockner, R. K. & Manning, J. A. (1976) Fatty acid binding protein: role in esterification of absorbed long chain fat in rat intestine. *Journal of Clinical Investigation,* **58,** 632.

Patton, J. S. & Carey, M. C. (1979) Watching fat digestion. *Science,* **204,** 145.

Rayford, P. L., Miller, T. A. & Thompson, J. C. (1976) Secretion of cholecystokinin and new gastrointestinal hormone. *New England Journal of Medicine,* **294,** 1093-1157.

Read, N. W., Leven, R. J. & Holdsworth, C. D. (1976) Measurement of the functional unstirred layer thickness in the human jejunum in vivo. *Gut,* **17,** 387.

Redgrave, T. G. & Small, D. M. (1979) Transfer of surface components of chylomicrons to the high density lipoprotein fraction during chylomicron catabolism in the rat. *Journal of Clinical Investigation,* **64,** 162.

Ross, C. A. C. & Sammons, H. C. (1955) Non-pancreatic lipase in children with pancreatic fibrosis. *Archives of Diseases in Childhood,* **30,** 428-431.

Smithson, K. W., Millar, D. B., Jacobs, L. R. & Gray, G. M. (1981) Intestinal diffusion barrier: unstirred water layer of membrane surface mucous coat? *Science,* **214,** 1241-1244.

Tall, A. R., Green, P. H. R. & Glickman, R. M. (1979) Metabolic fate of chylomicron phospholipids and apoproteins in the rat. *Journal of Clinical Investigation,* **64,** 977.

Theron, J. J., Wittmann, W. & Prinston, J. G. (1971) The fine structure of the jejunum in Kwashiorkor. *Experimental Molecular Pathology,* **14,** 184.

Trier, J. S. (1978) Whipples' disease. In *Gastrointestinal Disease* (Ed.) Sleisenger, M. H. & Fordtran, J. S. Chapter 64. p. 1104. Philadelphia: W. B. Saunders.

Weisgraber, K. H., Bersot, T. P. & Mahley, R. W. (1978) Isolation and characterization of an apoprotein from the d<1.006 lipoproteins of human and canine lymph homologous with the rat A-IV apoprotein. *Biochemical and Biophysical Research Communications,* **85,** 287.

Wilson, F. A. & Dietschy, J. M. (1971) Differential diagnostic approach to clinical problems of malabsorption. *Gastroenterology,* **61,** 911.

Wilson, F. A. & Dietschy, J. M. (1972) Characterization of bile acid absorption across the unstirred water layer and brush border of the rat jejunum. *Journal of Clinical Investigation,* **51,** 3015.

Wilson, F. A., Sallee, V. L. & Dietschy, J. M. (1971) Unstirred water layers in the intestine rate determinant of fatty acid absorption from micellar solutions. *Science,* **174,** 1031.

Windmeller, H. G., Herbert, P. N. & Levy, R. I. (1973) Biosynthesis of lymph and plasma lipoprotein apoproteins by isolated perfused rat liver and intestine. *Journal of Lipid Research,* **14,** 215.

Wu, A.-L. & Windmeller, H. G. (1978) Identification of circulating apolipoproteins synthesized by rat small intestine in vivo. *Journal of Biological Chemistry,* **253,** 2525.

2

Carbohydrate Absorption and Malabsorption

WILLIAM J. RAVICH
THEODORE M. BAYLESS

Carbohydrates provide most humans with the majority of their energy requirements. In the average western diet, approximately 50 per cent of absorbable carbohydrates are ingested as starch with lesser proportions of sucrose, lactose, and fructose. In addition, small amounts of the absorbable sugar trehalose and non-absorbable carbohydrates including stachyose, raffinose and cellulose are ingested (McMichael, 1976; Gray, 1981). Specific patterns of sugar intake are affected by a variety of cultural and economic factors. It has become apparent through epidemiological studies on lactose malabsorption that symptoms of sugar intolerance may exert an important influence on cultural habits, resulting in avoidance of certain sugars even when those foods are readily available (Simoons, 1981).

While normally most of an ingested carbohydrate load is completely absorbed before reaching the colon, a number of disorders can result in impairment of absorption by the small intestine. Symptoms of sugar malabsorption include abdominal distension, cramps, flatulence and diarrhoea. Whether sugar malabsorption produces symptoms depends not only on the absolute intestinal digestive and absorptive capacity, but also on additional factors such as the quantity of the ingested sugar load, the rate of gastric emptying, the response of the small intestine to an osmotic load, the metabolic activity of the colonic bacterial microflora and the compensatory capacity of the colon to absorb excess water and short chain fatty acids. Sugar malabsorption and sugar intolerance are, therefore, not synonymous. The physiology and pathophysiology of sugar absorption and malabsorption will be discussed as a basis for the consideration of specific disorders of carbohydrate absorption.

DEFINITIONS

The term 'sugar malabsorption' indicates that ingested carbohydrates are incompletely absorbed by the small intestine. 'Sugar intolerance' refers to symptoms that result from sugar malabsorption.

A number of objective tests are currently used to study the completeness

0300-5089/83/1202-335 $05.00© 1983 W. B. Saunders Company Ltd of sugar absorption for clinical purposes. The term sugar malabsorption frequently refers to an abnormal result of one or more of these tests. Disaccharidase activity can be measured in fragments of small intestinal tissue obtained by peroral biopsy. 'Disaccharidase deficiency' is therefore defined as a low level of mucosal disaccharidase activity. Aside from the invasive nature of the test, the measurement fails to consider the influence of other factors on the degree of malabsorption. It is also limited to use in abnormalities in oligosaccharide digestion, as no assays are readily available for measurement of monosaccharide transport systems.

Perhaps the most widely available test for assessing sugar malabsorption is the oral sugar tolerance test. In this test serial blood samples are obtained after ingestion of a defined, usually large, sugar load. A peak rise in serum glucose of less than 20-25 mg/dl is considered to represent sugar malabsorption. If symptoms also occur with the tolerance test, the term intolerance is usually applied to that individual.

In the last decade the breath hydrogen test has been popularized for the assessment of sugar malabsorption for both clinical and research purposes. Hydrogen is produced by bacterial fermentation of undigested sugar entering the colon. A portion of this hydrogen is absorbed and excreted by the lungs. Samples of expired air can be assessed for breath hydrogen concentration by gas chromatography. A peak rise in breath hydrogen of greater than 20 parts per million over the fasting baseline value is generally accepted as indicating sugar malabsorption. One advantage of the breath hydrogen test is that it can be applied to any ingested carbohydrate. Details of breath hydrogen technique are given in a separate chapter.

Much of our understanding of sugar malabsorption in man is based on application of these three tests to different situations. The assumption is that these measurements should correlate well with measurements of sugar content of aspirates from the ileo-caecal valve area. As we extend our observations it has become apparent that sugar malabsorption represents a continuum of incomplete absorption which any test depending on a sharp division between normal and abnormal will fail to appreciate.

PHYSIOLOGY

For absorption to occur, carbohydrates must be presented to the intestinal epithelium in monosaccharide form. As most sugars are ingested as polysaccharides (starch) and disaccharides (sucrose, lactose), digestion must precede absorption. There are three distinct phases in which carbohydrates are prepared for absorption and then transferred into the intestinal cell (Figure 1).

Phase of luminal digestion

Starch is a complex carbohydrate in which branching chains of glucose molecules are linked together by α-1,4 and α-1,6 bonds. Unbranched chains, in which the glucose moieties are linked by α-1,4 bonds only, are referred to as amylose, while those with branched chains connected by α-1,6 bonds are called amylopectin.

LUMEN   INTESTINAL CELL

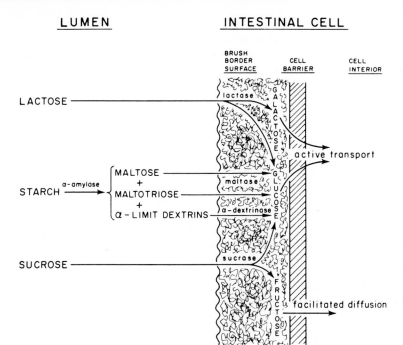

Figure 1. Carbohydrate absorption involves three distinct phases. In the luminal phase, ingested polysaccharides are hydrolysed into the oligosaccharides maltose, maltotriose, and α-limit dextrins. In the brush border phase, oligosaccharides are hydrolysed by specific brush border enzymes into their component monosaccharides. During the phase of cellular absorption, sugars are transported across the cell membrane by carrier proteins. From Gray (1978b), with kind permission of the author.

Digestion of starch begins during mastication and mixing of food with salivary α-amylase in the oral cavity. However, salivary α-amylase is rapidly inactivated in the acidic environment of the stomach. Digestion begins again in the duodenum by virtue of another α-amylase excreted by the exocrine pancreas in response to meal-stimulated secretin and cholecystokinin, released by the small intestine.

α-Amylase has a limited specificity. It is capable of hydrolysing the α-1,4 glucoside bond in starch. It cannot hydrolyse the α-1,6 bonds and has little activity against terminal α-1,4 bonds or those immediately adjacent to α-1,6 bonds. Because of this, little glucose is produced during the luminal phase of starch digestion. Instead oligosaccharides of variable length and structure are produced as end-products (Roberts and Whelan, 1960). Polysaccharides in which the link between subunits is not an α-1,4 bond (cellulose) escape luminal digestion in the small bowel altogether and reach the colon unabsorbed. These polysaccharides function as dietary fibre. The end-products of the luminal phase of starch digestion include maltose, maltotriose, and α-limit dextrins. Subsequent digestion of these oligosaccharides occurs at the intestinal cell surface.

Phase of brush border digestion

Oligosaccharides, including those produced as a consequence of luminal digestion of starch and those ingested as such (e.g., sucrose, lactose, trehalose), are not digested within the lumen by free hydrolytic enzymes but rather are hydrolysed on the brush border surface of the enterocyte (Miller and Crane, 1961) by oligosaccharidases which are attached to the extracellular surface of the cell membrane (Gray and Ingelfinger, 1965). Monosaccharides are thereby released in close proximity to the membrane across which they are subsequently to be transported.

The brush border enzymes are active against specific sugar bonds. Some enzymes have specificity for more than a single substrate. For example, the oligosaccharidase sucrase can hydrolyse both sucrose and maltose (Gray, Lally and Conklin, 1979). Conversely, some substrates are susceptible to hydrolysis by more than one enzyme. For example, maltose can be hydrolysed by both sucrase and glucoamylase. The branched chain oligosaccharides, the α-limit dextrins, require serial digestion into the component free monosaccharides by means of a number of different enzymes (Gray, 1981).

With the exception of lactose, the capacity for oligosaccharide digestion appears to exceed the capacity for absorption of the component monosaccharides. As a result, some accumulation of monosaccharides is noted in the intestinal lumen (Gray and Ingelfinger, 1965; McMichael, Webb and Dawson, 1967). Thus, for most oligosaccharides, hydrolysis is not the rate-limiting step in absorption. However, accumulation of monosaccharides in the lumen is limited as a result of end-product inhibition of oligosaccharidase activity (Alpers and Cote, 1971). Premature hydrolysis is therefore avoided. Such autoregulation would have the beneficial effect of limiting a local increase in osmotic load which would contribute to net fluid accumulation and thus alter passive diffusion and the rate of intestinal transit. In addition, monosaccharide release occurs at sites where local absorptive capacity is capable of handling the load. This type of auto-regulation of oligosaccharidase activity is rapid-acting and appears not to be related to changes in oligosaccharidase concentrations.

In contrast to other oligosaccharides, lactose hydrolysis is the rate-limiting step for lactose absorption. Even in apparently normal individuals mucosal lactase concentration is the lowest of any of the disaccharidases and the capacity for hydrolysis can be overloaded. Monosaccharide accumulation does not occur, indicating that the transport system for its component monosaccharides, glucose and galactose, is capable of completely absorbing all hydrolytic end-products presented to it (Gray and Santiago, 1966). In isolated lactase deficiency and in diseases involving damage to the small intestinal mucosa, lactase levels are further diminished and are incapable of completely hydrolysing even moderate lactose loads (Gray and Santiago, 1966; McMichael, Webb and Dawson, 1967).

In addition to end-product inhibition of oligosaccharidase activity, regulation of brush border enzyme concentrations does occur. Pancreatic and bacterial proteases, lysolecithin, and bile acids are all capable of reducing oligosaccharidase concentrations (Alpers and Tedesco, 1975;

Jonas, Krishnan and Forstner, 1978; Alpers, 1981). In the rat, 95 per cent pancreatectomy increases oligosaccharidase concentrations while levels return to normal with infusion of elastase (Alpers and Tedesco, 1975). Patients with pancreatic insufficiency due to chronic pancreatitis have increased concentrations of jejunal sucrase and maltase but not lactase (Arvanitakis and Olsen, 1974).

Fluctuations in oligosaccharidase concentrations may occur in normal individuals on a daily basis. In the rat relatively high concentrations of oligosaccharidases noted during the fasting state start to decline immediately prior to eating, with trough levels occurring about one hour postprandially. Levels gradually return toward basal levels (Kaufman, Korsmo and Olsen, 1980). Relatively low levels are sustained throughout the daytime when rats are allowed to eat ad lib. However, this pattern is reversed if feeding is restricted at night (Stevenson et al, 1975). Presumably pancreatic proteases, released as a result of neural and hormonal stimulation in anticipation of and in response to eating, are responsible. What practical significance such a meal-related decrease in brush border enzyme concentrations has on digestion is uncertain.

While feeding transiently decreases oligosaccharidase activity, prolonged fasting also diminishes oligosaccharidase activity in humans. This effect precedes any atrophic mucosal changes detectable by routine light microscopy. Therefore, feeding stimulates disaccharidase activity and prepares the bowel for absorption. This effect is not disaccharide-specific. Feeding either glucose or lactose increases activity of both sucrase and lactase (Knudson et al, 1968).

High (supranormal) levels of maltase and sucrase occur with high sucrose or fructose diets in man, a process referred to as 'adaptation'. However, this enhancement of activity does not occur with glucose feeding (Rosensweig and Herman, 1969). No change in lactase levels is noted.

It is generally held that lactase levels cannot be induced in lactase deficient individuals by high lactose diets (Cuatrecasas, Lockwood and Caldwell, 1965; Gilat et al, 1972). However, one recent study using serial breath hydrogen testing did find improvement in lactose absorption with high lactose ingestion (Kotlar, 1982). Studies in rats suggest that this improvement in lactose digestion was unrelated to any alteration in mucosal lactase levels (Kotlar, Holt and Rosensweig, 1981).

Normally, oligosaccharide digestion is nearly complete by the mid jejunum. In the light of the limited back-diffusion of monosaccharides after disaccharide hydrolysis, the ileum represents a surplus surface for sugar digestion. The distal small bowel provides a margin of safety which can compensate to some degree for incomplete sugar digestion proximally. However, the hydrolytic capacity of the ileum appears to be more limited than that of the jejunum (Gray and Ingelfinger, 1965).

Phase of cellular absorption

Absorption into the enterocyte requires prior digestion to free monosaccharide components. The major dietary monosaccharides (glucose, galactose, and fructose) are all absorbed at rates far in excess of those expected on the basis of simple passive diffusion (Cori, 1925). In addition, glucose and galactose are absorbed against concentration gradients, indicating the presence of an active transport system (Crane, 1960). Groen (1937) demonstrated the presence of a transport maximum for all three monosaccharides. This indicates that the mechanism of absorption for each is saturable and, therefore, that a carrier-mediated transport system is involved.

Holdsworth and Dawson (1964), using an intestinal intubation technique in humans, showed that the transport systems for glucose and galactose followed similar kinetics, while that for fructose followed a different kinetic pattern. On the basis of this study the absorptive capacity of these three sugars appeared to be prodigious. Extrapolating their data, Crane (1975) calculated a total absorptive capacity for glucose and galactose of over 5000 grams per day, while that of fructose was calculated to be over 4500 grams per day. Although these calculations rested on certain assumptions concerning bowel length and uniformity of absorptive capacity that Crane recognized as questionable, it appeared that the small intestinal absorptive capacity for the major monosaccharides was so great that the possibility of incomplete absorption of any likely dietary intake would be remote. More recent information suggests that the absorptive capacity for some mono-saccharides may be limited under physiological conditions (Ravich, Bayless and Thomas, 1983). The occurrence of a single inherited disorder of carbohydrate absorption in which both glucose and galactose absorption are impaired indicates that the transport system for these two sugars is identical.

Considerable research has been done on the characteristics of the glucose-galactose transport system. As mentioned, it is a saturable carrier-mediated transport system, capable of active transport against a concentration gradient, and the carrier is located at the brush border membrane. Eighty per cent of glucose absorption occurs by means of this transport system (Kimmich, 1981). Most of the rest probably occurs by passive diffusion along a concentration gradient, as postprandial luminal concentrations in the proximal small intestine exceed those found intracellularly (Crane, 1975).

Sodium appears to increase affinity of the carrier for glucose. High luminal sodium concentrations result in rapid sodium binding. This enhances glucose affinity, presumably by means of a conformational change in the carrier molecule (Crane, Fortner and Eichholz, 1965). The Na^+-bound carrier then is pulled along the electrochemical gradient set up by Na^+ to the intracellular border of the cell membrane, where sodium is released into the low Na^+ environment of the cell. This diminishes glucose affinity and the glucose molecule is therefore released in turn (Kimmich and Carter-Su, 1978).

Calculations indicate that a Na^+-mediated carrier system based on an electrochemical gradient alone in which sodium and glucose are transported in equal amounts is inadequate to explain the concentrating capacity of the glucose transport system. Some energy is derived from the potassium gradient. The K^+-bound carrier has the opposite effect of Na^+; in other words, K^+ diminishes glucose affinity (Bosackova and Crane, 1965). As the K^+ concentration is opposite to that of Na^+, its effect on the carrier protein's affinity for glucose is supplemental to that of Na^+.

The problem of adequate energy for the degree of glucose accumulation has apparently been resolved by the realization that the actual Na^+:glucose stoichiometric ratio is 2:1, rather than 1:1 (Kimmich and Randles, 1980). Free carrier protein appears to have a negative charge, and two molecules are required to alter the glucose affinity of the carrier. This means that the double Na^+-bound carrier at the external cell membrane surface has a positive charge which draws it along the transmembrane electrochemical gradient into the cell. On release of the Na^+ molecules the carrier, now negatively charged, is propelled back to the external surface, rather than drifting back passively. This means that the speed of transfer across the membrane is increased in both directions, with a resultant increase in the maximum rate of transfer. For a detailed review of this subject see Kimmich (1981).

While glucose-galactose transport has received considerable attention, less is known about the fructose carrier system. This system is also saturable. However, fructose follows its own chemical gradient and, therefore, is absorbed by facilitated diffusion (Crane, 1960). The carrier is distinct from that involved in the glucose-galactose system (Holdsworth and Dawson, 1964), and children with a defect in the glucose-galactose absorption are able to absorb fructose. Although Holdsworth and Dawson suggested a large capacity for fructose absorption, a recent study in normal subjects using the breath hydrogen technique indicated that most subjects incompletely absorb fructose if the dose and concentration are high enough (Ravich, Bayless and Thomas, 1983). The limits of fructose absorption in some individuals is not far in excess of the amounts and concentrations commonly ingested by individuals who drink moderately large amounts of fructose-sweetened soda and are far below the levels calculated on the basis of Holdsworth and Dawson's data.

Other Factors Influencing Sugar Absorption and Tolerance

If sugar intolerance were merely a matter of small bowel absorptive capacity, symptoms of sugar malabsorption would correlate well with objective measures of absorptive capacity. About a quarter of individuals with lactase deficiency by peroral mucosal biopsy failed to recognize that they have a limited absorptive capacity for milk sugar (Welsh, 1970; Bayless et al, 1975). Though lack of recognition was frequently due to self-restriction of milk ingestion or failure to properly attribute symptoms to milk intake, many lactose malabsorbers ingest substantial amounts of milk without symptoms (Welsh, 1970). This suggests that other factors must influence the symptomatic expression of carbohydrate intolerance.

Though to some degree resistance to symptoms may be related to pain threshold, other more objectively measurable factors are involved (Figure 2). Unabsorbed sugar causes net fluid accumulation in the intestinal lumen and decreases transit time (Launiala, 1968). Such an alteration in motility

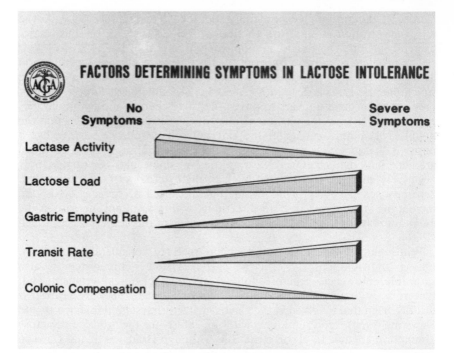

Figure 2. Factors determining symptoms in lactose intolerance. Factors influencing symptoms include not only lactase activity but also the ingested lactose load, the rate of gastric emptying, the rate of transit, and colonic handling of the non-absorbed sugar load. These factors are also involved with symptomatic response to malabsorption of other sugars. From the American Gastroenterology Association — Undergraduate Teaching Project, Unit VI, with kind permission of the editor (Henry L. Binder) and distributor.

would serve to decrease contact time available for hydrolysis and further impair absorption (Launiala, 1969). The degree to which fluid accumulation alters motility could be affected by neural and hormonal interactions which may vary significantly between individuals. The concentration at which sugars enter the small bowel is probably important. In one study, when normal subjects ingested fructose (50 g) as 10 per cent and 20 per cent solutions, the frequency of incomplete absorption measured by breath hydrogen rise increased from 41 per cent to 75 per cent (Ravich, Bayless and Thomas, 1983).

Regulation of gastric emptying appears to play a critical role in diminishing the effects of a high sugar load (Krasilnikoff, Gudmand-Hoyer and Moltke, 1975). The rate of gastric emptying is regulated by neural and hormonal feedback mechanisms initiated by chemoreceptors in the duodenum. Concentrated solutions are retained in the stomach longer than dilute solutions (Hunt and Knox, 1968). Gradual release diminishes the effect of a large ingested sugar load. Gastric drainage procedures damage this regulatory mechanism. Thus patients often develop symptoms of lactose intolerance for the first time after gastric surgery (Welsh, 1981). Despite the apparent enormous absorptive capacity for glucose, there is some data that even the glucose transport system can be overloaded after partial gastrectomy (Bond and Levitt, 1972).

All sugars are not emptied from the stomach at the same rate. Glucose is emptied more slowly than fructose. Whereas glucose slows gastric emptying linearly as the concentration of the ingested solution increases, fructose does not begin to slow gastric emptying until hypertonic solutions are ingested (Hunt and Knox, 1968). To some extent, then, fructose is handled in the intact stomach in a manner comparable to glucose in the partially-resected stomach. This may in part account for the high frequency of fructose malabsorption mentioned above.

At the other end of the alimentary tract, colonic function has an important effect on the clinical expression of sugar intolerance. Though the colon is impermeable to monosaccharides, the colonic bacterial flora metabolizes unabsorbed sugar into short-chain fatty acids. Most of these short-chain fatty acids do not appear in the stool in adults but rather are absorbed by the colonic mucosa, a process referred to as 'colonic salvage' (Bond et al, 1980; Ruppin et al, 1980). Such absorbed metabolites would theoretically be available for the metabolic requirements of the human host. In addition, most of the remaining sugar is altered into a non-dialysable form which is less osmotically active, thereby decreasing the effect of non-absorbed sugars on colonic fluid accumulation even further. Relatively little non-absorbed sugar is excreted in the faeces unaltered in the adult (Bond et al, 1980).

Colonic bacteria, therefore, alter non-absorbed sugar in ways that permit absorption and limit osmotic pressure. With absorption of sugar metabolites, water can be absorbed in turn. The colonic capacity for handling between 2.5 and 4 times the normal colonic water load is a major factor in limiting the diarrhoea that can occur with sugar malabsorption.

Most studies on sugar absorption deal with the effect of the absorption of a single sugar. The effect of concurrent ingestion of multiple foods has not received much attention. The fat content of milk appears to decrease the breath hydrogen rise of equivalent amounts of lactose in lactose-intolerant children (Solomons, Garcia-Ibanez and Viteri, 1979). The effect of fat in whole milk on adults is controversial. Leichter (1973) reported that lactose-intolerant adults were less symptomatic with whole milk than with either skim milk or aqueous milk. However, Solomons, Garcia-Ibanez and Viteri (1980) noted no difference between whole milk and aqueous lactose when studied with the breath hydrogen technique. It is assumed that the high fat content of whole milk results in delayed gastric emptying. Addition of dietary fibre delays gastric emptying and may delay small intestinal transit in the rat (Forman and Schneeman, 1982). Both effects may improve overall sugar absorption. A recent study indicates that addition of dietary fibre can decrease the rise in breath hydrogen after glucose ingestion found in patients with previous gastric surgery (Welsh et al, 1982). The mechanism of this effect is unclear but appears to be at least partially due to delayed gastric emptying (Ralphs et al, 1978). Whether fibre also slows glucose absorption by small intestine, and what effect this might have on total carbohydrate absorption, is controversial (Schwartz and Levine, 1980; Blackburn and Johnson, 1981). Lactase-deficient adults have fewer symptoms when lactose was taken after a meal as compared with fasting (Bedine and Bayless, 1973). The influence of dietary composition on the clinical expression of sugar malabsorption requires more study.

Pathophysiology of symptoms

Symptoms of sugar malabsorption include abdominal distension, cramps, flatulence, and watery diarrhoea. Though often temporally related to ingestion of specific foods, symptom onset can be delayed. This can cause the association with dietary intake to remain unappreciated, particularly when the sugar is ingested on a daily basis. Initially, distension and discomfort result from the osmotic effect of the sugar in the small intestine. This effect may cause nausea as well. Borborygmus is common due to increased peristaltic activity.

Colonic bacterial metabolism produces short-chain fatty acids which are osmotically active and may have a direct cathartic effect on the colon. Fortunately this effect is diminished by colonic absorption of these sugar metabolites. In addition, gas production occurs with release of hydrogen, carbon dioxide, and in some individuals, methane. Fluid accumulation and gas release account for colonic symptoms including cramping, pain, tenesmus, flatulence, and laxation. Though diarrhoea is often considered the most significant symptom for consideration of the diagnosis of sugar malabsorption, the most common symptoms patients complain of with small to moderate amounts of unabsorbed carbohydrates are probably distention and flatulence.

Though individual differences in bacterial microflora (Bond, Engel and Levitt, 1971) and colonic pH (Perman, Modler and Olson, 1981) account for variations in the type and proportion of gases released, the importance of these variations for the symptomatic expression of sugar intolerance is not well defined.

DISORDERS OF SUGAR ABSORPTION

Mucosal injury

Impaired absorption of a variety of ingested sugars can occur after a number of diseases which cause diffuse mucosal damage or dysfunction, including coeliac disease, tropical sprue, acute gastroenteritis, and protein-caloric malnutrition (Gray, 1978a). In these situations sugar malabsorption is often associated with fat malabsorption. Structural damage to the mucosa can cause decreases in absorptive surface area or in specific hydrolytic enzymes and carrier proteins. In some disorders physiological dysfunction occurs without detectable structural damage. Return to normal absorptive function may lag behind the clinical course of the initiating disease and cause prolongation of symptoms if sugars are introduced into the diet prematurely (Hirschhorn and Molla, 1969). With time, normal levels of absorptive proteins are seen on mucosal biopsy (James, 1971; Poley, Bhatia and Welsh, 1978). Because lactose hydrolysis is rate-limiting for absorption even in subjects with normal lactase levels, and perhaps because of its superficial location on the brush border membrane (Alpers, 1981), lactase is most sensitive to diffuse mucosal damage with resultant lactose malabsorption.

Starch malabsorption

Though malabsorption of starch is a theoretical possibility either on the basis of decreased pancreatic amylase secretion or low brush border maltase activity, no case of isolated starch intolerance has been described. The capacity of the pancreas to excrete sufficient amylase to digest dietary starch into oligosaccharide fragments is quite large and even in patients with fat malabsorption secondary to pancreatic insufficiency, only a moderate reduction in starch hydrolysis can be detected (Fogel and Gray, 1973). Because multiple brush border enzymes have maltase activity, isolated starch malabsorption due to maltase deficiency has not been reported. Nonetheless, starch absorption may be affected by the form in which it is ingested. Anderson, Levine and Levitt (1981) demonstrated a significant rise in breath hydrogen in healthy asymptomatic volunteers after ingestion of 100 grams of starch in the form of bread and macaroni made with wheat flour, but not with bread containing the same amount of starch made with low-gluten wheat flour or rice flour. Further studies, using the same technique, indicate incomplete absorption of large amounts of starch from corn or oat flour and from baked potato (Levine and Levitt, 1981). Recently 'starch blockers', isolated from legumes, have been advocated for dieting. These drugs are said to function by blocking starch hydrolysis. As might be expected, they appear to cause symptoms suggestive of sugar malabsorption in some individuals.

Lactose intolerance

Lactose malabsorption is the most common disorder of sugar absorption. Decreased brush border lactase levels occur in most mammals, including man, during the postweaning period (Kretschmer, 1981). By adulthood, the majority of humans worldwide are lactase-deficient (Huang and Bayless, 1968). There are three distinct disorders of lactose absorption.

Acquired lactase deficiency. Lactase deficiency should be considered a normal condition in adults. Postweaning declines in lactase levels are genetically determined and inherited as an autosomal recessive characteristic (Bayless, Christopher and Boyer, 1969; Sahi et al, 1973; Lisker, Gonzalez and Daltabrut, 1975). The decline in lactase levels in an individual is not influenced significantly by dietary intake of milk and will occur even if high levels of milk intake are sustained (Cuatrecasas, Lockwood and Caldwell, 1965; Keusch et al, 1969; Gilat et al, 1972). Conversely children with galactosaemia who never ingest lactose have normal lactase levels. Low lactase levels occur some time after infancy. It appears that the time of onset of the decline may vary between ethnic groups. Thus, most Thai children have low lactase levels by about two years of age (Keusch et al, 1969), while American whites begin to show declining levels only after five years of age (Welsh et al, 1978). Evidence of sugar malabsorption by oral lactose tolerance test or breath hydrogen technique suggest increasing prevalence of malabsorption with age with a substantial percentage of individuals demonstrating abnormal tests only as teenagers (Caskey et al, 1977; Newcomer et al, 1977; Paige, 1981). It is likely that steadily declining lactase levels into and throughout adolescence account for the frequent onset of lactose intolerance in teenagers and young adults.

Substantial variations in the prevalence of lactose malabsorption have been noted among different ethnic groups, with the prevalence of lactose malabsorption ranging from 0 to 100 per cent. In general, subjects of Northern European ancestry have low prevalences (⩽20 per cent), while subjects of African and Asian ancestry have high prevalences (⩾65 per cent) of lactose malabsorption. However, remarkable exceptions exist, with certain ethnic groups from Africa and the Indian subcontinent having low frequencies of lactose malabsorption comparable to those found in Northern Europeans (Simoons, 1978). These ethnic differences have been attributed to the early introduction of dairy practices of certain cultural groups — the 'geographic hypothesis' (Simoons, 1978). It is suggested that the ready availability of milk in certain cultures produced selective pressures for persistence of high lactase levels. Those with adequate lactase levels could utilize this valuable source of nutrition without adverse symptoms. As a result, they were better nourished, more productive, and more procreative. Over many generations, this genetic advantage produced a trend toward the high prevalence of lactose tolerance seen today in ethnic groups with long traditions of dairying. In non-dairy cultures, such selective pressures for the development of lactose tolerance would not be present and the prevalence of lactose malabsorption would remain high.

The reasons for intermediate prevalences of lactose malabsorption are not clear. It is possible that more recent exposure to dairy practices has resulted in a gradual increase in lactose tolerance and what is being witnessed is genetic selection in progress. However, it appears that in most cases where evidence is available, an intermediate prevalence results from genetic admixture between ethnic groups with different dairying traditions (Johnson, 1981).

As mentioned, the decline in lactase levels begins sometime after infancy and the frequency of symptomatic lactose malabsorption increases with age. However, even in those individuals with severe symptoms, some residual mucosal lactase is present and has the same physical characteristics as that found in lactose-tolerant individuals (Asp and Dahlquist, 1974; Lebenthal, Tsuboi and Kretschmer, 1974).

Diagnosis, once entertained, is most commonly confirmed by oral lactose tolerance test, breath hydrogen excretion test, or peroral mucosal biopsy. However, because of the high prevalence of lactase deficiency in some ethnic groups, and the occasional poor correlation between objective measures of sugar malabsorption and symptoms, results of such studies must be considered in light of actual dietary intake of milk products (Figure 3). Final confirmation of the clinical importance of milk intolerance in an individual patient requires resolution of symptoms on complete elimination of milk products from diet. Partial resolution of symptoms may suggest a coincidental problem of lactose malabsorption with another disorder, most often irritable bowel syndrome. Under this circumstance, undigested lactose may exacerbate the symptoms of the underlying disease.

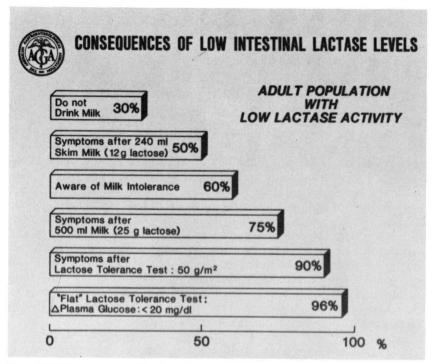

Figure 3. The consequences of low intestinal lactase activity in adults, given as the frequency of responses to varying amounts of milk and lactose. The data are derived from Bayless and Rosensweig, 1966; Welsh, 1970; Bedine and Bayless, 1973; Payne-Bose and Welsh, 1973; Bayless et al, 1975; Jones et al, 1976; Gudmand-Hoyer and Simony, 1977; Lisker et al, 1978; Cheng et al, 1979. From the American Gastroenterology Association — Undergraduate Teaching Project, Unit VI, with kind permission of the editor (Henry L. Binder) and distributor.

Lactose intolerance should be considered as a cause of flatulence, abdominal discomfort, bloating or diarrhoea when a patient is consuming one or two glasses of milk or a large portion of ice cream or commercial yogurt at a time. Some will be symptomatic with even less lactose. One's suspicion of lactose intolerance will be higher in a person with a family history of milk intolerance or in members of populations with a high prevalence of lactose intolerance, such as Blacks, Orientals, Jews, American Indians, Mexican Americans, South American Indians, Arabs or other Mediterranean peoples. Approximately 60 per cent of lactose-intolerant adults are aware that they are milk-intolerant and about half would be symptomatic with 1 or 2 glasses of skim milk taken on an empty stomach.

Milk intolerance may aggravate the symptoms of the irritable bowel syndrome or of organic intestinal disorders such as Crohn's disease or ulcerative colitis. Because of mucosal damage and secondary disaccharidase deficiency, milk intolerance may be one of the modes of presentation of coeliac disease or of giardiasis. The relationship of symptoms to milk ingestion is often so subtle that it is unrecognized by the patient. This was true in some older children and adolescents with recurrent abdominal pain who were found to be lactose intolerant and whose symptoms improved with lactose restriction. Recent studies have confirmed that milk intolerance is not the cause of most abdominal pain in teenagers but may be an aggravating factor which is quite treatable (Bayless, 1982).

Treatment involves decreasing the amount of lactose in the diet. However, complete elimination could have detrimental effects on nutrition, especially because milk is a major source of calcium. As individual sensitivity to milk varies considerably and some individuals with lactase deficiency can ingest substantial amounts of milk without symptoms, reintroduction of gradually increasing amounts of milk to tolerance may be desirable. Milk ingestion as part of a meal may be better tolerated than when taken alone. Milk in cheese and yogurt is partially pre-hydrolysed and is often tolerated better than equivalent amounts of lactose in other forms. Should the patient desire milk, the use of lactose-hydrolysed milk will permit milk ingestion without symptoms. Preparations of lactose-digesting enzymes can be added to milk which is then refrigerated for 24 hours to allow digestion of 60 - 90 per cent of the lactose. In some areas of the United States, pre-hydrolysed milk is commercially available.

Congenital lactase deficiency. This is a rare disorder in which mucosal lactase levels are low or even absent at birth. Lactase, when present, has physical characteristics identical to those found in acquired lactase deficiency (Asp and Dahlquist, 1974; Freiburghaus et al, 1975). Symptoms begin as soon as milk is introduced into the diet whether by breast-feeding or with milk-based formulae. Symptoms include irritability, presumably due to abdominal discomfort, failure to thrive, and frequent watery stools. The disorder has been noted in siblings, but not in parents, of involved individuals, suggesting an autosomal recessive transmission (Holzel, Schwarz and Sutcliffe, 1959).

Stools will have a low pH, and testing a stool sample with a Clinitest tablet will indicate the presence of glucose derived from undigested lactose by bacterial fermentation. Though lactase is the last of the oligosacchar-idases to achieve normal levels in the fetus (Dahlqvist and Lindberg, 1966), normal levels are usually achieved prenatally or soon after birth (Boellner, Beard and Panos, 1965). MacLean and Fink (1980) found a high prevalence lactose malabsorption by breath hydrogen testing in premature infants within the first month after birth. Such an apparently transient and common impairment of lactose absorption should be distinguished from congenital lactase deficiency, particularly as the prolonged restriction of milk ingestion with which the latter is treated would be unnecessary in the former. Therefore, while confirmation of the diagnosis is important, final objective assessment may have to be delayed till after the first few months. Diagnosis can be made by the oral lactose tolerance test or by breath hydrogen test, although peroral mucosal biopsy may be desirable to rule out secondary causes of lactose malabsorption. Congenital glucose-galactose malabsorption will mimic congenital lactase deficiency as lactose is composed of both malabsorbed sugars. The distinction can be suggested if the oral sugar tolerance test or breath hydrogen test are repeated with glucose in place of lactose, and is confirmed when normal lactase levels are seen on mucosal biopsy. Treatment involves elimination of milk from the diet with substitution of soy- or casein-based formulae.

A seemingly separate disorder of lactose tolerance has been described in a few infants. In this syndrome, severe symptoms suggestive of sugar intolerance occur. Children may become dehydrated. An unusual feature of this disorder is the presence of lactosuria, suggesting a mucosal abnormality permitting absorption of unhydrolysed disaccharides (Holzel, Mereu and Thomsen, 1962). The occurrence in related individuals suggests a possible genetic origin, probably autosomal recessive (Darling, Mortensen and Sondergaard, 1960). Though the presentation is suggestive of sugar intolerance, resolution with elimination of milk from diet is variable. In addition, oral lactose tolerance test and mucosal lactase levels have been normal in the few patients so studied (Holzel, Mereu and Thomsen, 1962; Berg et al, 1969). The diagnosis is made by virtue of a clinical picture suggestive of sugar intolerance in association with lactosuria.

Sucrase-isomaltase deficiency

A single hydrolytic enzyme is responsible for hydrolysis of sucrose and isomaltose (also called α-limit dextrin). It appears that sucrase and isomaltase activity are localized to different parts of the molecule (Cogoli et al, 1973). Sucrase-isomaltase deficiency is inherited as an autosomal recessive trait (Kerry and Townley, 1965) and occurs with different frequencies in various ethnic groups. In North Americans it is a rare disorder occurring in 0.2 per cent of the population (Peterson and Herber, 1967) while in some Eskimo tribes it occurs in as many as 10 per cent (McNair et al, 1972). Sucrase activity is more profoundly impaired, at least in some individuals (Hadorn et al, 1981), than isomaltase activity.

Symptoms of sugar malabsorption occur when sugar-sweetened foods are introduced into the diet and resolve with removal of table sugar from the diet. Symptoms of isomaltose malabsorption do not occur, in part because some isomaltase activity is usually present, and in part because of the limited osmotic activity of the undigested isomaltose molecule. Some individuals present in adulthood with symptoms suggestive of irritable bowel syndrome. Careful questioning of subject and parents, however, will usually reveal a life-long history of abdominal complaints.

Diagnosis is supported by a low stool pH. However, stool sampling with Clinitest tablets is often negative. Preheating the stool specimen will cause this test for glucose to become positive. Oral sucrose tolerance test or a breath hydrogen test after sucrose ingestion is usually used for diagnosis, but definitive diagnosis depends on finding low sucrase and normal maltase and lactase concentrations on mucosal biopsy. Treatment involves eliminating sucrose from the diet. Some reports suggest that sucrose tolerance improves with time and that some sucrose can be reintroduced into the diet in adolescence. Whether this apparent improvement in tolerance is due to adaptation or increase in enzyme activity is unknown.

Trehalase deficiency

Trehalose is a disaccharide found in insects and in most lower plants. However, it is ingested by man only in mushrooms. It is hydrolysed by a specific brush border enzyme. Trehalose ingestion has been implicated as a cause of symptoms of sugar malabsorption in only three patients. In one case, failure to absorb trehalose was confirmed by an oral trehalose tolerance test (Bergoz, 1971). In another report, a patient with symptoms of sugar malabsorption was found to have a flat glucose curve on oral trehalose tolerance test. Trehalase deficiency was confirmed by assay of a mucosal biopsy. Investigation of the patient's family subsequently revealed that the father also had a positive oral trehalose tolerance test and absent trehalase on mucosal biopsy (Madzerovova-Nohejlova, 1973). This family constellation suggests an inherited disorder. The rare occurrence of this disorder may be due more to the relatively limited intake of mushrooms than to the actual prevalence of low trehalase levels. Trehalose content is especially high in young mushrooms where it composes 1.4 per cent by weight. Substantial quantities of mushrooms must therefore be ingested to cause symptoms. Treatment involves simply decreasing the ingestion of mushrooms in the diet.

Glucose-galactose malabsorption

This rare disorder of monosaccharide transport is inherited as an autosomal recessive trait (Mellin and Meewisse, 1969). Symptoms of sugar malabsorption begin as soon as milk is introduced into the diet. Initially the diagnosis of congenital milk intolerance may be entertained, as the clinical picture is identical. However, symptoms occur with food containing glucose or galactose, whether ingested as free monosaccharide or as part of a disaccharide. Intestinal mucosal biopsies reveal normal levels of all disaccharidases. This disorder of monosaccharide transport affects other organ systems, including the renal tubules. Diagnosis can be confirmed by breath hydrogen technique or oral glucose tolerance test after ingestion of glucose. Studies have demonstrated poor mucosal binding of glucose (Meewisse and Dahlquist, 1968) and galactose (Schneider, Kinter and Stirling, 1966). Treatment involves the elimination of all lactose and sucrose from diet and substitution of fructose which is absorbed normally. As with sucrase-isomaltase deficiency, some observers report that glucose tolerance improves over time.

Fructose malabsorption

Four individuals with a specific disorder of fructose absorption have been described (Anderssen and Nygren, 1978). This was the first report of fructose malabsorption. These patients presented with symptoms consistent with sugar malabsorption after ingestion of fruit. Delayed fructose absorption was documented by means of a $^{14}CO_2$ excretion test. Symptoms resolved with elimination of fructose from the diet. Our recent report of limited fructose absorption in asymptomatic controls (Ravich, Bayless and Thomas, 1983) may mean that latent fructose malabsorption is more common than currently recognized, but that symptomatic expression is prevented by the relatively low amounts of fructose in the average western diet. However, the increasing use of fructose as a commercial food sweetener threatens to unmask this disorder. It is important to distinguish this disorder from hereditary fructose intolerance which is an abnormality of fructose metabolism and not a disorder of the fructose intestinal absorption of fructose (Cox et al, 1982).

THERAPEUTIC AND COMMERCIAL APPLICATIONS OF NON-ABSORBABLE SUGARS

Though we think of sugar malabsorption as a cause of distressing symptoms, some degree of incomplete absorption of carbohydrate is not only common but probably desirable. In our constipated society, it may be ingestion of milk or other sources of poorly absorbed carbohydrates that keeps us regular.

Certainly poorly absorbed carbohydrates are of value in this regard. Dietary fibre is predominantly composed of carbohydrates for which humans do not have the necessary digestive mechanisms. Lactulose, a non-digestible disaccharide initially used to lower absorption of ammonia from the colon in hepatic encephalopathy, is being advertised for its laxative effects. Bran cereal or psyllium is being prescribed for chronic constipation, diverticular disease and irritable bowel syndrome. Ingestion of guar gum has been recommended for treating diabetes, reactive hypoglycaemia and the dumping syndrome, all on the basis of its effect on delaying glucose absorption. The margin between sugar malabsorption and sugar intolerance is an important one for these therapeutic applications of non-absorbable foodstuff.

There is a trend in the food industry to substitute uncommon and often synthetic forms of sugar in food products. One motivation for this is the desire to find a cheaper source of food sweetener than table sugar. In addition, there are health advantages purported to derive from lowering intake of sucrose, including decreasing the incidence of overt diabetes and decreasing the incidence of cavities. Fructose-sweetened foods are now available, as are foods sweetened with sugar alcohols such as sorbitol and xylitol. As suggested by our study of the frequency of rise in breath hydrogen with fructose (Ravich, Bayless and Thomas, 1983), complete absorption of these substitute sweeteners should not be taken for granted. Dietetic candies containing sugar alcohol as sugar substitute have also been reported to produce diarrhoea in some individuals (Ravry, 1980).

REFERENCES

Alpers, D. H. (1981) Carbohydrate digestion: effects of monosaccharide inhibition and enzyme degradation on lactase activity. In *Lactose Digestion: Clinical and Nutritional Implications* (Ed.) Paige, D. M. & Bayless, T. M. pp. 58-68. Baltimore: Johns Hopkins University Press.

Alpers, D. H. & Cote, M. N. (1971) Inhibition of lactose hydrolysis by dietary sugars. *American Journal of Physiology,* **221,** 865-868.

Alpers, D. H. & Tedesco, F. J. (1975) The possible role of pancreatic proteases in the turnover of intestinal brush border proteins. *Biochimica et Biophysica Acta,* **401,** 28-40.

Anderson, I. H., Levine, A. S. & Levitt, M. D. (1981) Incomplete absorption of the carbohydrate in all-purpose wheat flour. *New England Journal of Medicine,* **304,** 891-892.

Anderssen, D. E. H. & Nygren, A. (1978) Four cases of long-standing diarrhoea and colic pains cured by fructose-free diet — a pathogenetic discussion. *Acta Medica Scandinavica,* **203,** 87-92.

Arvanetikis, C. & Olsen, W. A. (1974) Intestinal mucosal dissacharidases in chronic pancreatitis. *American Journal of Digestive Diseases,* **19,** 417-421.

Asp, N. & Dahlqvist, A. (1974) Intestinal β-galactosides in adult low lactase activity and in congenital lactase deficiency. *Enzyme,* **18,** 84-102.

Bayless, T. M. (1982) Lactose intolerance of the adolescent. *Journal of Adolescent Health Care,* **3,** 65-68.

Bayless, T. M. & Rosensweig, N. S. (1966) A racial difference in the incidence of lactase deficiency: a survey of milk tolerance and lactase deficiency in healthy males. *Journal of the American Medical Association,* **197,** 968-972.

Bayless, T. M., Christopher, N. L. & Boyer, S. H. (1969) Autosomal recessive inheritance of intestinal lactase deficiency: evidence from ethnic differences. *Journal of Clinical Investigation,* **48,** 6a.

Bayless, T. M., Rothfeld, B., Massa, C. et al (1975) Lactose and milk intolerance: clinical implications. *New England Journal of Medicine,* **294,** 1156-1159.

Bedine, M. S. & Bayless, T. M. (1973) Modification of lactose tolerance by glucose or a meal. *Clinical Research,* **20,** 448.

Berg, N. O., Dahlqvist, A., Lindberg, T. & Studnitz, W. V. (1969) Severe familial lactose intolerance — a gastrogen disorder. *Acta Paediatrica Scandinavica,* **58,** 525-527.

Bergoz, R. (1971) Trehalose malabsorption causing intolerance to mushrooms. *Gastroenterology,* **60,** 909-912.

Blackburn, N. A. & Johnson, J. T. (1981) The effect of guar gum on the viscosity of the gastrointestinal contents on glucose uptake from the perfused jejunum in the rat. *British Journal of Nutrition,* **46,** 239-246.

Boellner, S. W., Beard, A. G. & Panos, T. C. (1965) Impairment of intestinal hydrolysis of lactose in newborn infants. *Pediatrics,* **36,** 542-550.

Bond, J. H., Jr & Levitt, M. D. (1972) Use of pulmonary hydrogen (H_2) measurements to quantitate carbohydrate absorption: study of partially gastrectomized patients. *Journal of Clinical Investigation,* **51,** 1219-1225.

Bond, J. R., Engel, R. R. & Levitt, M. D. (1971) Methane production in man. *Journal of Experimental Medicine,* **133,** 572-588.

Bond, J. R., Currier, B., Buchwald, H. & Levitt, M. D. (1980) Colonic conservation of malabsorbed carbohydrates. *Gastroenterology,* **78,** 444-447.

Bosackova, J. & Crane, R. K. (1965) Studies on the mechanism of intestinal absorption of sugars. XIII. Cation inhibition of active sugar transport and ^{22}Na influx into hamster small intestine, in vitro. *Biochimica et Biophysica Acta,* **102,** 423-435.

Caskey, D. A., Payne-Bose, D., Welsh, J. D. et al (1977) Effects of age on lactose malabsorption in Oklahoma native Americans as determined by breath H_2 analysis. *American Journal of Digestive Diseases*, **22**, 113-116.

Chen, A. H. R., Brunsor, O., Espinoza, J. et al (1979) Long-term acceptance of low-lactose milk. *American Journal of Clinical Nutrition*, **32**, 1989-1993.

Cogoli, A., Eberle, A., Sigrist, H. et al (1973) Subunits of the small intestinal sucrase-isomaltase complex and separation of its enzymatically active isomaltase moiety. *European Journal of Biochemistry*, **33**, 40-48.

Cori, C. F. (1925) The fate of sugar in the animal body. I. The rate of absorption of hexoses and pentoses from the intestinal tract. *Journal of Biological Chemistry*, **66**, 691-715.

Cox, T. M., Camerilli, M., O'Donnell, M. W. & Chadwick, V. S. (1982) Pseudominant transmission of fructose intolerance in an adult and three offspring: heterozygote detection by intestinal biopsy. *New England Journal of Medicine*, **307**, 537-540.

Crane, R. K. (1960) Intestinal absorption of sugars. *Physiological Reviews*, **40**, 789-825.

Crane, R. K. (1975) The physiology of the intestinal absorption of sugars. In *Physiological Effects of Food Carbohydrates* (Ed.) Jeanes, A. & Hodges, J. pp. 2-19. Washington, DC: American Chemical Society.

Crane, R. K., Fortner, G. & Eichholz, A. (1965) Studies of the mechanism of the intestinal absorption of sugars. X. An effect of Na^+ concentration on the apparent Michaelis constants for intestinal sugar transport, in vitro. *Biochimica et Biophysica Acta*, **109**, 467-477.

Cuatrecasas, P., Lockwood, D. H. & Caldwell, J. R. (1965) Lactase deficiency in the adult: a common occurrence. *Lancet*, **i**, 14-21.

Dahlquist, A. & Lindberg, T. (1966) Development of the intestinal disaccharidase and alkaline phosphatase activities in the human foetus. *Clinical Science*, **30**, 517-528.

Darling, S., Mortensen, O. & Sondergaard, G. (1960) Lactosuria and amino aciduria in infancy: a new inborn error of metabolism. *Acta Paediatrica*. **119**, 281-290.

Fogel, M. R. & Gray, G. T. (1973) Starch hydrolysis in man: an intraluminal process not requiring membrane digestion. *Journal of Applied Physiology*, **35**, 263-267.

Forman, L. P. & Schneeman, B. O. (1982) Dietary pectin's effect on starch utilization in rats. *Journal of Nutrition*, **112**, 528-533.

Freiburghaus, A. U., Schmitz, J., Schindler, M. et al (1976) Protein patterns of brush border fragments in congenital lactose malabsorption and in specific hypolactasia in the adult. *New England Journal of Medicine*, **294**, 1030-1032.

Gilat, T., Russo, S., Gelman-Malachi, E. & Aldor, T. A. M. (1972) Lactase in man: a non-adaptable enzyme. *Gastroenterology*, **62**, 1125-1127.

Gray, G. M. (1978a) Intestinal disaccharidase deficiencies and glucose-galactose malabsorption. In *Metabolic Basis of Inherited Disease* (Ed.) Stanbury, J. B., Wyngaarden, J. B. & Frederickson, D. S. 4th Edition, pp. 1526-1535. New York: McGraw Hill.

Gray, G. M. (1978b) Mechanisms of digestion and absorption of food. In *Gastrointestinal Disease* (Ed.) Sleisenger, M. H. & Fordtran, J. S. 2nd Edition, Vol. I, pp. 241-250. Philadelphia: W. B. Saunders.

Gray, G. M. (1981) Carbohydrate absorption and malabsorption. In *Physiology of the Gastrointestinal Tract* (Ed.) Johnson, L. R. pp. 1063-1072. New York: Raven Press.

Gray, G. M. & Ingelfinger, F. J. (1965) Intestinal absorption of sucrose in man: the site of hydrolysis and absorption. *Journal of Clinical Investigation*, **44**, 390-398.

Gray, G. M. & Santiago, N. (1966) Disaccharide absorption in normal and diseased human intestine. *Gastroenterology*, **51**, 489-498.

Gray, G. M., Lally, B. C. & Conklin, K. A. (1979) Action of intestinal sucrase-isomaltase and its free monomers on an α-limit dextrin. *Journal of Biological Chemistry*, **254**, 6039-6043.

Groen, J. (1937) The absorption of hexoses from the upper part of the small intestine in man. *Journal of Clinical Investigation*, **16**, 245-255.

Gudmand-Hoyer, E. & Simony, K. (1977) Individual sensitivity to lactose in lactose malabsorption. *American Journal of Digestive Diseases*, **22**, 177-181.

Hadorn, B., Green, J. R., Sterchi, E. E. & Hauri, H. P. (1981) Biochemical mechanisms in congenital enzyme deficiencies of the small intestine. *Clinics in Gastroenterology*, **10**, 671-690.

Hirschhorn, N. & Molla, A. (1969) Reversible jejunal disaccharidase deficiency in cholera and other acute diarrhea diseases. Johns Hopkins Medical Journal, **125**, 291-300.

Holdsworth, C. D. & Dawson, A. M. (1964) The absorption of monosaccharides in man. *Clinical Science,* **27,** 371-379.

Holzel, A., Mereu, T. & Thomsen, M. L. (1962) Severe lactose intolerance in infancy. *Lancet,* **ii,** 1346-1348.

Holzel, A., Schwarz, V. & Sutcliffe, K. W. (1959) Defective lactose absorption causing malnutrition in infancy. *Lancet,* **i,** 1126-1128.

Huang, S. S. & Bayless, T. M. (1968) Milk intolerance in healthy orientals. *Science,* **160,** 83-84.

Hunt, J. N. & Knox, M. T. (1968) The regulation of gastric emptying. In *Handbook of Physiology: Alimentary Canal IV.* pp. 1917-1935. Washington, DC: American Physiological Society.

James, W. P. T. (1971) Jejunal disaccharidase activities in children with marasmus and with kwashiorkor: response to treatment. *Archives of Disease in Childhood,* **46,** 218-220.

Johnson, J. D. (1981) The regional and ethnic distribution of lactose malabsorption: adaptive and genetic hypotheses. In *Lactose Digestion: Clinical and Nutritional Implications* (Ed.) Paige, D. M. & Bayless, T. M. pp. 11-22. Baltimore: Johns Hopkins University Press.

Jonas, A., Krishnan, C. & Forstner, G. (1978) The pathogenesis of mucosal injury in the blind loop syndrome: release of disaccharidases from the brush border membranes by extracts of bacteria obtained from intestinal blind loops in rats. *Gastroenterology,* **75,** 791-795.

Jones, D. V., Latham, M. C., Kosikowski, F. V. & Woodward, G. (1976) Symptom response to lactose-reduced milk in lactose-intolerant adults. *American Journal of Clinical Nutrition,* **29,** 633-638.

Kaufman, M. A., Korsmo, H. A. & Olsen, W. A. (1980) Circadian rhythm of intestinal sucrase activity in rats: mechanism of enzyme change. *Journal of Clinical Investigation,* **65,** 1174-1181.

Kerry, K. R. & Townley, R. W. (1965) Genetic aspects of intestinal sucrase-isomaltase deficiency. *Australian Paediatric Journal,* **1,** 223-235.

Keusch, G., Troncale, F. J., Miller, L. H. et al (1969) Acquired lactose malabsorption in Thai children. *Pediatrics,* **43,** 540-545.

Kimmich, G. A. (1981) Intestinal absorption of sugar. In *Physiology of the Gastrointestinal Tract* (Ed.) Johnson, L. R. pp. 1035-1062. New York: Raven Press.

Kimmich, G. A. & Carter-Su, C. (1978) Membrane potentials and the energetics of intestinal Na^+-dependent transport systems. *American Journal of Physiology,* **235,** C73-C81.

Kimmich, G. A. & Randles, J. (1980) Evidence for an intestinal Na^+:sugar transport coupling stoichiometry of 2.0. *Biochimica et Biophysica Acta,* **596,** 439-444.

Knudson, K. B., Bradley, E. M., Lecocq, F. R. et al (1968) Effect of fasting and refeeding on the histology and disaccharidase activity of the human intestine. *Gastroenterology,* **55,** 46-51.

Kotlar, D. P. (1982) Lactose adaptation in man is adaptable. *Gastroenterology,* **82,** 1105.

Kotlar, D. P., Holt, P. R. & Rosensweig, N. S. (1981) Lactose absorption by rat intestine is adaptable. *Gastroenterology,* **80,** 1198.

Krasilnikoff, P. A., Gundmand-Hoyer, E. & Moltke, H. H. (1975) Diagnostic value of disaccaridase tolerance tests in children. *Acta Paediatrica Scandinavica,* **64,** 693-698.

Kretschmer, N. (1981) The significance of lactose intolerance: an overview. In *Lactose Digestion: Clinical and Nutritional Implications* (Ed.) Paige, D. M. & Bayless, T. M. pp. 3-7. Baltimore: Johns Hopkins University Press.

Launiala, K. (1968) The effect of unabsorbed sucrose and mannitol on small intestinal flow rate and mean transit time. *Scandinavian Journal of Gastroenterology,* **3,** 665-671.

Launiala, K. (1969) The effect of unabsorbed sucrose- or mannitol-induced accelerated transit on absorption in the human small intestine. *Scandinavian Journal of Gastroenterology,* **4,** 25-31.

Lebenthal, E., Tsuboi, K. & Kretschmer, N. (1974) Characterization of human lactase and hetero-β-galactosidases of infants and adults. *Gastroenterology,* **67,** 1107-1113.

Leichter, J. (1973) Comparison of whole milk and skim milk with aqueous lactose solution in lactose intolerance. *American Journal of Clinical Nutrition,* **26,** 393-396.

Levine, A. S. & Levitt, M. D. (1981) Malabsorption of starch moiety of oats, corn and potatoes. *Gastroenterology,* **80,** 1209.

Lisker, R., Aguilar, L. & Zavala, C. (1978) Intestinal lactase deficiency and milk drinking capacity in the adult. *American Journal of Clinical Nutrition,* **31,** 1499-1503.

Lisker, R., Gonzalez, B. & Daltabrut, M. (1975) Recessive inheritance of the adult type of intestinal lactose deficiency. *American Journal of Human Genetics,* **27,** 662-664.

MacLean, W. C. Jr & Fink, B. B. (1980) Lactose malabsorption by premature infants: magnitude and clinical significance. *Journal of Pediatrics,* **97,** 383-388.

Madzerovova-Nohejlova, J. (1973) Trehalose deficiency in a family. *Gastroenterology,* **65,** 130-133.

McMichael, H. B. (1976) Disorders of carbohydrate digestion and absorption. *Clinics in Endocrinology and Metabolism,* **5,** 627-649.

McMichael, H. B., Webb, J. & Dawson, A. M. (1967) The absorption of maltose and lactose in man. *Clinical Science,* **33,** 135-145.

McNair, A., Gudmand-Hoyer, E., Jarnum, S. & Orrild, L. (1972) Sucrose malabsorption in Greenland. *British Medical Journal,* **ii,** 19-21.

Meewisse, G. W. & Dahlqvist, A. (1968) Glucose-galactose malabsorption: a study with biopsy of the small intestinal mucosa. *Acta Paediatrica Scandinavica,* **57,** 273-280.

Mellin, K. & Meewisse, G. W. (1969) Glucose-galactose malabsorption: a genetic study. *Acta Paediatrica Scandinavica* (Supplement) **188,** 19.

Miller, D. & Crane, R. K. (1961) The digestive function of the epithelium of the small intestine. II. Localization of disaccharide hydrolysis in the isolated brush border portion of intestinal epithelial cells. *Biochimica et Biophysica Acta,* **52,** 293-298.

Newcomer, A. D., Thomas, P. T., McGill, D. & Hofmann, A. F. (1977) Lactose deficiency: a common genetic trait of the American Indian. *Gastroenterology,* **72,** 234-237.

Paige, D. M. (1981) Lactose malabsorption in children: prevalence, symptoms, and nutritional considerations. In *Lactose Digestion: Clinical and Nutritional Implications* (Ed.) Paige, D. M. & Bayless, T. M. pp. 151-161. Baltimore: Johns Hopkins University Press.

Payne-Bose, D. & Welch, J. D. (1973) Lactose malabsorption in Oklahoma Indians. *American Journal of Clinical Nutrition,* **26,** 1320-1322.

Perman, J. A., Modler, S. & Olson, A. C. (1981) Role of pH in production of hydrogen from carbohydrates by colonic bacterial flora. *Journal of Clinical Investigation,* **67,** 643-650.

Peterson, M. L. & Herber, R. (1967) Intestinal sucrase deficiency. *Transactions of the Association of American Physicians,* **80,** 275-283.

Poley, J. R., Bhatia, M. & Welsh, J. D. (1978) Disaccharidase deficiency in infants with cow's milk protein intolerance. *Digestion,* **17,** 97-107.

Ralphs, D. N. L., Lawaetz, O., Brown, N. J. G. & Leeds, A. R. (1978) Effect of a dietary fibre on gastric emptying in dumpers. *Gut,* **19,** A986-A987.

Ravich, W. J., Bayless, T. M. & Thomas, M. E. (1983) Fructose: limited intestinal absorption in man. *Gastroenterology,* **84,** 26-29.

Ravry, M. J. R. (1980) Dietetic food diarrhea. *Journal of the American Medical Association,* **244,** 270.

Roberts, P. J. P. & Whelan, W. J. (1960) The mechanism of carbohydrase action. 5. Action of human salivary α-amylase on amylopectin and glycogen. *Biochemical Journal,* **76,** 246-253.

Rosensweig, N. S. & Herman, R. H. (1969) Timed response of jejunal sucrase and maltase activity to a high sucrose diet in normal man. *Gastroenterology,* **56,** 500-505.

Ruppin, H., Bar-Meir, S., Soergel, K. H. et al (1980) Absorption of short-chain fatty acids by the colon. *Gastroenterology,* **78,** 1500-1507.

Sahi, T., Isokoski, M., Jussila, J. et al. (1973) Recessive inheritance of adult type lactose malabsorption. *Lancet,* **ii,** 823-826.

Schneider, A. J., Kinter, W. B. & Stirling, C. E. (1966) Glucose-galactose malabsorption. *New England Journal of Medicine,* **274,** 305-312.

Schwartz, J. E. & Levine, G. D. (1980) Effects of dietary fiber on intestinal glucose absorption and glucose tolerance in rats. *Gastroenterology,* **79,** 833-836.

Simoons, F. J. (1978) Geographic hypothesis and lactose malabsorption: a weighing of the evidence. *American Journal of Digestive Diseases,* **23,** 963-980.

Simoons, F. J. (1981) Geographic patterns of primary adult lactose malabsorption: a further interpretation of evidence for the old world. In *Lactose Digestion: Clinical and Nutritional Implications* (Ed.) Paige, D. M. & Bayless, T. M. pp. 23-48. Baltimore: Johns Hopkins University Press.

Solomons, N. H., Garcia-Ibanez, R. & Viteri, F. E. (1979) Reduced rate of breath hydrogen (H_2) excretion with lactose tolerance tests in young children using whole milk. *American Journal of Clinical Nutrition,* **32,** 783-786.

Solomons, N. H., Garcia-Ibanez, R. & Viteri, F. E. (1980) Hydrogen (H_2) breath tests of lactose malabsorption in adults: the application of physiological doses and whole cow's milk sources. *American Journal of Clinical Nutrition,* **33,** 545-554.

Stevenson, N. R., Ferrigni, F., Parnicky, K. et al (1975) Effect of changes in feeding schedule on the diurnal rhythms and daily activity levels of intestinal brush border enzymes and transport systems. *Biochimica et Biophysica Acta,* **406,** 131-145.

Welsh, J. D. (1970) Isolated lactase deficiency in humans: report on 100 patients. *Medicine,* **49,** 257-277.

Welsh, J. D. (1981) Causes of isolated low lactase levels and lactose intolerance. In *Lactose Digestion: Clinical and Nutritional Implications* (Ed.) Paige, D. M. & Bayless, T. M. pp. 69-79. Baltimore: Johns Hopkins University Press.

Welsh, J. D., Poley, J. R., Bhatia, M. & Stevenson, D. E. (1978) Intestinal disaccharidase activities in relation to age, race and mucosal damage. *Gastroenterology,* **75,** 847-855.

Welsh, J. D., Manion, C. V., Griffith, W. J. & Bird, P. C. (1982) Effect of psyllium hydrophilic mucilloid on oral glucose tolerance and breath hydrogen in postgastrectomy patients. *Digestive Diseases and Sciences,* **27,** 7-12.

3

Human Protein Digestion and Absorption: Normal Mechanisms and Protein-energy Malnutrition

HUGH J. FREEMAN
MARVIN H. SLEISENGER
YOUNG S. KIM

Protein is an essential nutrient for continued health and homeostasis (Hellier and Holdsworth, 1975; Freeman et al, 1978, 1979; Sleisenger and Kim, 1979). It has been estimated that a 70 kg man requires approximately 45 g of protein daily to remain in positive nitrogen balance (Heller and Holdsworth, 1975). Among industrialized countries, this amounts to about 10 to 15 per cent of the average caloric intake. A number of factors determines the nutritive value of dietary protein. These include: quantity and quality of constituent amino acids in food protein, and digestibility of whole proteins in food complexed to other non-protein nutrients. In addition to exogenous dietary sources, a considerable amount of endogenous protein is available. In recent years, normal mechanisms involved in the assimilation of dietary protein have been exensively reviewed (Weinstein, 1974; Hellier and Holdsworth, 1975; Matthews and Adibi, 1976; Freeman et al, 1978, 1979, 1981; Sleisenger and Kim, 1979; Adibi and Kim, 1981; Munck, 1981). In the present paper, this information is synthesized along with alterations that occur in disease states. Finally, protein-energy malnutrition is discussed to place some of this data into clinical and nutritional perspective.

EXOGENOUS DIETARY PROTEIN SOURCES

Essential and non-essential amino acids

Dietary protein must supply essential amino acids since their carbon skeletons cannot be formed in man. The essential amino acids include leucine, isoleucine, lysine, tryptophan, phenylalanine, methionine, threonine and valine. Cystine and tyrosine are also considered essential as these are derived from methionine and phenylalanine, respectively. Arginine is thought to be an essential nutrient for children (Freeman and Kim, 1978).

Clinics in Gastroenterology — Vol. 12, No. 2, May 1983

0300-5089/83/1202-357 $05.00© 1983 W. B. Saunders Company Ltd

Non-essential amino acids derive their carbon skeletons from intermediary products of carbohydrate and fat metabolism, while amino groups result from transamination. Both an adequate supply of essential amino acids and ready availability of non-essential amino acids are required to maintain positive nitrogen balance and effective protein synthesis.

Digestibility of food protein

Except for rare examples, such as egg albumen, most natural and processed foods contain protein complexed to fat or carbohydrate. Digestibility probably varies because fat or carbohydrate complexed to protein may limit efficient proteolysis. With modern food processing techniques, changes in the chemical composition of food proteins may occur. Heating and storage can lead to interactions between functional groups, creating new amide or ester linkages within and between peptide bonds or causing conditions resistant to enzymatic hydrolysis. It can be anticipated that other adverse effects on the nutritional value of food protein will be observed with the further evolution of food processing methods (Freeman and Kim, 1978).

ENDOGENOUS PROTEIN SOURCES

In addition to dietary proteins, endogenous sources may provide a significant pool of usable protein. These include secretions from salivary glands, stomach, intestine, biliary tract and pancreas. It has been estimated that this source amounts to at least 20 to 30 g daily and consists primarily of hydrolytic enzymes, glycoproteins or mucins shed into the bowel lumen (Freeman and Kim, 1978). In addition, desquamated cells, derived from active renewal of the lining epithelium, contribute approximately 30 g of protein daily. In disease states characterized by accelerated kinetic parameters of epithelial cell renewal, such as in coeliac sprue (Wright et al, 1973a,b; Weinstein, 1974), this source of endogenous protein may be even more substantial. Finally, small amounts of plasma proteins are normally secreted into the intestinal tract at a rate of about 1 to 2 g daily. Albumin, gamma globulin and other serum proteins have been amply demonstrated in the bowel luminal contents of normal subjects by both electrophoretic and immunological methods (Freeman and Kim, 1978). In several diseases that involve the stomach or small or large bowel serum protein loss by this route may be excessive, leading to hypoproteinaemia (i.e., protein-losing gastro-enteropathy) (Jeffries, 1978). While the amount of endogenous protein from each source probably varies in a given individual, endogenous proteins probably undergo extensive hydrolysis within the intestine before being reused by the host as a nitrogen source.

ASSIMILATION EFFICIENCY

The healthy adult ordinarily excretes 1 to 2 g of faecal nitrogen per day, equivalent to approximately 6 to 12 g of protein. This implies that under normal conditions, processes involved in digestion and absorption of both dietary exogenous protein (70 to 100 g daily) and endogenous protein (30 to 200 g daily) are highly efficient.

Mechanisms of protein digestion and absorption

Digestion is initiated in the stomach by a group of gastric proteases or pepsins that function optimally at an acid pH. These are activated from precursor zymogens or pepsinogens following selective enzymatic cleavage of a small basic peptide. Peptic digestion results in polypeptides with N-terminal amino acids (i.e., phenylalanine, leucine), some oligopeptides, and a small number of single amino acids. Some individual L-amino acids, especially phenylalanine and tryptophan, appear to be potent stimulants of acid secretion as well as gastrin and pancreatic polypeptide release (Taylor et al, 1982), implying that modulation of the gastric response to a protein-containing meal may occur depending on the effectiveness of peptic digestion and composition of resultant peptic digestion products. In previous years, the role of gastric digestion in the overall process of protein assimilation has been considered limited since positive nitrogen balance is possible and well documented even after total gastrectomy. Recent studies, however, indicate that, under certain conditions, gastric digestion may be critical. In an animal model of pancreatic exocrine insufficiency, for example, intestinal absorption of dietary protein was enhanced significantly by pre-incubation of protein with acid or pepsin (Curtis, Gaines and Kim, 1979).

Digestion products resulting from gastric peptic activity are more potent mucosal endocrine cell secretagogues than whole protein. Hormone peptides secreted by these cells cause acinar cell release of pancreatic exocrine enzyme precursors or zymogens. Cholecystokinin (CCK) and secretin are potent and weak stimulants, respectively, of an enzyme-protein-rich pancreatic secretion (Meyer, 1981). The role of other peptides is not as clearly delineated. Gastrin, having the carboxyl terminal of CCK, may have similar, albeit less potent, effects (Stening and Grossman, 1969). Vasoactive intestinal peptide (VIP), structurally related to secretin, shares some of the actions of secretin but is less potent (Meyer, 1981). Bombesin, structurally unrelated to CCK or gastrin, stimulates an enzyme-rich pancreatic juice (Meyer, 1981). Bombesin may act indirectly through release of endogenous CCK or gastrin, although evidence accumulated from studies on isolated acinar cells in vitro also suggests that bombesin may act directly (Uhlemann, Rottman and Gardner, 1979). Finally, some peptide extracts, such as chymodenin, appear to cause selective secretion of chymotrypsinogen (Adelson and Rothman, 1975), raising the possibility of selective secretory control of individual pancreatic enzymes by peptide hormones (Meyer, 1981). Moreover, some peptides appear to act synergistically so that enzyme or protein outputs are augmented if secretin and CCK are administered together (Meyer, Spingola and Grossman, 1971). Similar observations are reported with secretin and gastrin as well as VIP and CCK (Meyer, 1981). Finally, some peptides, like somatostatin or VIP released in response to feeding, may function locally within the pancreas in association with neural stimuli (Chariot et al, 1978; Mitchell and Bloom, 1978). Besides the direct modulating role of these peptides in causing release and secretion of an enzyme-rich pancreatic juice, hormones may liberate several hydrolytic glycoprotein enzymes from the intestinal brush border membrane, including enteropeptidase (i.e., enterokinase).

Enterokinase selectively cleaves a hexapeptide from the amino terminus of trypsinogen to yield trypsin. Trypsin then activates several pancreatic zymogens and autocatalyses trypsinogen activation. The resultant pancreatic enzymes act intraluminally to cleave peptide bonds internally (i.e., endopeptidases: trypsin, chymotrypsin, elastase) and at the carboxyl terminus (i.e., exopeptidases: carboxypeptidase A and B) (Gray and Cooper, 1971). Aminopeptidase activity can also be detected in trace amounts in activated pancreatic juice. The combined action of these enzymes causes the intraluminal release of several small peptides of two to six amino acid residues as well as single amino acids. In proximal jejunum, the peptide fraction accounts for about 60 to 70 per cent of luminal alpha-amino nitrogen, whereas the remainder is associated mainly with single amino acids (Nixon and Mawer, 1970a,b; Adibi and Mercer, 1973; Chung et al, 1974). Further information regarding the chain length and amino acid composition of these oligopeptides in different regions of the small intestine is still required.

The final stages in the process of protein assimilation are directly associated with the small intestinal mucosa. Examination of postprandial blood reveals that essentially all amino nitrogen is present as free amino acids. However, some exceptions occur. For example, small peptides containing proline and hydroxyproline can be detected in portal blood after intake of gelatin (Matthews and Adibi, 1976), and both carnosine and anserine have been observed after ingestion of poultry (Matthews and Adibi, 1976). In addition, some large macromolecules that may be antigenically, although not nutritionally, important can be transported into mucosal cells of fetal and neonatal small intestine in certain mammalian species (Lev and Orlic, 1973; Walker and Isselbacher, 1974; Walker, 1981). The serum of newborns contains bovine serum albumin after oral feeding (Rothberg, 1969) and, compared to the serum of adults, a higher ratio of antibodies to food antigens (Walker and Isselbacher, 1974). Immunoglobulin from colostrum appears also to be absorbed intact by the neonate, affording passive immunity for the newborn (Walker and Isselbacher, 1974). The process of intact transport of significant amounts of protein appears confined to the first 48 hours after birth. Studies in mature mammalian gut with ferritin (Bockman and Winborn, 1966) and horseradish peroxidase (Cornell, Walker and Isselbacher, 1971) indicate that uptake of small amounts of intact macromolecules may occur. In addition, several studies (Wilson and Walzer, 1935, Grusky and Cook, 1955; Korenblat, Rothberg and Minden, 1968) suggest that limited amounts of macromolecules can cross the mature mucosal barrier under normal physiological conditions. For example, milk antibodies are found in the serum after milk protein is ingested orally (Korenblat, Rothberg and Minden, 1968).

Mucosal cells contain abundant enzymatic activities for hydrolysis of luminal oligopeptides (Heizer and Laster, 1969). Aminopeptidase, for example, can be localized at a subcellular level to cytosol and particulate fractions, including the brush border of human small intestinal mucosa (Kim et al, 1972, 1974). In rats, different physicochemical properties in substrate specificities suggest that enzyme activities found in these two subcellular fractions are distinct (Kim et al, 1972, 1974). Aminopeptidases cleave peptide bonds from the amino terminus of small peptides, releasing free amino-terminal amino acid. The type and chain length of the oligopeptide substrate appear to influence the subcellular site of this hydrolytic activity (Kim et al, 1972, 1974; Nicholson and Peters, 1977). For dipeptides, only a small amount of the total activity found in mucosal cells is localized to the brush border. For tripeptides, however, aminopeptidase activities appear to be approximately evenly distributed between the cytosol and brush border. Longer peptides appear to be hydrolysed almost exclusively by the brush border fraction (Nicholson and Peters, 1977).

The brush border aminopeptidases that have been solubilized, purified and characterized have been shown to be integral transmembrane glycoproteins with two domains (Kim and Brophy, 1976; Louvard, Semiriva and Maroux, 1976; Maroux and Louvard, 1976). The active site and the carbohydrate-rich hydrophilic portion of the enzyme molecule are externally oriented on the microvillus membrane of the epithelial cell with a small hydrophobic peptide sequence anchoring the protein to the membrane. Studies from different laboratories (Wojnarowska and Gray, 1975; Kim et al, 1976; Shoaf et al, 1976; Gray and Santiago, 1977; Kanra et al, 1977) indicate that the aminopeptidases in rat small intestine are high in molecular weight and have differing electrophoretic mobilities. The specificity for the amino terminal residue of the substrate appears to be broad; however, dipeptides containing proline or D-amino acids at the carboxyl terminus or amino terminus of the peptide are not hydrolysed. Thus, a free alpha-amino group and the L-configuration for the first two amino acid residues are required substrate characteristics for these enzymes. Three to four active subsites in the aminopeptidases have been postulated through correlations of substrate structure with kinetic parameters (Kanra et al, 1977).

The biosynthesis of intestinal brush border glycoproteins, such as aminopeptidase, have been demonstrated using ultrastructural autoradiographic and biochemical methods (Bennett et al, 1974; Weiser et al, 1974; Quaroni et al, 1979a,b) to follow a similar intracellular route as for most cell surface membrane glycoproteins (Rothman and Lenard, 1977). They are synthesized in the rough endoplasmic reticulum of enterocytes, pass through the Golgi apparatus and are inserted into the plasma membrane. Some of these glycoproteins may be first inserted into the enterocyte basolateral membrane before reaching the brush border. Earlier immunohistological methods suggested the presence of inactive aminopeptidase precursors in the apical cytoplasm of enterocytes (Wachsmuth and Torhorst, 1974); however, recent immunofluorescent and histochemical labelling studies employing ultrathin sections have localized aminopeptidase in the brush border and a possibly inactive partially glycosylated form of the enzyme in the Golgi region (Feracci et al, 1982). In addition, some active aminopeptidase may be present in a structure located under the terminal web and the upper part of the lateral membrane (Feracci et al, 1982).

Other intestinal mucosal enzymes may play a role in peptide hydrolysis.

Cytoplasmic dipeptidase and aminotripeptidase activities have been detected (Kim et al, 1974, 1979). Glycyl-L-leucine dipeptidase is one of the major cytoplasmic enzymes with broad specificity for dipeptides containing neutral amino acids. Cytoplasmic aminotripeptidase has broad substrate specificity for tripeptides with a free alpha-amino group and for tripeptides containing proline at the amino terminus. Cytoplasmic proline dipeptidase (prolidase or imidopeptidase) has recently been purified (Baksi and Radhakrishnan, 1974; Sjostrom and Noren, 1974). It is a glycoprotein containing two subunits of equal molecular weight with a narrow substrate specificity. It appears to be active on dipeptides containing proline or sarcosine in the penultimate position. Dipeptidyl peptidase IV, capable of cleaving two amino acid residues from the amino terminus of a peptide substrate, can be found in the brush border (Adibi and Kim, 1981). It is an intrinsic membrane glycoprotein consisting of two identical subunits. High activities are observed for peptides with proline in the penultimate position, and it is this enzyme that probably plays a substantial role in hydrolysis of proline-containing oligopeptides. Moreover, this enzyme seems to be widely distributed including the renal microvillus membranes (Kenny et al, 1976). Jejunal mucosal cells in the rat contain gamma-glutamyl-transpeptidase, an enzyme capable of catalysing the transfer of a gamma-glutamyl moiety (of glutathione or other gamma-glutamyl-containing compounds) to an amino acid or peptide acceptor to form the corresponding gamma-glutamyl amino acid or peptide derivative (Garvey, Hyman and Isselbacher, 1976). Although it shares the substrate specificity and kinetic properties of those detected in the renal brush border membrane (Tata and Meister, 1974), its precise physiological role and importance, if any, in human intestinal protein assimilation is unknown. Other peptidases may be present but require further study. A prolyl carboxypeptidase has been localized to the brush border membrane of rabbit small intestine (Auricchio et al, 1978). Intrinsic brush border endopeptidases may be present (Adibi and Kim, 1981) which are capable of hydrolysing dietary proteins or polypeptides, but a clear distinction from pancreatic enzymatic activities is still needed.

The products that arise from intestinal hydrolysis undergo transport by distinct mechanisms. For amino acids, the following observations have been made in human subjects: first, higher absorption rates for some amino acids are observed in the jejunum compared to ileum (Adibi and Gray, 1967); second, amino acids with longer side chains and lower net positive or negative electrical charges (i.e., neutral amino acids) have higher affinities for jejunal absorption sites, greater rates of absorption, and are able to competitively inhibit absorption of amino acids with lower affinities (Adibi and Gray, 1967); and third, different transport systems for amino acids are present that appear shared to some degree with mechanisms operative in the renal tubules (Freeman et al, 1978, 1979). Several rare amino acid transport defects have been described, and their clinical features are summarized in Table 1 (Freeman and Kim, 1979). Symptoms referable to the central nervous system or genitourinary tract predominate in these patients. Gastrointestinal symptoms and signs are generally uncommon. However, in

Table 1. *Intestinal amino acid transport disorders*

Disorder	Substrate(s)	Clinical features
Hartnup disease	Neutral amino acids	Pellagra-like rash, cerebellar ataxia, neuropsychiatric disorder, neutral aminoaciduria
Blue diaper disease (tryptophan malabsorption)	Tryptophan	Indigo blue discolouration of diapers, no tryptophanuria, growth retardation, hypercalcaemia
Oasthouse urine disease (methionine malabsorption)	Methionine	Seizures, mental retardation, episodic hyperpnoea, diarrhoea, urinary odour with increased alpha-hydroxybutryric acid
Cystinuria	Cystine, ornithine, arginine, lysine	Recurrent urinary tract calculi, hereditary pancreatitis, cerebral dysfunction, cystine-dibasic aminoaciduria
Hyperdibasic aminoaciduria	Lysine	Familial protein intolerance, diarrhoea, failure to thrive, hepatosplenomegaly, dibasic aminoaciduria (ornithine, arginine, lysine)
Joseph's syndrome (iminoglycinuria)	Proline, hydroxy-proline, glycine	No reproducible clinical picture, aminoaciduria (imino acids, glycine)

patients with cystinuria, recurrent episodes of abdominal pain may be associated with a hereditary form of chronic relapsing pancreatitis as well as urinary tract lithiasis. Intestinal uptake and renal tubular reabsorption of cystine and certain dibasic amino acids are impaired. Cystine may be insoluble in acid urine and can precipitate in the renal parenchyma to produce renal failure and stone formation. Stones are often radio-opaque and high in sulphur content. Diagnosis of cystinuria is aided by detection of flat hexagonal crystals in the urine with a positive cyanide nitroprusside test; confirmation may be sought by high voltage urinary electrophoresis. Homocystinuria, the only other disorder giving a positive cyanide nitro-prusside test, can readily be distinguished clinically and excluded definitively by urinary electrophoretic methods (Schriver and Rosenberg, 1973). Complications of cystinuria can include pancreatic insufficiency, pseudo-cyst formation, abdominal venous thrombosis, ductal calcification and carcinoma of the pancreas. Although the therapy is no different from that used in other types of pancreatitis, detailed screening of family members, even if asymptomatic, is indicated following discovery of the propositus.

Although the clinical impact of disordered intestinal amino acid transport is minimal, substantial evidence for independent mechanisms of amino acid and peptide uptake has resulted following detailed studies of these patients as reviewed elsewhere (Hellier and Holdsworth 1975; Matthews and Adibi, 1976; Freeman et al, 1978, 1979, 1981; Sleisenger and Kim, 1979). In Hartnup disease, for example, severe nutritional disturbance is uncommon despite a serious defect in the transport of neutral amino acids and continued nitrogen loss. This maintenance of normal nutrition is due to adequate protein intake with transport of intact dipeptides providing adequate amino acid uptake. Similar observations have been made in cystinuria.

For small peptides, more than one mode of intestinal mucosal uptake is evident (Hellier and Holdsworth, 1975; Matthews and Adibi, 1976; Freeman et al, 1978, 1979, 1981; Sleisenger and Kim, 1979; Adibi and Kim, 1981). In one, dipeptides and tripeptides poorly hydrolysed at the brush border can be absorbed intact, bypassing brush border aminopeptidases, with subsequent cytoplasmic hydrolysis. This mechanism of peptide transport appears distinct from the uptake mechanism for single amino acids. Alternatively, dipeptides and tripeptides may undergo initial hydrolysis at the brush border, and the resultant hydrolytic products, including both amino acids and dipeptides, are then absorbed by their respective transport mechanisms. Information regarding the limiting size of the peptide that can undergo intact absorption in human subjects is incomplete. Tetraglycine, the only tetrapeptide studied in vivo to date, appears to be initially hydrolysed into glycine and triglycine prior to transport. For large peptides present evidence, although limited in human subjects, suggests that the major site of hydrolysis is the brush border (Adibi et al, 1971, 1975). In experimental animals, absorption of a tetrapeptide may occur by a mechanism distinct from that for amino acids or for dipeptides and tripeptides (Chung, Silk and Kim, 1983).

Dipeptides can be absorbed well from both jejunum and ileum although greater mucosal hydrolytic activities for most peptide substrates are found distally. At present, the existence of more than one peptide transport system, analogous to different carriers proposed for amino acids, is controversial and remains unproved. To date, an isolated primary defect in peptide transport has not been reported.

Developmental changes

The mechanisms involved in protein assimilation appear to undergo maturation during fetal and neonatal life (Grand, Watkins and Torti, 1976). Studies on these developmental changes have been limited. Human fetal gastric peptic activity may be detected during the sixteenth week of gestation and increases substantially from the twenty-eighth to fortieth week (Werner, 1948). A 'fetal pepsinogen' has also been demonstrated by immunochemical methods in fetal gastric mucosa. Pepsin and acid secretions in the fetal stomach have not been well studied. In the neonatal period up to the age of two years, pepsin and acid secretions occur in parallel to reach adult levels. In the premature infant, it is thought that low gastric pepsin and acid content may produce detrimental nutritional effects but there are no firm supportive data available. Pancreatic zymogen granules may be observed in the fetus during the fifth month of gestation (Conklin, 1962; Liu and Potter, 1962). Tryptic activity, however, is measurable as early as sixteen weeks and increases with advancing gestational age, particularly after the twenty-eighth week (Lieberman, 1966). CCK and secretin administration produce stimulation of exocrine secretion in the neonate (Zoppi, Andreotti and Pajno-Ferrara, 1972). Maximal stimulation of pancreatic trypsin activity, if measured, appears to be low in the first 24 hours after birth but increases markedly by nine months (Grand, Watkins and Torti, 1976). Recent studies examining the development of intestinal regulatory peptides in the human fetus indicate that many, including secretin, can be detected as early as eight weeks with adult distribution patterns established by twenty weeks of age (Bryant et al, 1982). The functional significance of these observations remains to be defined. Absorption of intact protein occurs in both fetal and neonatal intestine, however, only limited information is available regarding in utero protein digestion and utilization. Transport of L-alanine has been documented in human fetus (Levin et al, 1968) but detailed studies on amino acid and peptide uptake are still required. The development of small intestinal enzyme activities has been examined with histochemical and analytical methods. Leucine aminopeptidase has been shown histochemically in the seven to eight week fetus and higher specific activities are found in proximal compared to distal small bowel early in fetal life. With increasing gestational age, activities increase more distally with the development of a proximal-to-distal gradient. After 16 weeks gestation, distal values are twice proximal values (Jirosva et al, 1966; Lindberg, 1966; Lev, Siegel and Bartman, 1972). In the fetus, the colon may also play a significant absorptive role in utero possibly because of some similarities to fetal small intestine.

Protein-energy malnutrition

Protein-energy malnutrition may result from reduced protein intake or inability to consume sufficient amounts of dietary proteins, ingestion of poor quality protein, impaired digestion and/or absorption of ingested protein, or excessive gastrointestinal protein loss, i.e., protein-losing gastro-enteropathy. Moreover, requirements may be significantly increased in patients due to growth, pregnancy, tissue injury or a superimposed disease. In some individuals with chronic debilitating disease there may be multiple contributing factors present. This is especially true in hospitalized patients where net nitrogen loss frequently develops. In turn, protein-energy malnutrition may itself change the structure and/or function of several tissues critical to the assimilation process, including the intestinal tract and pancreas.

Protein-energy malnutrition may occur at any age, although most observations are based on studies conducted in underdeveloped nations. Separation of protein-energy malnutrition into a predominately protein-depleted (i.e., kwashiorkor) or calorie (i.e., energy) starved (i.e., marasmus) state may be artificial since features attributed to either condition usually coexist. In addition, changes observed have poorly defined limits and may be dominated by the results of other nutrient/vitamin deficiency syndromes, disturbances in fluid-electrolyte balance and the frequent occurrence of viral, bacterial and parasitic infections in these patients.

Clinical and laboratory features of protein-energy malnutrition have been previously reviewed (Freeman et al, 1979) and vary depending on the severity and duration of nutrient deficiency, age at onset, and the presence or absence of other contributing factors. Clinical findings are not specific and may be caused by other non-nutritional factors. Despite this limitation, their identification may indicate the presence of protein-energy malnutrition and permit the formulation of an index of nutritional status. With minimal deficiency, abnormalities may be subtle, especially in adults where growth requirements are minimal. Muscle wasting, loss of subcutaneous fat, weakness and psychomotor changes may develop. Non-tender parotid enlargement occurs. Patchy brown pigmentation appears, especially over the malar eminences of the face. The hair becomes lacklustre with thinning and increased shedding, especially from the sides of the head. Bradycardia is observed. In some, variable degrees of hepatic enlargement occur associated with steatosis on liver biopsy. In adults with severe malnutrition, or in growing children, clinical features are more significant. Muscle wasting, subcutaneous fat loss, dependent oedema and weight loss may be marked. Severe mental apathy and reduced physical activity occur. Abnormalities in the hair, especially in children, may be striking with severe dyspigmentation. Hair may be removed without discomfort and nails become brittle with horizontal grooves. An asymmetrical confluent pattern of skin hyperpigmentation may develop, particularly over perineal as well as exposed areas such as the face. Extensive skin desquamation results in areas of depigmentation and superficial ulceration, particularly on the buttocks and posterior aspects of the thighs. Gastrointestinal symptoms are common. These include marked constipation to severe diarrhoea, anorexia or hyperphagia, nausea, vomiting and dehydration. Laboratory features also vary. There may be a significant reduction in serum proteins, including serum albumin and some higher molecular weight transport proteins such as transferrin, ceruloplasmin, lipoproteins, and thyroxin- and cortisol-binding proteins. Serum amino acid anlysis may show a decrease in essential amino acids (i.e., leucine, isoleucine, valine, methionine) and either normal or depressed levels of non-essentials (i.e., glycine, serine, glutamine). The urinary excretion of urea, creatinine and hydroxyproline may be decreased. Severe electrolyte abnormalities develop although serum levels may be normal.

Structural and functional changes in the gastrointestinal tract and pancreas may result from protein-energy malnutrition which, in turn, may further aggravate nutritional status (Viteri and Schneider, 1973). Pancreatic acinar cell atrophy may occur with reduced numbers of zymogen granules detectable in exocrine cells (Barbezat and Hansen, 1968). The pancreatic response to stimulation with CCK and/or secretin is reduced (Barbezat and Hansen, 1968), with a reduced content of enzyme activities (i.e., trypsin, chymotrypsin, lipase, amylase) recorded for pancreatic juice (Viteri and Schneider, 1973). Reversibility appears possible with return to normal nutritional state, but this may require several weeks (Barbezat and Hansen, 1968). The stomach and small bowel mucosal thickness appears reduced (Schneider and Viteri, 1972), resembling observations in 'starved' self-emptying blind intestinal segments after experimental jejunoileal bypass (Garrido et al, 1981). This change also appears to be reversible with protein repletion (Schneider and Viteri, 1972). With light microscopy marked changes may develop, including a severely abnormal 'flat' small intestinal mucosa (Perera et al, 1974). In contrast to changes seen in coeliac sprue, reduced numbers of crypt mitoses may be seen and the mucosa may appear hypoplastic (Brunser et al, 1966; Rose et al, 1971; Hopper et al, 1972). Protein repletion may cause a complete reversion to normal mucosal structure (Barbezat and Hansen, 1968; Duque, Bolanos and Lotero, 1975). Non-specific ultrastructural changes have been observed, including the presence of lipid droplets in epithelial cells that disappear with protein repletion (Duque, Lotero and Bolanos, 1975). Changes may be present throughout the small bowel in an irregular 'patchy' distribution, although the jejunum appears most severely affected in protein-deficient monkeys (Deo and Ramalingaswami, 1963). Qualitative and quantitative changes in the intestinal microflora, particularly anaerobes, occur in protein-energy malnutrition (Mata et al, 1972). However, their role in altering mucosal structure and function in these patients remains to be defined. Activities of several mucosal enzymes (i.e., disaccharidases) (Bowie et al, 1965; Dahlquist and Lindquist, 1971) are reduced reflecting, in part, reduced numbers of mucosal cells similar to alterations reported in rats after experimental jejunoileal bypass in the blind loop (Garrido et al, 1981). As a result, mal-absorption of various substances (i.e., lactose) may be observed. Reversion of changes to normal can follow protein repletion. In such patients, however, the precise relationship to ethnic enzymatic deficiencies (i.e., lactase) remains unclear. Altered uptake of glucose and D-xylose is reported (James, 1968; Viteri et al, 1973). Steatorrhoea may be present with impaired absorption of fat and some fat-soluble vitamins (Viteri et al, 1973). Faecal nitrogen may be increased both in human subjects and in experimental animals with protein-depletion (Viteri and Schneider, 1973). Serum protein loss into the gastrointestinal tract may be increased (Cohen et al, 1962). Studies in patients with protein-energy malnutrition associated with chronic infection or jejunoileal bypass for obesity suggest that both peptide and amino acid uptake may be significantly reduced (Fogel et al, 1976). However, peptide transport is less severely altered (Fogel et al, 1976). Aminopeptidase activities have been studied only to a limited extent in humans and appear to be reduced but increased with protein repletion (Gjessing et al, 1977). In experimental animals deprived of protein, peptidase activities of the brush border fraction are reduced whereas activities in the cytoplasmic fraction are increased (Nicholson et al, 1974). Treatment of protein-energy malnutrition requires administration of high quality protein with sufficient calories and supplemented with other essential minerals and vitamins. During therapy, attention to fluid-electrolyte imbalances and to the threat of infections are critical.

Protein-energy malnutrition is a frequent accompaniment of cancer. Progressive wasting, weakness and anorexia develop and a multitude of metabolic changes occur as the tumour enlarges and becomes more advanced (Lawson et al, 1982). Initially, total body protein may be unchanged, although there is a redistribution of nitrogen from muscle to tumour. Subsequently, with severe anorexia, total body protein declines with depletion of essential nutrients (Fenninger and Mider, 1954). Such changes are not unique to malignant disease but occur to some degree in 30 to 50 per cent of hospitalized patients, including those with chronic non-neoplastic disorders (e.g., chronic disseminated infections, cardiopulmonary or renal failure) (Heymsfield et al, 1980). The mechanisms associated with the development of cancer cachexia are poorly understood, and probably reflect multiple causes including reduced intake as well as impaired mechanisms for digestion and/or absorption. A number of other metabolic factors, however, play a role, some appearing unique for neoplasia.

Hypophagia is prominent in advanced malignancy. Although contributing mechanical factors (e.g., malignant oesophageal stricture, ascites) and anorexigenic therapy (e.g., radiotherapy, chemotherapy) are responsible in part, food aversion may occur in the absence of such factors and is poorly correlated with tumour bulk (Garathini et al, 1980). In experimental animals, feeding activity may be initiated normally but may be terminated earlier, suggesting that responsiveness to normal neural signals of feeding and satiety are altered (Lawson et al, 1982). In addition, taste sensation may be abnormal (DeWys, 1979). A variety of mechanisms have been postulated, including the release of bioactive factors from the tumour. Impaired digestion and absorption of protein in cancer patients frequently results, with direct neoplastic involvement of the pancreas or small bowel, enteropathic effects of treatment (i.e., especially with radiation or chemotherapy), mesenteric lymphatic infiltration by tumour or mucosal atrophy imposed by starvation. Metabolic studies indicate that anorexia can only partially explain the wasting process associated with cancer. It appears that metabolic disturbances within the tumour or within host tissues, or both, also play a significant role. Metabolic changes in cancer cells have been extensively reviewed by others (Lawson et al, 1982). Carbohydrate, lipid and amino acid metabolism in cancer cells are substantially altered and may contribute to the growth advantage of malignant cells as well as the overall picture of cancer cachexia. Consumption of glucose and production of lactate are increased. Hexoses utilized by malignant cells may support proliferation as well as energy production. Significant changes in fatty acid and cholesterol metabolism occur and disproportionate amounts of amino acids are preferentially used by tumour cells with a significant impact on the host as well as having a regulatory role in cell division. Wasting of muscle and adipose tissue occurs, in part, because protein synthesis and carbohydrate utilization are suppressed in skeletal muscle. Some of these features are shared in individuals without cancer while hepatic alterations in glucose/amino acid metabolism may reflect the response of the liver to release of bioactive products by the tumour. Thus, protein-energy malnutrition in the cancer patient shares many of the features seen in non-neoplastic disorders. However, relatively unique metabolic derangements occur, contributing to anorexia and hypermetabolism, that require further elucidation.

PROTEIN MALDIGESTION AND MALABSORPTION

The principal causes of impaired assimilation of dietary protein are diseases of the exocrine pancreas and small intestine. Severe protein-energy malnutrition may result. However, even after total pancreatectomy, significant absorption may occur. In animals with pancreatic duct ligation, 37 per cent of administered protein was absorbed despite the absence of luminal trypsin activity (Curtis et al, 1979). This suggests that the intestine is rate-limiting although pancreatic enzymes remain critical to the process.

Pancreatic exocrine insufficiency

Deficient luminal proteolytic activity can result directly from diseases involving the exocrine pancreas. The reserve capacity of this organ appears to be considerable and nitrogen loss is significant only if trypsin is less than 10 per cent of normal (DiMagno et al, 1973). Low intraluminal trypsin concentrations are observed after peptic ulcer surgery (MacGregor et al, 1977). In this situation, the pancreas can respond normally to exogenous stimuli, and reduced proteolytic enzyme levels result primarily from rapid gastric emptying and subsequent intraluminal dilution of pancreatic enzymes (MacGregor et al, 1977).

Reduced pancreatic proteolytic activity may result indirectly from intestinal enterokinase deficiency (Hadorn et al, 1969). This is a rare disorder characterized by vomiting, diarrhoea, hypoproteinaemia, anaemia and failure to thrive. Diagnosis can be made by detection of absent trypsin, chymotrypsin and carboxypeptidase activities in small intestinal juice followed by increased activities after addition of enterokinase, i.e., a zymogen activation test. In the limited number of patients with detailed studies, the small intestinal biopsy is reportedly normal and enterokinase activity deficient. In isolated trypsinogen deficiency (Townes, 1965), the clinical presentation is similar to enterokinase deficiency. However, addition of enterokinase to duodenal fluid fails to cause an increase in tryptic activity.

Several methods are available to examine the function of the exocrine pancreas (Arvanitakis and Cooke, 1978). The analysis of duodenal contents after direct hormonal stimulation with secretin (and/or CCK), or indirectly, after a test meal (i.e., Lundh meal) remains the most useful at present. These require duodenal intubation under fluoroscopic guidance with care taken to prevent contamination with gastric content. Enzymatic activities (including trypsin and chymotrypsin) can be measured before and after pancreatic exocrine stimulation; however, it is generally thought that enzyme response measurements provide a less accurate assessment of functioning acinar cells compared to electrolyte (especially bicarbonate) response (Arvanitakis and Cooke, 1978). Wide ranges in normal subjects occur, and difficulties are evident in defining abnormal limits (Goldberg and Wormsley, 1970). Intraduodenal pancreatic enzyme concentrations may not accurately reflect concentrations in pancreatic secretions owing to differing activation rates of proenzymes, calcium ion concentrations required for trypsinogen activation, as well as dilutional and luminal pH effects. Caerulein and bombesin have also been recorded as hormonal stimulants (Goldberg and Wormsley, 1970) but standardization is still required. In patients with more advanced pancreatic disease sufficient to cause significant steatorrhoea and or azotorrhoea, feeding of a liquid test meal with measurement of duodenal trypsin activity can provide an inexpensive, technically easy and reliable test of pancreatic function (Lundh, 1962). Generally, this is performed after an overnight fast followed by ingestion of a meal containing 6 per cent fat, 15 per cent carbohydrate and 5 per cent protein. This indirect test has additional disadvantages. Normal gastroduodenal anatomy is required along with intact small bowel mucosa. In coeliac sprue, for example, the test may not be valid because of impaired hormonal release from the intestinal epithelium (DiMagno et al, 1972). Similar enzyme responses may be measured after different test meals of varying composition. A meal of essential amino acids has been advocated to provide as great a response as direct stimulation with CCK (Go et al, 1970). Following oral ingestion of gelatin or casein, digestion products in serum, in intestinal content and in urine have been measured, although the clinical value of this test remains to be determined (Cerda et al, 1968). Recently, a new approach has been advocated employing a synthetic peptide, N-benzoyl-L-tyrosyl-p-aminobenzoic acid (Bz-Ty-PABA). This peptide is specifically cleaved by chymotrypsin to Bz-Ty and PABA. PABA is absorbed and undergoes urinary excretion. The urinary PABA concentration is thought to reflect intraluminal chymotrypsin activity. Some drugs — including sulphonamides, thiazide and furosemide diuretics, acetominophen, and antimicrobials like chloramphenicol, as well as hippurate precursor-containing foods — may interfere with the test. In this investigation, the need for intubation is eliminated; however, gastric emptying, intestinal absorption and renal function must be normal (Arvanitakis and Greenberger, 1976).

Duodenal fluid is a mixture of secretions from different sources. For this reason, pure pancreatic juice collected at the time of endoscopic ductal cannulation may be valuable because of the potential opportunity to localize more precisely a digestive defect. Several problems are apparent, however, that may restrict its usefulness. These include the need for local anaesthetics and sedatives, technical problems in cannulation, and finally, leakage around the cannula, particularly during long collections. Measurements of faecal trypsin and chymotrypsin levels are of limited value but may be useful in children in whom intubation may be more difficult. Tests of therapy, such as a favourable reduction in azotorrhoea with oral pancreatic enzymes, may potentially provide a further index of exocrine pancreatic function. Although a variety of imaging methods are available, most provide information regarding organ structure rather than function. In the future, however, modern imaging methods employing radioisotopes in positron emission tomographic scanners or nuclear magnetic resonance may find some applicability in the study of pancreatic function.

Small intestinal disease

Mucosal diseases may lead to defective protein assimilation. In patients with coeliac sprue, several mechanisms appear to be present. First, jejunal absorption of free amino acids and dipeptides may be reduced, although peptide absorption appears to be less severely altered (Adibi, Fogel and Agrawal, 1974). Second, intestinal digestion of peptides is impaired due to reduced numbers of mucosal cells and peptidase activities (Heizer and Laster, 1969). Third, increased endogenous protein from accelerated turnover and desquamation of lining epithelium as well as excessive intestinal loss of serum proteins may further protein deficiency (Waldman, 1966; Freeman, Kim and Sleisenger, 1979). Finally, the effects of protein-energy malnutrition may be superimposed. With gluten restriction, all these abnormalities are usually reversed.

In patients with significantly reduced intestinal absorptive surface following surgical resection or jejunoileal bypass, the ability to assimilate dietary protein may be markedly reduced. Precise quantitative information in human subjects following massive resection is not available. However, in rats able to maintain their body weight, 70 per cent removal of the proximal jejunoileum results in increased absorption of amino acids and dipeptides as well as aminopeptidase activities in the residual ileal segment (Garrido et al, 1979). Although the intestinal mucosa in human subjects can compensate to a limited degree, this may be insufficient in the long term to prevent malnutrition. Furthermore, other factors may contribute to a continued state of negative nitrogen balance, the most important of which is residual mucosal disease. Moreover, altered motility and stasis of intestinal content following surgery may lead to overgrowth of bacteria, and this, in itself, may lead to nitrogen wasting. Following jejunoileal bypass for severe obesity, protein-energy malnutrition frequently develops, in large part, due to exclusion of a major portion of the absorptive surface. In the rat, intestinal amino acid and peptide absorption in vivo as well as mucosal aminopeptidase activities are reduced in the bypassed segment (Garrido et al, 1981). Similar reductions in amino acid and peptide transport in vivo in the non-bypassed segment have been reported in humans (Fogel, Rawich and Adibi, 1976). In these patients relative sparing of peptide transport was observed (Fogel, Rawich and Adibi, 1976), suggesting that peptide diets might provide a nutritional advantage over equivalent amino acid mixtures in these patients (Fogel, Rawich and Adibi, 1976; Matthews and Adibi, 1976). In recent years, the use of intravenous dipeptides and tripeptides in experimental animals have been tested. Although other tissues besides intestine appear capable of assimilating some peptides, their effectiveness and safety will require more detailed evaluation before their use in humans can be recommended.

In small intestinal bacterial overgrowth or stasis syndrome significant evidence of protein wasting may be present, sometimes severe enough to resemble protein-energy malnutrition (Isaacs and Kim, 1974; King and Toskes, 1979). In addition, reduced serum albumin concentrations and excessive faecal nitrogen excretion occurs. The pathogenesis for these phenomena are probably multifactorial. Reduced output of enterokinase may be present (Rutgeerts, Mainguet and Tytgat, 1974). Uptake of L-leucine is impaired in experimental animals with self-filling blind loops, suggesting that amino acid transport may be altered in this condition

(Giannella, Rout and Toskes, 1974). Increased intraluminal endogenous protein may be present in rats with self-filling blind loops (Curtis, Prizont and Kim, 1979). In addition, amino acids from both exogenous and endogenous sources may be converted to unusable forms by bacteria. Organisms in the small intestine may elaborate enzymes that deaminate or decarboxylate amino acids. A patient with blind loop syndrome and marked hypoproteinaemia was observed to have reduced albumin and fibrinogen synthesis (Jones et al, 1968). This was thought to result from bacterial deamination of dietary protein with subsequent ammonia formation and utilization of ammonia for urea synthesis. Several microbes produce tryptophanase which converts tryptophan to indole derivatives. These may be absorbed and metabolized to indicans and subsequently excreted. Following intake of oral antimicrobials, urinary tryptophan metabolites decrease and stool tryptophan increases. This has also been observed in Hartnup disease, underlining the importance of the intestinal microflora in this disorder. However, urinary indican excretion may also increase in patients with small intestinal mucosal disease. This appears to be related to delivery of increased amounts of unabsorbed tryptophan to the colon where indole compounds are formed prior to being absorbed and excreted in the urine. Enteric loss of protein also occurs, especially if intestinal stricture or inflamed small bowel is present. In addition to morphological alterations, significant faecal protein loss is demonstrable. Protein loss appears to reflect functionally significant mucosal injury in the contaminated non-stagnant small bowel as well as the stagnant part of the small intestine affected by bacterial overgrowth. Antimicrobial therapy may partially or completely reverse protein loss after prolonged therapy, but surgical extirpation of the bowel loop may be necessary (King and Toskes, 1981).

Protein-losing gastroenteropathy

This disorder may be suspected in any patient with hypoproteinaemia or hypoalbuminaemia, particularly if hepatic and renal function are normal. The gastrointestinal tract plays a small but significant role in the normal metabolism and degradation of serum proteins (Waldman, 1966). Studies using radioactively labelled albumin indicate that this tissue accounts for about 10 per cent of normal turnover (Waldman, 1966). With disease, excessive loss occurs from the inflamed or ulcerated mucosa associated with altered intestinal cell permeability. In some disorders, lymphatic pressure may be increased due to 'downstream' obstruction, and lymphatic rupture has been postulated. To date, the precise route of loss under normal in vivo conditions remains to be elucidated. Several clinical conditions have been described with protein loss as a complication (Waldman, 1966). In part, the development of more refined quantitative methods for the identification of plasma proteins in gastrointestinal secretions and excreta has been instrumental.

To document enteric protein loss, the patient is given an intravenous injection of a labelled protein (e.g., albumin). Over a four-day period less than 1 per cent of ^{51}Cr-albumin will be detected in stools of normal subjects, although higher levels may be observed if there is urinary contamination of the collection. In most patients with protein-losing gastroenteropathy, excessive levels above 2 per cent are observed (Waldman, 1966). Studies with labelled globulins reveal a reduced intravascular pool along with an increased fractional catabolic rate comparable to rates observed for albumin catabolism. These results suggest that bulk loss of all serum proteins occurs rather than selective loss. Although diagnosis depends on documentation of excessive enteric protein loss, lymphangiectasia may be observed in some patients on mucosal biopsy. However, caution is advised in overinterpretation of apparent lymphatic dilatation, particularly if the remainder of the biopsy is completely normal (Perera et al, 1975). Furthermore, mucosal biopsy cannot be used to distinguish between primary and secondary forms of lymphangiectasia (Perera et al, 1975). In the primary form, children or young adults are usually affected. Asymmetrical oedema, lymphocytopenia, impaired cell-mediated immune responsiveness (i.e., delayed hypersensitivity, homograft survival) and deficient or abnormal lymphatic drainage at other sites (i.e., chylothorax, chylous ascites, chyluria) occur. Malabsorption, particularly of fat, may be present since long-chain fatty acids require lymphatic transport. Chylous fluid may be detected in the duodenum whereas lymphangiograms may show hypoplastic peripheral and visceral lymphatics. A low-fat diet or a diet containing medium-chain triglycerides may reduce lymphatic flow. For patients with secondary forms of enteric protein loss therapy should be directed to the underlying condition if a specific cause can be defined.

To a large extent, the methods available for documentation of enteric protein loss are cumbersome, involve the use of expensive radiochemicals, and prohibit other diagnostic procedures from being performed. Recently, faecal clearance measurements of alpha-1-antitrypsin have been advocated as a sensitive marker of endogenous protein loss (Florent et al, 1981) and studies suggest a significant correlation with ^{51}Cr-plasma protein clearance. Further studies are needed to confirm these observations.

ACKNOWLEDGEMENTS

Supported by research grants from the Medical Research Council of Canada (MA 6918) and the National Cancer Institute of Canada to Dr Freeman, US Public Health Service grant AM 17938 through the National Institutes of Health (Dr Kim) and the Veterans Administration Medical Research Service (Drs Kim and Sleisenger). Dr Freeman is a Research Scholar supported by the British Columbia Health Care Research Foundation.

REFERENCES

Adelson, J. W. & Rothman, S. S. (1975) Chymodenin, a duodenal peptide: specific stimulation of chymotrypsinogen secretion. *American Journal of Physiology,* **229**, 1680-1686.
Adibi, S. A. & Gray, S. J. (1967) Intestinal absorption of essential amino acids in man. *Gastroenterology,* **52**, 837.
Adibi, S. A. & Kim, Y. S. (1981) Peptide absorption and hydrolysis. In *Physiology of the Gastrointestinal Tract* (Ed.) Johnson, L. R., Christensen, J., Grossman, M. I. et al. Volume, 2. pp. 1073-1095.
Adibi, S. A. & Mercer, D. W. (1973) Protein digestion in human intestine as reflected in luminal, mucosal and plasma amino acid concentrations after meals. *Journal of Clinical Investigation,* **52**, 1586-1594.

Adibi, S. A. & Morse, E. L. (1971) Intestinal transport of dipeptides in man: relative importance of hydrolysis and intact absorption. *Journal of Clinical Investigation,* **50,** 2266-2275.

Adibi, S. A. & Morse, E. L. (1979) The number of glycine residues which limits intact absorption of glycine oligopeptides in human jejunum. *Journal of Clinical Investigation,* **60,** 1008-1016.

Adibi, S. A., Fogel, M. R. & Agrawal, R. M. (1974) Comparison of free amino acid and dipeptide absorption in the jejunum of sprue patients. *Gastroenterology,* **67,** 586-591.

Adibi, S. A., Morse, E. L., Masilamani, S. S. & Amin, P. M. (1975) Evidence for two different modes of tripeptide disappearance in human intestine. *Journal of Clinical Investigation,* **56,** 1355-1363.

Arvanitakis, C. & Greenberger, N. J. (1976) Diagnosis of pancreatic disease by a synthetic peptide — a new test of pancreatic function. *Lancet,* **i,** 663-666.

Arvanitakis, C. & Cooke, A. R. (1978) Diagnostic tests of exocrine pancreatic function and disease. *Gastroenterology,* **74,** 932-948.

Auricchio, S., Greco, L., DeVizia, B. & Buonocore, V. (1978) Dipeptidyl amino peptidase and carboxypeptidase activities of the brush border of rabbit small intestine. *Gastroenterology,* **75,** 1073-1079.

Baksi, K. & Radhakrishnan, A. N. (1974) Purification and properties of prolidase (imidodipeptidase) from monkey small intestine. *Indian Journal of Biochemistry and Biophysics,* **11,** 7-11.

Barbezat, G. O. & Hansen, J. D. L. (1968) The exocrine pancreas and protein calorie malnutrition. *Pediatrics,* **42,** 77.

Bennett, G., Leblond, C. P. & Haddad, A. (1974) Migration of glycoprotein from the Golgi apparatus to the surface of various cell types as shown by radioautography after labelled fucose injection into rats. *Journal of Cell Biology,* **60,** 258-284.

Bockman, D. E. & Winborn, W. B. (1966) Light and electron microscopy of intestinal ferritin absorption. Observations in sensitized and non-sensitized hamsters. *Anatomical Record,* **155,** 603-622.

Bowie, M. D., Brinkman, G. L. & Hansen, J. D. L. (1965) Acquired disaccharide intolerance in malnutrition. *Journal of Pediatrics,* **66,** 1083.

Brunser, O., Reid, A. & Monckeberg, F. (1966) Jejunal biopsies in infant malnutrition: with special reference to mitotic index. *Pediatrics,* **38,** 605.

Bryant, M. G., Buchan, A. M. J., Gregor, M. et al (1982) Development of intestinal regulatory peptides in the human fetus. *Gastroenterology,* **83,** 47-54.

Cerda, J. J., Brooks, F. P. & Prockup, D. J. (1968) Intraduodenal hydrolysis of gelatin as a measure of protein digestion in normal subjects and in patients with malabsorption of syndromes. *Gastroenterology,* **54,** 358-365.

Chariot, J., Roze, C., Vaille, C. & Debray, C. (1978) Effects of somatostatin on the external secretion of the pancreas of the rat. *Gastroenterology,* **75,** 832-837.

Chung, Y. C., Silk, D. B. A. & Kim, Y. S. (1983) Intestinal transport of a tetrapeptide. L-leucyl-glycyl-glycyl-glycine in rat small intestine in vivo. *Clinical Science and Molecular Medicine,* in press.

Chung, Y. C., Kim, Y. S., Scadchehr, A., Garrido, A., McGregor, I. L. & Sleisenger, M. H. (1979) Protein digestion and absorption in human small intestine. *Gastroenterology,* **76,** 1415-1421.

Cohen, J., Metz, J. & Hart, D. (1962) Protein-losing gastroenteropathy in Kwashiorkor. *Lancet,* **i,** 725.

Conklin, J. L. (1962) Cytogenesis of human fetal pancreas. *American Journal of Anatomy,* **11,** 181-203.

Cornell, R., Walker, W. A. & Isselbacher, K. J. (1971) Small intestinal absorption of horse-radish peroxidase. A cytochemical study. *Laboratory Investigation,* **25,** 42-48.

Curtis, K. J., Gaines, H. D. & Kim, Y. S. (1979) Protein digestion and absorption in rats with pancreatic duct occlusion. *Gastroenterology,* **74,** 1271-1276.

Curtis, K. J., Prizont, R. & Kim, Y. S. (1979) Protein digestion and absorption in the blind loop syndrome. *Digestive Diseases and Sciences,* **24,** 929-933.

Dahlquist, A. & Lindquist, B. (1971) Lactose intolerance and protein malnutrition. *Acta Paediatrica Scandinavica,* **60,** 488.

Deo, M. G. & Ramalingaswami, V. (1963) Absorption of [58]Co-labeled cyanocobalamin in protein deficiency. *Gastroenterology,* **44,** 167.

DeWys, W. D. (1979) Anorexia as a general effect of cancer. *Cancer*, **43**, 2013-2019.

DiMagno, E. P., Go, V. L. W. & Summerskill, W. H. J. (1972) Impaired cholecystokinin-pancreozymin secretion, intraluminal dilution and maldigestion of fat in sprue. *Gastroenterology*, **63**, 25-32.

DiMagno, E. P., Go, V. L. W. & Summerskill, W. H. J. (1973) Relations between pancreatic enzyme outputs and malabsorption in severe pancreatic insufficiency. *New England Journal of Medicine*, **288**, 813-815.

Duque, E., Bolanos, O. & Lotero, H. (1975) Enteropathy in adult protein malnutrition: light microscopic findings. *American Journal of Clinical Nutrition*, **28**, 901.

Duque, E., Lotero, H. & Bolanos, O. (1975) Enteropathy in adult protein malnutrition: ultrastructural findings. *American Journal of Clinical Nutrition*, **28**, 914.

Fenninger, L. D. & Mider, G. B. (1954) Energy and nitrogen metabolism in cancer. *Advances in Cancer Research*, **2**, 229-253.

Feracci, H., Bernadac, A., Gorvel, J. P. & Maroux, S. (1982) Localization by immunofluorescence and histochemical labelling of aminopeptidase N in relation to its biosynthesis in rabbit and pig enterocytes. *Gastroenterology*, **82**, 317-324.

Florent, C., L'Hirondel, C., Desmazures, C. et al (1981) Intestinal clearance of alpha-1-antitrypsin. A sensitive method for the detection of protein-losing enteropathy. *Gastroenterology*, **81**, 777-780.

Fogel, M. R., Rawitch, M. M. & Adibi, S. A. (1976) Absorptive and digestive functions of the jejunum after jejunoileal bypass for treatment of human obesity. *Gastroenterology*, **71**, 729-733.

Freeman, H. J. (1981) Digestion and absorption of carbohydrate, protein and fat. *Medicine North America*, **18**, 1763-1769.

Freeman, H. J. & Kim, Y. S. (1978) Digestion and absorption of protein. *Annual Review of Medicine*, **29**, 99-116.

Freeman, H. J., Kim, Y. S. & Sleisenger, M. H. (1979) Protein digestion and absorption in man. Normal mechanisms and protein-energy malnutrition. *American Journal of Medicine*, **67**, 1030-1036.

Garathini, S., Bizzi, A., Donelli, M. G. et al (1980) Anorexia and cancer in animals and man. *Cancer Treatment Reviews*, **7**, 115-140.

Garrido, A. B., Freeman, H. J. & Kim, Y. S. (1981) Amino acid and peptide absorption in bypassed jejunum following jejunoileal bypass in rats. *Digestive Diseases and Sciences*, **26**, 107-112.

Garrido, A. B., Freeman, H. J., Chung, Y. C. & Kim, Y. S. (1979) Amino acid and peptide absorption after proximal small intestinal resection, *Gut*, **20**, 114-120.

Garvey, I. Q., Hyman, P. E. & Isselbacher, K. J. (1976) Gamma-glutamyl transpeptidase of rat intestine: localization and possible role in amino acid transport. *Gastroenterology*, **71**, 778-785.

Giannella, R. A., Rout, W. R. & Toskes, P. O. (1974) Jejunal brush border injury and impaired sugar and amino acid uptake in the blind loop syndrome. *Gastroenterology*, **67**, 965-974.

Gjessing, E. C., Villanewa, D. & Duque, E. (1977) Dipeptide hydrolase activity of the intestinal mucosa from protein-malnourished adult patients and controls. *American Journal of Clinical Nutrition*, **30**, 1044.

Go, V. L. W., Hofmann, A. F. & Summerskill, W. H. J. (1970) Pancreozymin bioassay in man based on pancreatic enzyme secretion: potency of specific amino acids and other digestive products. *Journal of Clinical Investigation*, **49**, 1558-1564.

Goldberg, D. M. & Wormsley, K. G. (1970) The interrelationship of pancreatic enzymes in human duodenal asperate. *Gut*, **11**, 859-866.

Grand, R. J., Watkins, J. B. & Torti, F. M. (1976) Development of the human gastrointestinal tract. *Gastroenterology*, **70**, 790-810.

Gray, G. M. & Cooper H. L. (1971) Protein digestion and absorption. *Gastroenterology*, **61**, 535.

Gray, G. M. & Santiago, N. A. (1977) Intestinal surface amino-oligopeptidases. 1. Isolation of two weight isomers and their subunits from rat brush border. *Journal of Biological Chemistry*, **252**, 4922-4928.

Grusky, F. C. & Cooke, R. C. (1955) The gastrointestinal absorption of unaltered protein in normal infants and in infants recovering from diarrhea. *Pediatrics*, **16**, 763-768.

Hadorn, B., Tarlow, M. J., Lloyd, J. D. & Wolff, O. H. (1969) Intestinal enterokinase deficiency. *Lancet,* **i,** 812-813.

Heizer, W. D. & Laster, L. (1969) Peptide hydrolase activities of the mucosa of human small intestine. *Journal of Clinical Investigation,* **48,** 210-228.

Hellier, M. D. & Holdsworth, C. D. (1975) Digestion and absorption of proteins. In *Intestinal Absorption in Man* (Ed.) McColl, I. & Sladen, G. E. pp. 143-186. London: Academic Press.

Heymsfield, S. B., Horowitz, J. & Lawson, D. H. (1980) Enteral hyperalimentation. In *Developments in Digestive Diseases* (Ed.) Berk, J. E. Volume **3,** 59-83. Philadelphia: Lea and Febiger.

Hopper, A. F., Rose, P. M. & Wannemacher, R. W. (1972) Cell population changes in the intestinal mucosa of protein-depleted or starved rats. II. Changes in cellular migration in rats. *Journal of Cell Biology,* **53,** 225.

Isaacs, P. E. T. & Kim, Y. S. (1974) The contaminated small bowel syndrome. *American Journal of Medicine,* **67,** 1049-1057.

James, W. P. T. (1968) Intestinal absorption in protein caloric malnutrition. *Lancet,* **i,** 333.

Jeffries, G. H. (1978) Protein metabolism and protein-losing enteropathy. In *Gastrointestinal Disease* (Ed.) Sleisenger, M. H. & Fordtran, J. S. Second Edition. pp. 354-367. Philadelphia: W. B. Saunders.

Jirosva, V., Koldovsky, O., Heringova, A. et al (1966) The development of the functions of the small intestine of the human fetus. *Biology of the Neonate,* **9,** 44-49.

Jones, E. A., Craigie, A., Taville, A. S. et al (1968) Protein metabolism in the intestinal stagnant loop syndrome. *Gut,* **9,** 466-469.

Kanra, R. K., Santiago, N. W. & Gray, G. M. (1977) Intestinal surface oligoaminopeptidases. II. Substrate kinetics and topography of the active site. *Journal of Biological Chemistry,* **252,** 4929-4934.

Kenny, A. J., Booth, A. C., George, S. G. et al. (1976) Dipeptidyl peptidase IV, a kidney brush border serine peptidase. *Biochemical Journal,* **157,** 169-182.

Kim, Y. S., Birtwhistle, W. & Kim, Y. (1972) Peptide hydrolases in the brush border and soluble fractions of small intestinal mucosa of rat and man. *Journal of Clinical Investigation,* **51,** 1419-1430.

Kim, Y. S. & Brophy, E. J. (1976) Rat intestinal brush border membrane peptidases. 1. Solubilization, purification and physicochemical properties of two different forms of the enzyme. *Journal of Biological Chemistry,* **251,** 3199-3205.

Kim, Y. S., Brophy, E. J. & Nicholson, J. A. (1976) Rat intestinal brush border membrane peptidases. 2. Enzymatic properties, immunochemistry and interactions with lectins of two different forms of the enzyme. *Journal of Biological Chemistry,* **251,** 3206-3212.

Kim, Y. S., Kim, Y. & Sleisinger, M. H. (1974) Studies on the properties of peptide hydrolases on the brush border and soluble fractions of small intestinal mucosa of rat and man. *Biochimica et Biophysica Acta,* **370,** 283-296.

Kim, Y. S., Kim, Y., Gaines, H. D. & Sleisinger, M. H. (1979) Zymogram studies of human intestinal bush border and cytoplasmic peptidases. *Gut,* **20,** 987-991.

King, C. E. & Toskes, P. P. (1979) Small intestine bacterial overgrowth. *Gastroenterology,* **76,** 1035-1055.

King, C. E. & Toskes, P. P. (1981) Protein-losing enteropathy in the human and experimental rat blind-loop syndrome. *Gastroenterology,* **80,** 504-509.

Korenblat, R. E., Rothberg, R. M. & Minden, P. (1968) Immune response of human adults after oral and parenteral exposure to bovine serum albumin. *Journal of Allergy,* **41,** 226-235.

Lawson, D. H., Richmond, A., Nixon, D. W. & Rudman, D. (1982) Metabolic approaches to cancer cachexia. *Annual Review of Nurition,* **2,** 277-301.

Lev, R. & Orlic, D. (1973) Uptake of proteins in swallowed amniotic fluid by monkey fetal intestine in utero. *Gastroenterology,* **65,** 60-68.

Lev, R., Siegel, H. I. & Bartman, J. (1972) Histochemical studies of developing human fetal small intestine. *Histochemie,* **29,** 103-119.

Levin, R. J., Koldovsky, O., Hoskova, J. et al (1968) Electrical activity across human foetal small intestine associated with absorption processes. *Gut,* **9,** 206-213.

Lieberman, J. (1966) Proteolytic enzyme activity in fetal pancreas and meconium. *Gastroenterology,* **50,** 183-190.

Lindberg, T. (1966) Intestinal dipeptidases, characterization, development and distribution of intestinal dipeptidases of the human foetus. *Clinical Science,* **30,** 505-515.

Liu, H. M. & Potter, E. L. (1962) Development of human pancreas. *Archives of Pathology,* **74,** 439-452.

Louvard, D., Semeriva, M. & Maroux, S. (1976) The brush border intestinal aminopeptidase, a transmembrane protein as probed by macromolecular photolabelling. *Journal of Molecular Biology,* **106,** 1025-1035.

Lundh, G. (1962) Pancreatic exocrine function in neoplastic and inflammatory disease: a simple and reliable new test. *Gastroenterology,* **42,** 275-280.

MacGregor, I. L., Parent, J. & Meyer, J. H. (1977) Gastric emptying of liquid meals and pancreatic and biliary secretion after gut total gastrectomy or truncal vagotomy and pyloroplasty in man. *Gastroenterology,* **72,** 195-205.

Maroux, S. & Louvard, D. (1976) On the hydrophobic part of aminopeptidase and maltases which bid the enzyme to the intestinal brush border membrane. *Biochimica et Biophysica Acta,* **419,** 189-195.

Mata, L. J., Jiminez, F. & Cordon, M. (1972) Gastrointestinal flora of children with protein calorie malnutrition. *American Journal of Clinical Nutrition,* **25,** 1118.

Matthews, D. M. & Adibi, S. A. (1976) Peptide absorption. *Gastroenterology,* **71,** 151-161.

Meyer, J. H. (1981) Control of pancreatic exocrine secretion. In *Physiology of the Gastro-intestinal Tract* (Ed.) Johnson, L. R., Christensen, J., Grossman, M. I. et al. Volume 2, pp. 821-829. New York: Raven Press.

Meyer, J. H., Spingola, C. J. & Grossman, M. I. (1971) Endogenous cholecystokinin potentiates exogenous secretin on pancreas of dog. *American Journal of Physiology,* **221,** 742-747.

Mitchell, S. J. & Bloom, S. R. (1978) Measurement of fasting and postpriandial plasma VIP in man. *Gut,* **19,** 1043-1048.

Munck, B. G. (1981) Intestinal absorption of amino acids. In *Physiology of the Gastro-intestinal Tract* (Ed.) Johnson, L. R., Christensen, J., Grossman, M. I., Jacobson, E. D. & Schultz, S. G. Volume 2, pp. 1097-1122. New York: Raven Press.

Nicholson, J. A. & Peters, T. J. (1977) Subcellular distribution of di- and tripeptidase activity in human jejunum. *Clinical Science and Molecular Medicine,* **52,** 168.

Nicholson, J. A., McCarthy, D. M. & Kim, Y. S. (1974) The responses of rat intestinal brush border and cytosol peptide hydrolase activity to variation in dietary protein content. *Journal of Clinical Investigation,* **54,** 890.

Nixon, S. E. & Mawer, G. E. (1970a) The digestion and absorption of protein in man. I. The site of absorption. *British Journal of Nutrition,* **24,** 227-240.

Nixon, S. E. & Mawer, G. E. (1970b) The digestion and absorption of protein in man. II. The form in which digested protein is absorbed. *British Journal of Nutrition,* **24,** 241-258.

Perera, D. R., Weinstein, W. M. & Rubin, C. E. (1975) Small intestinal biopsy. *Human Pathology,* **6,** 157-217.

Quaroni, A., Kirsh, K. & Weiser, M. M. (1979a) Synthesis of membrane glycoproteins in rat small intestinal cells. Redistribution of L(1,5,6-^{3}H)fucose-labelled membrane glycoproteins among Golgi, lateral basal and microvillus membrane in vivo. *Biochemical Journal,* **182,** 203-212.

Quaroni, A., Kirsh, K. & Weiser, M. M. (1979b) Synthesis of membrane glycoproteins in rat small intestinal villus cells. Effect of colchicine on the redistribution of L(1,5,6-^{3}H)fucose-labelled membrane glycoproteins among Golgi, lateral basal and microvillus membrane. *Biochemical Journal,* **182,** 213-221.

Rose, P. M., Hopper, A. F. & Wannemacher, R. W. (1971) Cell population changes in the intestinal mucosa of protein depleted or starved rats. I. Changes in mitotic cycle time. *Journal of Cell Biology,* **50,** 887.

Rothberg, R. M. (1969) Immunoglobulin and specific antibody synthesis during the first weeks of life of premature infants. *Journal of Pediatrics,* **75,** 391-399.

Rothman, J. E. & Lenard, J. (1977) Membrane asymmetry. The nature of membrane asymmetry provides clues to the puzzle of how membranes are assembled. *Science,* **195,** 743-753.

Rutgeerts, L., Mainguet, P. & Tytgat, G. (1974) Enterokinase in contaminated small-bowel syndrome. *Digestion,* **10,** 249-254.

Schneider, R. E. & Viteri, F. E. (1972) Morphological aspects of the duodenojejunal mucosa in protein-calorie malnutrition and during recovery. *American Journal of Clinical Nutrition,* **25,** 1091.

Schriver, C. R. & Rosenberg, L. E. (1973) *Amino Acid Metabolism and Its Disorders.* Philadelphia: W. B. Saunders. 491 pp.

Shoaf, C., Berko, R. M. & Heizer, W. D. (1976) Isolation and characterization of four peptide hydrolases from the brush border of rat intestinal mucosa. *Biochimica et Biophysica Acta,* **445,** 694-719.

Sjostrom, H. & Noren, O. (1974) Structural properties of pig intestinal proline dipeptidase. *Biochimica et Biophysica Acta,* **359,** 177-185.

Sleisenger, M. H. & Kim, Y. S. (1979) Protein digestion and absorption. *New England Journal of Medicine,* **300,** 659-663.

Stening, G. F. & Grossman, M. I. (1969) Gastrin related peptides as stimulants of pancreatic and gastric secretion. *American Journal of Physiology,* **217,** 262-266.

Tata, S. S. & Meister, A. (1974) Interaction of gamma-glutamyl transpeptidase with amino acids, dipeptides and derivatives and analogs of glutathione. *Journal of Biological Chemistry,* **249,** 7593-7602.

Taylor, I. L., Byrne, W. J., Christie, D. L. et al (1982) Effect of individual L-amino acids on gastric acid secretion and serum gastrin and pancreatic polypeptide release in humans. *Gastroenterology,* **83,** 273-278.

Townes, P. L. (1965) Trypsinogen deficiency disease. *Journal of Pediatrics,* **66,** 275-285.

Uhlemann, E. E. R., Rottman, H. A. & Gardner, J. D. (1979) Actions of peptides isolated from amphibian skin on amylase release from dispersed pancreatic acini. *American Journal of Physiology,* **236,** E571-E576.

Viteri, F. E. & Schneider, R. E. (1973) Gastrointestinal alterations in protein-calorie malnutrition. *Medical Clinics of North America,* **58,** 1487-1505.

Viteri, F. E., Flores, J. M. & Alvarado, J. (1973) Intestinal malabsorption in malnourished children before and during recovery. *American Journal of Digestive Diseases,* **18,** 201.

Wachsmuth, E. D. & Torhorst, A. (1974) Possible precursors of aminopeptidase and alkaline phosphatase in the proximal tubule of kidney and the crypts of small intestine of mice. *Histochemistry,* **38,** 43-46.

Waldman, T. A. (1966) Protein-losing enteropathy. *Gastroenterology,* **50,** 422.

Walker, W. A. (1981) Intestinal transport of macromolecules. In *Physiology of the Gastrointestinal Tract* (Ed.) Johnson, L. R., Christensen, J., Grossman, M. I. et al. Volume **2,** pp. 1271-1289. New York: Raven Press.

Walker, W. A. & Isselbacher, K. J. (1974) Uptake and transport of macromolecules by the intestine: possible role in clinical disorders. *Gastroenterology,* **67,** 531-550.

Weinstein, W. M. (1974) Epithelial cell renewal of the small intestinal mucosa. *Medical Clinics of North America,* **58,** 1375-1386.

Weiser, M. M., Neumeier, M. M., Quaroni, A. & Kirsh, K. (1978) Synthesis of plasmalemmal glycoproteins in intestinal epithelial cells. *Journal of Cell Biology,* **77,** 722-734.

Werner, B. (1948) Peptic and tryptic capacity of the digestive glands in newborns. *Acta Paediatrica Scandinavica,* **35** (supplement 70), 1-80.

Wilson, S. J. & Walzer, M. (1935) Absorption of undigested proteins in human beings. *American Journal of Diseases of Children,* **50,** 49-57.

Wojnarowska, F. & Gray, G. M. (1975) Intestinal surface peptide hydrolases, identification and characterization of three enzymes from rat brush border. *Biochimica et Biophysica Acta,* **403,** 147-160.

Wright, N., Watson, A., Morley, A. et al (1973a) The cell cycle time in the flat (avillous) mucosa of the human small intestine. *Gut,* **14,** 603-606.

Wright, N., Watson, A., Morley, A. et al (1973b) Cell kinetics in flat (avillous) mucosa of the human small intestine. *Gut,* **14,** 701-710.

Zoppi, G., Andreotti, G. & Pajno-Ferrara, F. (1972) Exocrine pancreas function in premature and fullterm neonates. *Pediatric Research,* **6,** 880-886.

4

Calcium Absorption and Vitamin D Metabolism

DANIEL D. BIKLE

Vitamin D, acting through its metabolite 1,25-dihydroxyvitamin D $(1,25(OH)_2D)$, is the principal regulator of intestinal calcium transport (Bikle et al, 1981). The mechanism(s) by which this regulation occurs remains the subject of lively investigation. Calcium transport through the intestinal epithelium involves functionally different plasma membranes (the brush border and the basolateral membranes), subcellular organelles (mitochondria, endoplasmic reticulum, and Golgi), and a cytosol protein (calcium binding protein). Each has its own characteristics of and thermodynamic requirements for calcium binding and transport. $1,25(OH)_2D$ affects these various components of the cell differently, as will be discussed in more detail in a later section.

The interrelationship between vitamin D and the intestine is not limited to the stimulation of calcium tranpsort by $1,25(OH)_2D$. Vitamin D is absorbed by the intestine (as well as produced in the skin). This absorption takes place in the distal small bowel and requires bile salts for maximum efficiency. Intrinsic small bowel and liver disease reduce vitamin D absorption. In addition to vitamin D absorption from foodstuffs, vitamin D and its metabolites undergo an active enterohepatic circulation. Disruption of this enterohepatic circulation by disease or drugs will deplete the body of vitamin D.

The liver is the principal organ metabolizing vitamin D to 25-hydroxyvitamin D (25OHD). The 25OHD is the major circulating form of vitamin D and the principal substrate for the renal enzymes converting 25OHD to more biologically active metabolites. The liver also produces the carrier or transport protein for vitamin D and its metabolites. The small intestine may play a role in metabolizing vitamin D and its metabolites, although the significance of such metabolism in man is not established.

Clearly the relationship between the intestine, vitamin D, and calcium transport has many facets. In this review I will first describe the basic physiological and molecular components of intestinal calcium transport and its regulation by vitamin D. I will then review the metabolism of vitamin D, emphasizing the aspects of particular relevance to gastroenterology. Finally, I will examine the impact of various gastrointestinal diseases on the vitamin

0300-5089/83/1202-379 $05.00©1983 W. B. Saunders Company Ltd

D endocrine system. I hope to demonstrate the significance of such diseases on calcium metabolism and provide a rationale for the treatment of such disorders to minimize their impact on calcium metabolism.

CALCIUM ABSORPTION — GENERAL

Calcium transport from the lumen to the blood appears to occur principally by the transcellular route, although a careful study of the paracellular route of calcium absorption has not been made. The transcellular route can be divided into three steps: transport of calcium into the cell, through the cell, and out of the cell (Figure 1). Calcium concentrations in the extracellular fluids are in the millimolar range. Calcium concentrations in the cytosol are in the submicromolar range. Therefore, calcium entry into the cell proceeds down a steep concentration gradient, whereas its removal from the cell occurs against a steep concentration gradient. Furthermore, the potential difference across the plasma membrane (the potential inside the cell is approximately −50 mV) increases the electrochemical driving force for calcium entry into the cell. The absorption of calcium from lumen to blood occurs against a transmural potential difference of approximately 5 mV (Walling and Rothman, 1969).

Much of our recent understanding of the mechanisms by which calcium is transported from the lumen to the blood has resulted from studies utilizing purified subcellular fractions of plasma membranes (brush border and basolateral membranes) and organelles (mitochondria, Golgi). These membrane fractions and organelles differ in both structure (lipid composition, protein profiles) and function (specific enzyme and ion transport properties). Calcium transport across these different membranes differs.

Calcium entry across the brush border membrane into the cell does not require the expenditure of energy; calcium enters the cell down a steep electrochemical gradient. The mechanisms regulating calcium permeability at the brush border membrane are beginning to be understood (Rasmussen et al, 1979; Miller and Bronner, 1981). The lipid composition of the brush border membrane has a high cholesterol : phospholipid ratio which results in a high viscosity of the membrane. Reductions in membrane viscosity by increases in temperature or unsaturated fatty acid content increase the permeability of the brush border membrane to calcium (Bikle et al, 1982, unpublished observations). Such data suggest that one mechanism controlling calcium permeability of the brush border membrane is the lipid composition of the membrane. In this regard, the brush border membranes from different regions of the small intestine differ both in their viscosity (Schachter and Shinitzky, 1977) and calcium permeability (Bikle, 1982, unpublished observations). The duodenal brush border membranes have the greatest calcium permeability and lowest viscosity, whereas the ileal brush border membranes have the lowest calcium permeability but the greatest viscosity. However, evidence for a calcium carrier mediating calcium movement through the brush border membrane also exists.

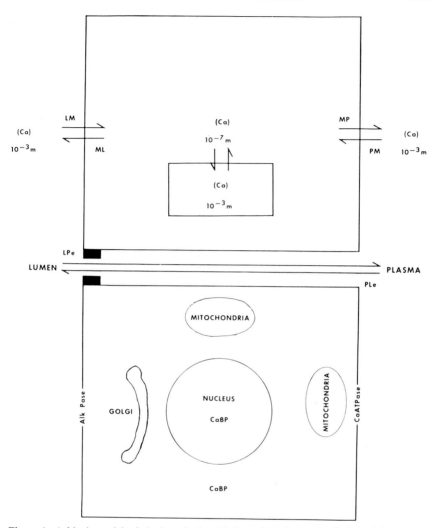

Figure 1. A block model of the intestinal epithelium depicting two cells joined by a tight junction. The brush border faces left, and basolateral membrane faces right. The upper cell depicts the transcellular pathway of calcium across the brush border membrane, through the cell — presumably inside a subcellular organelle such as mitochondrion — then out again at the basolateral membrane. The paracellular pathway is depicted as that occurring between the cells. The lower cell depicts subcellular organelles and the calcium binding protein (CaBP) thought to be involved in transcellular calcium transport. The symbols L, M, P refer to lumen, mucosa, and plasma, respectively.

Calcium transport into brush border membrane vesicles is at least partially saturable. Sodium and lanthanum block calcium entry. A calcium binding protein has been identified in the brush border membrane which may serve as the calcium carrier (Schachter and Kowarski, 1982). Most likely both mechanisms — lipid modulation of membrane permeability to calcium and protein-mediated calcium movement — play roles in regulating calcium movement across the brush border.

After calcium enters the cell it must be moved from the brush border region to the basolateral membrane without disrupting the cellular machinery. Several subcellular organelles and at least one cytosol protein appear to play a role in this process. The mitochondria have a large capacity for calcium accumulation (Bikle et al, 1980). However, the K_m of their calcium pump for calcium (approximately 10^{-6} to 10^{-5} M) appears to be too high for the mitochondria to play a substantial role in the intracellular movement of calcium at what is believed to be the normal levels of free calcium inside the cell (10^{-7} to 10^{-6} M). The Golgi fraction of the intestinal epithelium can accumulate large amounts of calcium, but the K_m of this process for calcium has not yet been determined (Freedman, Weiser and Isselbacher, 1977). This subcellular fraction may contain the lysosome-like organelle, observed in electron micrographs of intestinal epithelium, which appears to accumulate calcium (Morrissey et al, 1980). One cytosol protein thought to play a role in calcium transport is the vitamin D-induced calcium binding protein (CaBP). Another calcium binding protein, calmodulin, has also been found in the intestinal epithelium. Unlike CaBP, calmodulin does not appear to be influenced by the vitamin D status of the cell. Considerable evidence links CaBP to vitamin D-stimulated calcium transport through the cell, but its molecular role in this process remains undefined.

At the basolateral membrane calcium must be pumped out of the cell against a steep electrochemical gradient. ATP provides the energy (Murer and Hildmann, 1981; Nellans and Popovitch, 1981). Calmodulin stimulates the calcium pump in the basolateral membrane (Nellans and Popovitch, 1981) in a fashion similar to its effects on calcium pumps in other cell membranes. The calcium pump in the basolateral membrane must operate at the submicromolar concentrations of calcium found in the cytosol. The calcium ATPase located in basolateral membranes may be a component of the calcium pump and is stimulated by submicromolar concentrations of calcium (Ghijsen, DeJong and Van Os, 1980). Thus, the concept that the basolateral membrane contains a calmodulin-activated calcium ATPase capable of pumping calcium from the cell is gaining credence. However, this pump is not the only means by which calcium is removed from the cell. Sodium stimulates calcium efflux. This suggests that the calcium pump works in parallel with a Na-Ca exchange mechanism similar to that of other membranes.

REGULATION OF CALCIUM ABSORPTION BY VITAMIN D

Considering the variety of mechanisms required to transport calcium through the cell from the lumen to the blood stream, it is not surprising that vitamin D regulates calcium transport by multiple mechanisms (Figure 2). Our studies in chicks indicate that the following sequence of events occurs when $1,25(OH)_2D$ is administered to a vitamin D-deficient animal (Bikle, Zolock and Morrissey, 1981). Within two hours the permeability of the

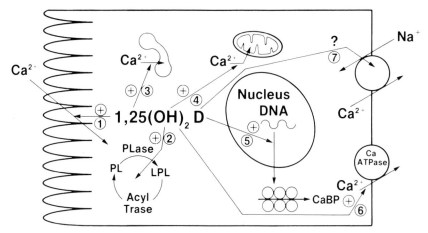

Figure 2. 1,25(OH)$_2$D regulates calcium transport by multiple mechanisms. (1) It increases calcium entry at the brush border by a mechanism not requiring new protein synthesis. (2) It stimulates the turnover of phospholipids in the membrane by activating phospholipase (PLase) and acyltransferase (Acyl Trase). This restructuring of the membrane could change its permeability to calcium. (3) It stimulates calcium uptake by the Golgi fraction. (4) It stimulates calcium uptake by mitochondria. (5) It induces calcium binding protein production. (6) It stimulates calcium efflux and Ca ATPase activity at the basolateral membrane. (7) A Na-Ca exchange mechanism also appears to be present, but it is not clear whether 1,25(OH)$_2$D alters this mechanism.

brush border membrane to calcium increases, resulting in an influx of calcium into the cell. This increased intracellular calcium parallels the initial increase in transcellular calcium transport. The calcium inside the cell is accumulated primarily by mitochondria. After eight hours the intracellular levels of calcium start to decline, reaching the prestimulated levels by 24 hours despite a continued increase in transcellular calcium transport. Inhibition of protein synthesis fails to block either the initial increase in intracellular calcium or the stimulation of calcium transport following 1,25(OH)$_2$D administration. However, the subsequent decline in intracellular calcium after eight hours does not occur when protein synthesis is inhibited. We interpret these results to mean that the initial actions of 1,25(OH)$_2$D to increase calcium entry at the brush border and the accumulation of calcium by mitochondria do not need new protein synthesis. However, stimulation by 1,25(OH)$_2$D of the normal movement of calcium through the cell and the efflux of calcium at the basolateral membrane do require protein synthesis. One such candidate protein is CaBP. This protein is induced de novo by 1,25(OH)$_2$D. CaBP could function to facilitate the removal of calcium from the cell by mediating a transfer of calcium from the mitochondria (or other subcellular organelles transporting calcium through the cell) to the calcium pump in the basolateral membrane.

This model is in keeping with several recent observations of 1,25(OH)$_2$D action using purified membrane and subcellular organelle preparations. Brush border membranes isolated from animals given 1,25(OH)$_2$D accumulate more calcium than brush border membranes isolated from vitamin D-deficient animals. This effect of 1,25(OH)$_2$D is not prevented by cycloheximide, a protein synthesis inhibitor, given prior to the administration of 1,25(OH)$_2$D (Rasmussen et al, 1979). A mechanism by which 1,25(OH)$_2$D could alter brush border membrane permeability to calcium without inducing new proteins is by altering the lipid composition of the membrane (O'Doherty, 1979; Matsumoto, Fontaine and Rasmussen, 1981). Such changes could alter either the activity of a preexisting calcium carrier or the permeability of the calcium channel via changes in membrane viscosity. Data showing a rapid effect (within two hours) of 1,25(OH)$_2$D on lipid turnover have been reported (Matsumoto, Fontaine and Rasmussen, 1981) and interpreted to indicate a change in membrane viscosity. The effects of 1,25(OH)$_2$D on calcium binding by subcellular organelles (mitochondria and Golgi) appear to be both direct and indirect. 1,25(OH)$_2$D can directly stimulate isolated mitochondrial preparations to accumulate calcium (Bikle et al, 1980). Changes in a mitochondrial protein have been observed following 1,25(OH)$_2$D treatment, but the significance of this observation is not clear (Hobden, Harding and Lawson, 1980) since cycloheximide does not block the ability of mitochondria to accumulate calcium. One of the most rapid events described in the intestinal epithelial cell following 1,25(OH)$_2$D treatment is the stimulation of calcium uptake by the Golgi fraction (Freedman, Weiser and Isselbacher, 1977; MacLaughlin, Weiser and Freedman, 1980). Stimulation of calcium uptake by this fraction occurs within 15 min, reaches a peak by 1 h, declines to pre-stimulated levels, then reemerges after 24 h. Using electron microscopy we have identified a lysosome-like organelle that is stimulated by 1,25(OH)$_2$D to accumulate calcium within 18 h but not at 12 h (Morrissey et al, 1980). The effect of 1,25(OH)$_2$D on calcium uptake by this organelle is blocked by cycloheximide. Most likely, the Golgi fraction isolated by MacLaughlin et al (1980) contains the organelle we observed morphologically. The stimulation of calcium efflux from the cell at the basolateral membrane has received limited study (Van Os and Ghijsen, 1982). Basolateral membranes isolated from animals receiving 1,25(OH)$_2$D accumulate calcium more readily than basolateral membranes isolated from vitamin D-deficient animals. Furthermore, the Ca ATPase activity is higher in basolateral membranes from animals given 1,25(OH)$_2$D. The dependency of these processes on new protein synthesis has not been established but seems likely.

Thus, the picture emerging for the regulation of calcium transport by 1,25(OH)$_2$D is complex but fascinating. The change in brush border membrane permeability to calcium occurs early and does not require new protein synthesis; perhaps 1,25(OH)$_2$D-mediated changes in lipid structure provide the mechanism. Several subcellular organelles appear to be involved in intracellular calcium transport and are affected differently by 1,25(OH)$_2$D; the effect on calcium uptake by the lysosome-like organelle appears to require protein synthesis, whereas the effect on mitochondrial calcium uptake does not. The mechanism by which 1,25(OH)$_2$D enhances calcium efflux at the basolateral membrane is not clear but probably involves an effect on the Ca ATPase. Therefore, $1,25(OH)_2D$ acts on the cell in part by receptor-mediated changes in protein synthesis and in part by actions not requiring new protein synthesis.

VITAMIN D BIOAVAILABILITY AND METABOLISM

Perhaps the single most important discovery in the vitamin D field within the past twenty years was the realization, initially by DeLuca (1969), that vitamin D needed to be converted enzymatically to a variety of different metabolites before its full biological activity could be expressed. Vitamin D, then, is really a prohormone of precursor for a family of biologically active metabolites. Two forms of vitamin D are available: vitamin D_3(cholecalciferol) and vitamin D_2 (ergocalciferol). Vitamin D_3 is the form produced in the skin; vitamin D_2 is a product of irradiated plant sterols. Vitamin D_2 is the most common vitamin D supplement in foodstuffs and the most common vitamin D in pharmaceutical preparations. Chemically, vitamin D_2 differs from vitamin D_3 in possessing a double bond (C22—C23) and an additional methyl group (C24) in the side chain. Biologically, vitamin D_2 and its metabolites appear to have comparable, if not equivalent, properties to vitamin D_3 and its metabolites in humans. Assays which measure the vitamin D metabolites generally do not distinguish between the vitamin D_2 and the vitamin D_3 forms, so the approximate biological equivalence of the two forms is assumed when interpreting the results of these assays.

The production of vitamin D from 7-dehydrocholesterol in the skin is a non-enzymatic process (Holick and Clark, 1978). Under the influence of ultraviolet irradiation, 7-dehydrocholesterol is converted to previtamin D which then undergoes isomerization to vitamin D. The capacity of the skin to produce vitamin D is enormous if given a little sunlight. However, in our modern society adequate sunlight exposure cannot be taken for granted and a variety of foodstuffs, dairy products in particular, are fortified with vitamin D.

Intestinal absorption of vitamin D can account for a considerable percentage of the circulating levels of vitamin D and its metabolites. For example, in a recent study of normal individuals in San Francisco we observed $25OHD_2$ levels that ranged up to 50 per cent of the total $25OHD$ concentrations (mean 23 ± 4 per cent, SEM) (Bikle and Halloran, 1982, unpublished data). Since vitamin D_2 is not made in the skin, the $25OHD_2$ originated exclusively from intestinal absorption of vitamin D_2. Vitamin D absorption occurs principally in the jejunum (Hollander and Muralidhara, 1978). Vitamin D is absorbed through the mucosa into the lymphatics by a process facilitated by bile salts, fatty acids, and monoglycerides (Hollander and Muralidhara, 1978). In addition to the absorption of vitamin D from exogenous sources the enterohepatic circulation of vitamin D and its metabolites plays an important role in vitamin D bioavailability. In one study in man (Arnaud et al, 1975), over 30 per cent of the dose of tritium-labelled $25OHD$ given intravenously was recovered in the bile within 24 h. The label appeared in polar compounds, presumably glucuronide and/or sulphate conjugates. Only 3 per cent was recovered in the faeces. This indicates that nearly all of the label secreted in bile was subsequently reabsorbed. More recent studies demonstrate a similar enterohepatic circulation for $1,25(OH)_2D$ and $24,25(OH)_2D$ (Kumar, 1982). Clearly, gastrointestinal disease, which interferes with vitamin D absorption and/or the enterohepatic circulation of its metabolites, could deplete body stores of these compounds.

Besides its involvement in the enterohepatic circulation and absorption of vitamin D and its metabolites, the liver plays two additional important roles in the vitamin D endocrine system. First, the liver converts vitamin D to its major circulating form, 25OHD (DeLuca, 1969). 25OHD has intrinsic biological activity, but, more importantly, serves as the substrate for $24,25(OH)_2D$ and $1,25(OH)_2D$ production in the kidney and elsewhere. The hepatic vitamin D 25-hydroxylase is not closely regulated. Circulating levels of 25OHD generally reflect the bioavailability of vitamin D from the skin and gut more than the regulation of the 25-hydroxylase. However, in severe liver disease this enzyme could become rate limiting. Second, the liver produces the transport protein for the vitamin D metabolites, vitamin D binding protein (DBP) (Haddad, 1979). Serum DBP concentrations are approximately 0.5×10^{-6} M, are increased during pregnancy or by oestrogens (like other steroid transport proteins), and are decreased in patients with liver disease. The affinity of DBP for the vitamin D metabolites differs: $25OHD = 24(R),25(OH)_2D = 25(R),26(OH)_2D > 25(S),26(OH)_2D > 1,25(OH)_2D \simeq D$. Although the affinity constant of DBP for these metabolites as reported by different groups varies, the results cluster around 10^8 M^{-1} for 25OHD and 10^7 M^{-1} for $1,25(OH)_2D$ (Haddad, 1979; Bouillon and Van Ballen, 1981). The total circulating levels of the vitamin D metabolites are considerably lower than that of DBP (approximately 50×10^{-9} M, 5×10^{-9} M, and 8×10^{-12} M for 25OHD, $24,25(OH)_2D$ and $1,25(OH)_2D$, respectively). Because of the high affinity of DBP for the metabolites and the huge excess of DBP relative to that of the metabolites, the unbound concentrations of the vitamin D metabolites are very low (less than 1 per cent of the total circulating levels) (Boullion and Van Ballen, 1981). Currently available assays for the vitamin D metabolites measure the total circulating levels, not the potentially physiologically more important unbound concentrations. At this time it is not clear whether DBP simply transports the vitamin D metabolites in blood or whether it is involved in the regulation of transport of the vitamin D metabolites into the cell.

The critical regulation of vitamin D metabolism occurs in the kidney (Fraser, 1980). In the renal mitochondria 25OHD is converted principally to $24,25(OH)_2D$ and $1,25(OH)_2D$. Because of the unequivocal biological importance of $1,25(OH)_2D$, especially for the regulation of intestinal calcium transport, the regulation of $1,25(OH)_2D$ production has received the most attention. Under normal conditions (except during pregnancy) little or no $1,25(OH)_2D$ is produced outside the kidney. Production of $1,25(OH)_2D$ is closely regulated by a variety of hormones and ions, the most important of which are parathyroid hormone, calcium, and phosphate. Increased parathyroid hormone levels or decreased calcium and/or phosphate levels result in increased $1,25(OH)_2D$ production. Once formed, $1,25(OH)_2D$ is delivered to its target tissues by the same serum protein (DBP) which transports 25OHD. The disposition kinetics of $1,25(OH)_2D$ indicate a rapid clearance from the blood ($T_{1/2}$ in minutes to hours) with rapid accumulation by the target tissues, including gut (Gray et al, 1978; Bikle et al, 1982). Therefore, unlike 25OHD, most of the $1,25(OH)_2D$ is found in receptor-containing target tissues such as the gut, or in tissues like the liver where it may be further metabolized and excreted.

We have come full cycle. We have discussed how $1,25(OH)_2D$ produced from vitamin D, much of which was absorbed from the intestine, returns to the intestinal epithelium to regulate calcium transport. Diseases of the gastrointestinal tract and liver disrupt this cycle. The clinical implications of such diseases for calcium homeostasis are discussed next.

GASTROINTESTINAL DISEASES AFFECTING VITAMIN D METABOLISM AND ACTION

Disease states affecting the vitamin D endocrine system can be categorized into one or more of three levels: vitamin D bioavailability, vitamin D metabolism, and target tissue response to vitamin D metabolites (Figure 3). Circulating levels of 25OHD serve as a good marker for the bioavailability of vitamin D for three reasons: blood is a major storage pool of 25OHD, the half life of 25OHD in blood is several weeks, and the production of 25 OHD from vitamin D by the liver is more a function of substrate availability than any other regulating factor. However, in interpreting measured values of 25OHD, one must remember that changes in the vitamin D binding protein, DBP, can alter total 25OHD levels without affecting the unbound 25OHD levels. If only the unbound 25OHD is available to cells and is, therefore, the physiologically important fraction (an issue not yet settled) then total 25OHD levels may be misleading. For example, the alcoholic with cirrhosis has several reasons to have a low 25OHD level: poor nutrition, limited sunlight exposure, limited production of DBP, and reduced 25-hydroxylase activity. It is not clear in such an individual whether a low total 25OHD level really reflects limited bioavailability when the unbound 25OHD levels could be normal.

Intrinsic small bowel disease such as sprue and regional enteritis, or surgical removal or revision of the small bowel such as jejunal-ileal bypass and gastrectomy, lead to lowered 25OHD levels and bone disease in many patients (Compston et al, 1978; Schoen et al, 1978). Although it seems likely that the low 25OHD levels contribute to the bone disease, studies to date have not convincingly demonstrated a clear association between low 25OHD levels and disordered calcium homeostasis in these diseases. Conceivably, even low levels of 25OHD are adequate to provide sufficient substrate for normal $1,25(OH)_2D$ and $24,25(OH)_2D$ production. Data on $1,25(OH)_2D$ and $24,25(OH)_2D$ levels in patients with intrinsic bowel disease or surgical rearrangements of the small bowel are limited.

More information exists linking chronic cholestatic disorders such as primary biliary cirrhosis to disordered calcium homeostasis and bone

Vitamin D Endocrine System

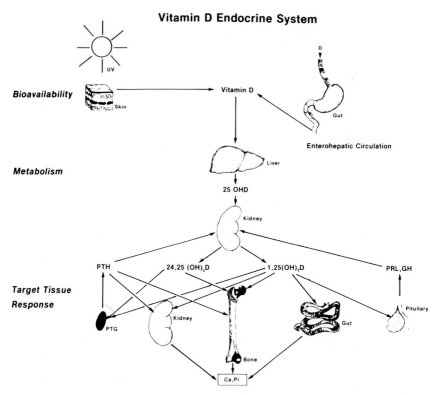

Figure 3. The vitamin D endocrine system. Vitamin D is made available to the body by photogenesis in the skin and absorption from the intestine. Part of the intestinal absorption involves endogenous vitamin D products secreted in bile (enterohepatic circulation). The vitamin D must then be hydroxylated first in the liver to 25OHD, then in the kidney to 1,25(OH)$_2$D and 24,25(OH)$_2$D. The active vitamin D metabolites act on different tissues to produce a variety of responses. The three principal target tissues responsible for calcium (Ca) and phosphate (Pi) homeostasis are kidney, bone and intestine. Endocrine tissues such as the parathyroid gland (PTG) and anterior pituitary also are target tissues. Their hormone products, parathyroid hormone (PTH), prolactin (PRL), and growth hormone (GH), help regulate vitamin D metabolism in the kidney in addition to direct effects, at least of PTH, on bone and kidney regulation of calcium and phosphate homeostasis. From Bikle (1982), with kind permission of the author and the publisher, Year Book Medical Publishers, Inc.

disease. The bone disease has been termed hepatic osteodystrophy (Long, 1980). Primary biliary cirrhosis affects the vitamin D endocrine system on at least two levels: bioavailability and metabolism. Abnormal bile production reduces vitamin D absorption and disrupts the normal enterohepatic circulation of the vitamin D metabolites. The malabsorption of vitamin D and its metabolites is aggravated by drugs such as cholestyramine often used in cholestatic disorders, since such bile acid-binding resins probably bind vitamin D conjugates as well. The cirrhotic liver may produce less 25OHD than normal. However, malabsorption of vitamin D and its metabolites appears to contribute more to the pathophysiology of the bone disease than does reduction of the liver 25-hydroxylase. This concept is supported by the observation that parenteral but not oral vitamin D administration has been successful in treating the osteomalacic component of the bone disease (Compston, Horton and Thompson, 1979).

The bone disease associated with primary biliary cirrhosis has two components: osteomalacia and osteoporosis (Long, 1980). Osteomalacia is best detected on bone biopsy specimens. The radiological assessment of osteomalacia is neither sensitive nor accurate. Osteomalacia is characterized morphologically as a reduction in mineralization front and widened osteoid seams. Osteoporosis is characterized by a reduction in total bone volume, but the remaining bone is normal morphologically. The secondary hyperparathyroidism that can accompany malabsorption disorders does not seem to result in bone disease (osteitis fibrosa) in patients with primary biliary cirrhosis. The osteoporotic component of hepatic osteodystrophy appears to dominate in the bones of patients living in the United States (Horlong, Recker and Maddrey, 1982; Mattoff et al, 1982); patients in England have more osteomalacia. The vitamin D metabolites used to treat the disease appear to reverse only the osteomalacic component (Long, 1980; Mattoff et al, 1982). At the moment our ability to arrest the progressive loss of bone (osteoporosis) in patients with primary biliary cirrhosis is limited.

Alcoholics with liver disease generally have low circulating 25OHD levels (Hepner, Roginsky and Moo, 1976). It is not clear whether this is a problem in bioavailability, metabolism, or low DBP levels. Clinical impression suggests an increased incidence of bone disease in such patients, but convincing data are limited (Nilsson and Westley, 1973; Dalen and Lamke, 1976). However, the likelihood that such patients are predisposed to bone disease for a number of reasons obligates the physician to evaluate 25OHD and calcium levels and to treat as appropriate.

Drugs can alter vitamin D metabolism and lead to bone disease. The best studied drugs are the anticonvulsants phenytoin and phenobarbitone (Hahn, 1980). These drugs alter the hepatic metabolism of vitamin D, resulting in lower circulating levels of 25OHD. This explanation is not complete, however, since anticonvulsant therapy does not reduce $1,25(OH)_2D$ levels (Jubiz et al, 1977). More recent evidence indicates a direct effect of anticonvulsants on bone (Hahn, 1980).

The clearest example of disordered vitamin D metabolism leading to disordered calcium metabolism is renal failure (Coburn and Massry, 1980). The clinical experience in treating renal osteodystrophy has made one point clear; loss of vitamin D metabolism by the kidney is devastating to bones. One form of renal osteodystrophy (pure osteomalacia) is refractory to $1,25(OH)_2D$ therapy alone. However, this form of bone disease appears to respond to 25OHD in high doses (Frost et al, 1981) or to a combination of $1,25(OH)_2D$ and $24,25(OH)_2D$ (Sherrard et al, 1982). Thus, the concept that $1,25(OH)_2D$ mediates all the biological actions of vitamin D needs to be reexamined. The lesson to be learned from the clinical experience in treating renal osteodystrophy is that different vitamin D metabolites have different biological functions: optimal therapy may require several different metabolites. This lesson must be kept in mind when patients with gastro-intestinal disease are to be treated with vitamin D.

The third level of vitamin D endocrine system, target tissue response, brings our attention back to the intestine. The paradigm for abnormal target tissue response to vitamin D is the rare genetic syndrome, vitamin D-dependent rickets type II (VDDR II). Most of the families studied with this recessive disorder have a lack or diminished number of functioning receptors for $1,25(OH)_2D$ in skin fibroblasts (Eil et al, 1981). Presumably the intestinal epithelial cell shares this defect. Therefore, despite high circulating levels of $1,25(OH)_2D$ in these patients, intestinal calcium absorption is low and does not respond to vitamin D treatment in any form.

Although VDDR type II is rare, a variety of other conditions associated with intestinal calcium absorption exist which are not rare and need to be recognized. Probably the most common such problem is age. As one ages, the dietary intake of calcium must be increased to compensate for a diminished ability to absorb calcium (Gallagher et al, 1979). This decline in intestinal calcium absorption with age may be related to a decline in $1,25(OH)_2D$ production with age, although this relationship is not clearly established. Chronic uraemia also is associated with diminished calcium absorption which is partially refractory to $1,25(OH)_2D$ treatment (Brickman et al, 1974). Such patients require higher doses of $1,25(OH)_2D$ to stimulate calcium transport than normal subjects.

The malabsorption syndromes can lead to a negative calcium balance by a variety of mechanisms in addition to the previously discussed reduction in bioavailability of vitamin D and its metabolites. Lack of acid production can result in decreased solubility of calcium salts in the lumen and reduced calcium absorption. Rapid transit through the small intestine can reduce the opportunity for calcium to be absorbed. Either of these mechanisms could explain the calcium malabsorption associated with partial gastrectomy (Harvald, Krogsgaard and Lous, 1962). Failure of fat hydrolysis and absorption due to inadequate pancreatic and/or biliary secretion can result in chelation of calcium to the fat and a reduction in calcium absorption (Agnew, Kehaoglou and Holdsworth, 1969). Intrinsic small bowel disease, such as non-tropical sprue associated with steatorrhoea, can lead to a reduction in calcium absorption. However, non-tropical sprue can also result in increased calcium secretion into the lumen with loss of endogenous calcium (Melvin et al, 1970). Glucocorticoids antagonize the ability of $1,25(OH)_2D$ to stimulate calcium absorption (Travis, Walling and Kimberg, 1973). The mechanism is not clear. The osteoporosis that develops in such patients is difficult to treat and may reflect this antagonism between glucocorticoids and $1,25(OH)_2D$. Ethanol, presumably by a direct toxic effect on the intestinal epithelium, reduces calcium absorption in a manner not reversed by $1,25(OH)_2D$ (Krawitt, Sampson and Katagini, 1975). The role this plays in the bone disease of alcoholics has not been determined.

In summary, a wide variety of gastrointestinal diseases and drugs can adversely affect calcium homeostasis by a variety of mechanisms. These mechanisms include a reduction in vitamin D bioavailability by diseases and drugs altering vitamin D absorption and enterohepatic circulation, disordered vitamin D metabolism by hepatic and renal disease, and disruption of the digestive processes required for normal calcium absorption. Frequently several mechanisms complicate a given disease.

THERAPEUTIC CONSIDERATIONS

Treatment of the various conditions leading to abnormal calcium absorption is simple in concept but often frustrating in practice. One example of the frustration is the newly recognized bone disease associated with total parenteral nutrition (TPN). Some patients treated with TPN develop a painful bone disease which morphologically has the characteristics of osteomalacia. One group (Klein et al, 1980) has concluded that vitamin D excess (not deficiency) is the cause of the osteomalacia. This point is controversial as other aetiological factors such as aluminium have been implicated (Shike et al, 1981).

In general, gastrointestinal disease results in a deficiency of both calcium and vitamin D. In the steady state, 24-hour urine collections provide a good indicator of intestinal calcium absorption. Serum 25OHD measurements provide a good indicator of the vitamin D status. Serum parathyroid hormone measurements by a reliable laboratory provide a sensitive indicator of physiologically important changes in serum calcium. Less readily available but of proven value is bone biopsy assessment by quantitative histomorphometry. Bone biopsy assessment permits the quantification of the extent of osteomalacia. Serum alkaline phosphatase levels are a less certain way of detecting osteomalacia and evaluating its treatment, especially in patients with liver disease.

The goal of therapy is to restore to normal the calcium and vitamin D levels with the hope of preventing or reversing the bone disease. From a practical standpoint this involves adding calcium to the diet (calcium carbonate is ideal because it is cheap, readily available, and has a high percentage of elemental calcium) to raise the urine and serum calcium into the high normal range and to decrease the serum PTH into the low normal range. Vitamin D itself is often successful in raising serum 25OHD levels into the mid to high normal range. Vitamin D is cheap and should be tried first for this reason. If vitamin D is not successful in raising 25OHD levels, then 25OHD itself (calcifediol) can be tried. Presumably because of its greater polarity, 25OHD is better absorbed from the intestine than vitamin D especially in the presence of steatorrhoea. There appears to be little justification for the use of $1,25(OH)_2D$ (calcitriol) or dihydrotachysterol in the treatment of gastrointestinal disease in the patients with normal renal function. Neither of these drugs can be metabolized to $24,25(OH)_2D$, a metabolite of 25OHD which may be important for normal bone mineralization. However, in the absence of data from comparative trials of these drugs no definitive statements can be made.

At this point, however, the use of any of the vitamin D metabolites in preventing or treating the bone disease of gastrointestinal disorders is of more heuristic than proven practical value. The experience in treating the bone disease of primary biliary cirrhosis indicates that only the osteomalacic component responds to vitamin D. The osteoporotic component prevails in patients in the United States. Nevertheless, until definitive studies are performed to indicate a different approach, it seems prudent to maintain normal calcium and vitamin D levels in patients with gastrointestinal disease with the judicious use of calcium and vitamin D supplements.

REFERENCES

Agnew, J. E., Kehayoglou, A. K. & Holdsworth, C. D. (1969) Comparison of three isotopic methods for the study of calcium absorption. *Gut,* **10,** 540-597.
Arnaud, S. B., Goldsmith, R. S., Lambert, P. W. & Go, V. L. W. (1975) 25-Hydroxyvitamin D_3: evidence of an enterohepatic circulation in man. *Proceedings of the Society for Experimental and Biological Medicine,* **149,** 570-572.
Bikle, D. D., Zolock, D. T. & Morrissey, R. L. (1981) Action of vitamin D on intestinal calcium transport. *Annals of the New York Academy of Sciences,* **372,** 481-501.
Bikle, D. D., Askew, E. W., Zolock, D. T. et al (1980) Calcium accumulation by chick intestinal mitochondria: regulation by vitamin D_3 and 1,25-dihydroxyvitamin D_3. *Biochimica et Biophysica Acta,* **598,** 561-574.
Bikle, D. D., Morrissey, R. L., Zolock, D. T. & Rasmussen, H. (1981) The intestinal response to vitamin D. *Reviews of Physiology, Biochemistry and Pharmacology,* **89,** 63-142.
Bikle, D. D., Peck, C. C., Holford, N. H. G. et al (1982) Pharmacokinetics and pharmaco-dynamics of 1,25-dihydroxyvitamin D_3 in the chick. *Endocrinology,* **111,** 939-946.
Bouillon, R. & Van Ballen, H. (1981) Transport of vitamin D: significance of free and total concentrations of the vitamin D metabolites. *Calcified Tissue International,* **33,** 451-453.
Brickman, A. S., Coburn, J. W., Massry, S. G. & Norman, A. W. (1974) 1,25-dihydroxy-vitamin D_3 in normal man and patients with renal failure. *Annals of Internal Medicine,* **80** (2), 161-168.
Coburn, J. W. & Massry, S. G. (Ed.) (1980) Uses and actions of 1,25 dihydroxyvitamin D_3 in uremia. *Control Nephrology,* **18,** 1-217.
Compston, J. E., Horton, L. W., Laker, M. F. et al (1978) Bone disease after jejuno-ileal bypass for obesity. *Lancet,* **ii,** 1-4.
Compston, J. E., Horton, L. W. L. & Thompson, R. P. H. (1979) Treatment of osteomalacia associated with primary biliary cirrhosis with parenteral vitamin D_2 or oral 25-hydroxyvitamin D_3. *Gut,* **20,** 133-136.
Dalen, N. & Lamke, B. (1976) Bone mineral losses in alcoholics. *Acta Orthopaedica Scandinavica,* **47,** 469-471.
DeLuca, H. J. (1969) 25-hydroxycholecalciferol, the probable metabolically active form of vitamin D. Isolation, identification, and subcellular localization. *American Journal of Clinical Nutrition,* **22,** 412-424.
DeLuca, H. J. & Schnoes, H. K. (1976) Metabolism and mechanism of action of vitamin D. *Annual Review of Biochemistry,* **45,** 631-666.
Eil, C., Liberman, U. A., Rosen, J. F. & Marx, S. J. (1981) A cellular defect in hereditary vitamin D-dependent rickets type II: defective nuclear uptake of 1,25 dihydroxyvitamin D in cultured skin fibroblasts. *New England Journal of Medicine,* **304,** 1588-1591.
Fraser, D. R. (1980) Regulation of the metabolism of vitamin D. *Physiological Reviews,* **60,** 551-613.
Freedman, R. A., Weiser, M. M. & Isselbacher, K. J. (1977) Calcium translocation by Golgi and lateral basal membrane vesicles from rat intestine: decrease in vitamin D deficient rats. *Proceedings of the National Academy of Sciences, USA,* **74,** 3612-3616.
Frost, H. M., Griffith, D. L., Jee, W. S. S. et al (1981) Histomorphometric changes in trabecular bone of renal failure patients treated with calcifediol. *Metabolic Bone Disease and Related Research,* **2,** 285-295.
Gallagher, J. C., Riggs, B. L., Eisman, J. et al (1979) Intestinal calcium absorption and serum vitamin D metabolites in normal subjects and osteoporotic patients: effect of age and dietary calcium. *Journal of Clinical Investigation,* **64,** 729-736.

Ghijsen, W. E. J. M., De Jong, M. D. & Van Os, C. H. (1980) Dissociation between Ca^{2+}-ATPase and alkaline phosphatase activities in plasma membranes of rat duodenum. *Biochimica et Biophysica Acta,* **599,** 538-551.

Gray, R. W., Caldas, A. E., Wily, D. R. et al (1978) Metabolism and excretion of ^3H-1,25(OH)$_2$ vitamin D$_3$ in healthy adults. *Journal of Clinical Endocrinology and Metabolism,* **46,** 756-765.

Haddad, J. G., Jr (1979) Transport of vitamin D metabolites. *Clinical Orthopaedics and Related Research,* **142,** 249-261.

Hahn, T. J. (1980) Drug-induced disorders of vitamin D and mineral metabolism. *Clinics in Endocrinology and Metabolism,* **9,** 107-129.

Harvald, B., Krogsgaard, A. R. & Lous, P. (1962) Calcium deficiency following partial gastrectomy. *Acta Medica Scandinavica,* **172,** 497-503.

Hepner, G. W., Roginsky, M. & Moo, H. F. (1976) Abnormal vitamin D metabolism in patients with cirrhosis. *Digestive Diseases and Sciences,* **21,** 527-532.

Hobden, A. N., Harding, M. & Lawson, D. E. M. (1980) 1,25-Dihydroxycholecalciferol stimulation of a mitochondrial protein in chick intestinal cells. *Nature,* **288,** 718-720.

Holick, M. F. & Clark, M. B. (1978) The photobiogenesis and metabolism of vitamin D. *Federation Proceedings,* **37,** 2567-2574.

Hollander, D. & Muralidhara, K. S. (1978) Vitamin D$_3$ intestinal absorption in vivo: influence of fatty acids, bile salts and perfusate pH on absorption. *Gut,* **19,** 267-272.

Horlong, H. J., Recker, R. R. & Maddrey, W. C. (1982) Bone disease in primary biliary cirrhosis: histologic features and response to 25-hydroxyvitamin D. *Gastroenterology,* **83,** 103-108.

Jubiz, W., Haussler, M. R., McCain, T. A. & Tolman, K. G. (1977) Plasma 1,25-dihydroxy-vitamin D levels in patients receiving anticonvulsant drugs. *Journal of Clinical Endocrinology and Metabolism,* **44,** 617-621.

Klein, G. L., Arment, M. E., Bluestone, R. et al (1980) Bone disease associated with total parenteral nutrition. *Lancet,* **ii,** 1041-1044.

Krawitt, E. L., Sampson, H. W. & Katagini, C. A. (1975) Effect of 1,25-dihydroxychole-calciferol on ethanol-mediated suppression of calcium absorption. *Calcified Tissue Research,* **18,** 119-124.

Kumar, R. (1982) Enterohepatic physiology of dihydroxylated vitamin D$_3$ metabolites. In *Vitamin D: Chemical, Biochemical and Clinical Endocrinology of Calcium Metabolism* (Ed.) Norman, A. W., Schaefer, K., Herrath, D. V. & Grigoleit, H. G. pp. 635-640. New York: Walter de Gruyter.

Long, R. S. (1980) Hepatic osteodystrophy: outlook good but some problems unsolved. *Gastroenterology,* **78,** 644-647.

MacLaughlin, J. A., Weiser, M. M. & Freedman, R. A. (1980) Biphasic recovery of vitamin D-dependent Ca^{2+} uptake by rat intestinal Golgi membranes. *Gastroenterology,* **78,** 325-332.

Matsumoto, T., Fontaine, O. & Rasmussen, H. (1981) Effect of 1,25-dihydroxyvitamin D$_3$ on phospholipid metabolism in chick duodenal mucosal cell: relationship to mechanism of action. *Journal of Biological Chemistry,* **256,** 3354-3360.

Mattoff, D. S., Kaplan, M. M., Neer, R. M. et al (1982) Osteoporosis in primary biliary cirrhosis: effects of 25-hydroxyvitamin D$_3$ treatment. *Gastroenterology,* **83,** 97-102.

Melvin, K. E. W., Hepner, G. W., Bordier, P. et al (1970) Calcium metabolism and bone pathology in adult coeliac disease. *Quarterly Journal of Medicine,* **39,** 83-113.

Miller, A., III & Bonner, F. (1981) Calcium uptake in isolated brush-border vesicles from rat small intestine. *Biochemical Journal,* **196,** 391-401.

Morrissey, R. L., Empsom, R. N., Jr, Zolock, D. T. et al (1978) Intestinal response to 1α, 25-dihydroxycholecalciferol. II. A timed study of the intracellular localization of calcium binding protein. *Biochimica et Biophysica Acta,* **538,** 34-41.

Morrissey, R. L., Zolock, D. T., Mellick, P. W. & Bikle, D. D. (1980) Influence of cycloheximide and 1,25-dihydroxyvitamin D$_3$ on mitochondrial and vesicle mineralization in the intestine. *Cell Calcium,* **1,** 69-79.

Murer, H. & Hildmann, B. (1981) Transcellular transport of calcium and inorganic phosphate in the small intestinal epithelium. *American Journal of Physiology,* **240,** G409-416.

Nellans, H. N. & Popovitch, J. E. (1981) Calmodulin regulated, ATP-driven calcium transport by basolateral membranes of rat small intestine. *Journal of Biological Chemistry,* **256,** 9932-9936.

Nilsson, B. E. & Westley, N. E. (1973) Changes in bone mass in alcoholics. *Clinical Orthopaedics and Related Research,* **90,** 229-232.

O'Doherty, P. J. A. (1979) 1,25-Dihydroxyvitamin D_3 increases the activity of the intestinal phosphatidylcholine deacylation-reacylation cycle. *Lipids,* **14,** 75-77.

Rasmussen, H., Fontaine, O., Max, E. E. & Goodman, D. B. P. (1979) The effect of 1α-hydroxyvitamin D_3 administration on calcium transport in chick intestine brush border membrane vesicles. *Journal of Biological Chemistry,* **254,** 2993-2999.

Schachter, D. & Kowarski, S. (1982) Isolation of the protein IMCal, a vitamin D dependent membrane component of the intestinal transport mechanism for calcium. *Federation Proceedings,* **41,** 84-87.

Schachter, D. & Shinitzky, M. (1977) Fluorescence polarization studies of rat intestinal microvillus membranes. *Journal of Clinical Investigation,* **59,** 536-548.

Schoen, M. S., Lindenbaum, J., Roginsky, M. S. & Holt, P. R. (1978) Significance of serum level of 25-hydroxycholecalciferol in gastrointestinal disease. *American Journal of Digestive Diseases,* **23,** 137-142.

Sherrard, D. J., Mott, S., Maloney, N. A. & Coburn, J. W. (1982) Use of 24,25-dihydroxy-vitamin D in the refractory osteomalacia form of renal osteodystrophy. In *Vitamin D: Chemical, Biochemical and Clinical Endocrinology of Calcium Metabolism* (Ed.) Norman, A. W., Schaefer, K., Herrath, D. V. & Grigoleit, H. G. pp. 169-172. New York: Walter de Gruyter.

Shike, M., Sturtridge, W. C., Stam, C. et al (1982) A possible role of vitamin D in the genesis of parenteral-nutrition-induced metabolic bone disease. *Annals of Internal Medicine,* **95,** 560-568.

Travis, M. J., Walling, M. W. & Kimberg, D. V. (1973) Effects of 1,25-dihydroxychole-calciferol on intestinal calcium transport in cortisone-treated rats. *Journal of Clinical Investigation,* **52,** 1680-1685.

van Os, C. H. & Ghijsen, W. E. J. M. (1982) Calcium transport mechanisms in rat duodenal basolateral plasma membranes: effects of $1,25(OH)_2D_3$. In *Vitamin D: Chemical, Biochemical and Clinical Endocrinology of Calcium Metabolism* (Ed.) Norman, A. W., Schaefer, K., Herrath, D. & Grigoleit, H. G. pp. 295-297. New York: Walter de Gruyter.

Walling, M. W. & Rothman, S. S. (1969) Phosphate independent carrier mediated active transport of calcium by rat intestine. *American Journal of Physiology,* **217,** 1144-1148.

5

Blind Loop Syndrome and Small Bowel Bacterial Contamination

PETER E. T. ISAACS
YOUNG S. KIM

The classic experiments in rats by Cameron, Watson and Witts (1949), in which jejunal blind loops were created, showed that weight loss and anaemia due to malabsorption of B_{12} rapidly ensued. The blind loop itself showed little mucosal damage and contained large numbers of bacteria with a predominance of anaerobes. B_{12} malabsorption and an abnormal duodenal luminal flora with anaerobic overgrowth has also been described in man in association with a variety of predisposing causes (Table 1) and is termed the blind loop syndrome, stagnant bowel syndrome, or bacterial overgrowth syndrome (King and Toskes, 1981). Gracey (1979) has proposed that, because various syndromes of bacterial contamination of the small intestine have some similarities with blind loop syndrome, the term contaminated small bowel syndrome should be adopted. However, not all clinical situations in which bacteria contaminate the small bowel present the typical malabsorptive abnormalities of the blind loop syndrome. There are several syndromes in which bacterial contamination of the small intestine occur; blind loop syndrome is one of them, kwashiorkor, tropical sprue and tropical malabsorption syndrome are others.

THE BACTERIOLOGY OF THE NORMAL AND ABNORMAL SMALL INTESTINE

Bacterial microecology

The gut of every species forms a habitat for bacteria, and often the ecology of the gut flora is extremely complex (Savage, 1977). Within the gut is a variety of niches distributed along the axis of the gut (Figure 1), and in each of these levels there may be a radial distribution of habitats and of flora. Thus, in addition to the luminal mixed flora, there may be a typical flora adherent to the mucosal surface and a deep flora permanently resident within the mucosal crypts. In the small intestine of a healthy man there is no permanent resident or autochthonous flora, but the bacteria present are both ingested species and oral residents which are survivors of the gastric acid bath. They are transient or allochthonous flora (Savage, 1977).

0300-5089/83/1202-395 $05.00©1983 W. B. Saunders Company Ltd

Table 1. *Causes of blind loop syndrome*

Abnormal gut anatomy:
  strictures
  diverticulosis
  internal fistulation
  surgical complications — afferent loop
  jejunoileal bypass

Abnormal intestinal motility
  intestinal pseudo-obstruction
  scleroderma
  drugs

Defective defence mechanisms
  hypochlorhydria
  immunodeficiency
  tropical sprue

The autochthonous flora of a gastrointestinal niche has been defined by Savage (1977) as (a) able to grow anaerobically, (b) always found in normal adults and able to sustain stable populations in particular areas of the gut — which they do in successive generations of infant animals. The autochthonous species are usually anaerobic or facultatively anaerobic and are closely associated with the mucosal epithelium in particular areas.

The typical anaerobic organisms of the colon are species of *Bacteroides*. These obligate anaerobic organisms constitute the most important genus of the family Bacteroidacae. *Bacteroides* species are distinguished from the other members of this family by the production of succinic, acetic, formic, lactic and propionic acids from peptone or glucose broth, while the other members of the family produce only butyric acid *(Fusobacterium)* or lactic acid *(Leptotrichia)* (Holdeman and Moore, 1977).

Anaerobic organisms derive their energy from fermentation of organic compounds and are themselves sensitive to the presence of oxygen because their metabolism produces organic peroxides which are toxic to them (Hentges and Maier, 1972). There is marked variation in sensitivity of various species or strains of anaerobic organisms. *Bacteroides fragilis* is very rapidly killed on exposure to air. Oxygen tolerance, however, can vary within this species, and strains isolated from faecal samples tend to be less tolerant of oxygen than strains isolated from urine infections (Rolfe, 1977). *Bacteroides* species tend to be resistant to penicillin, kanamycin and neomycin, but 98 per cent of strains are sensitive to erythromycin and clindamycin, and 80 per cent are sensitive to tetracycline (Holdeman and Moore, 1977). The bacterial flora of both the experimental blind loop of rats and that of patients with blind loop syndrome are very similar. There is a prolific population of bacteria of a multitude of species. Large numbers of anaerobic organisms are present and these may exceed the number of aerobic organisms. The interactions between aerobic and anaerobic species are complex. The lowering of oxygen tension and maintenance of a low oxidation-reduction potential (E_h) is probably achieved by the aerobic species, thus allowing the anaerobes to thrive. Essentially, in the blind loop syndrome the lumen of the intestine has been converted into a septic tank filled with the saprophytic species which ordinarily are immediately removed from the intestine. Unlike specific bacterial infections in which adhesion to the mucosa is an essential part of the disease, all the species are free-living and merely scavenging in the stagnant lumen. Mechanisms normally responsible for the removal of bacteria entering the intestine after surviving the gastric acid bath may be impaired in a variety of situations, and blind loop syndrome may then supervene.

A wide variety of conditions may lead to an increase in the small bowel flora, but it is frequently difficult for the clinician to decide whether the degree of bacterial overgrowth which has been demonstrated is really contributing to the functional disturbance of the intestine.

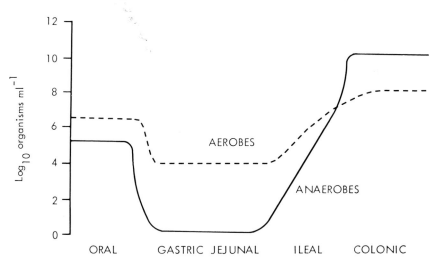

Figure 1. Schematic profile of normal gut flora. (Adapted from data of Gorbach, 1971, King and Toskes, 1981, and Tabaqchali, 1970.)

Regional quantitative bacteriology

Improvements in bacteriological techniques in the last ten years, especially for the culture of anaerobic species, have led to a continuous revision of our quantitative concepts of normality for small bowel flora. Because the numbers of bacteria recoverable from the small intestine are dependent upon the techniques employed to obtain samples and to culture them, a universal normal range cannot be laid down. However, in healthy normal subjects aged between 20 and 60, living in temperate climates and ingesting food and drink only lightly contaminated with microorganisms, most investigators recover up to 10^4 organisms/ml of aerobes and usually no anaerobic organisms from jejunal samples. Total numbers are greater in ileal samples, which also contain some anaerobes (see Figure 1). Such figures are usually obtained by intestinal aspiration using peroral intubation, but similar figures result when direct needle aspiration of intestinal segments is made at laparotomy of traumatized healthy young subjects (Thadepalli et al, 1979). Using a rigorous anaerobic technique, it was found that 82 per cent of patients had no detectable bacteria in the duodenal contents. In those from whom bacteria could be cultured, total aerobic bacteria range from 10^4 to 10^6 organisms/ml and facultative anaerobic bacteria up to 5×10^2/ml. Obligate anaerobes were absent.

In the mid jejunum 69 per cent of samples were sterile. Cultures yielded coliforms in four patients with counts between 10^2 and 10^{10} organisms/ml. Cocci and diphtheroids were also isolated, but in only one of 26 samples was an obligate anaerobe (*Clostridium*, 10/ml) isolated.

In the mid ileum only 55 per cent of the samples were sterile. Again the most common isolates were coliforms (10^4-10^9 organisms/ml). Other species such as *Enterobacter, Hafnia, Proteus* and *Citrobacter diversus* made their appearance. In this study of trauma patients there were no isolates of *Bacteroides*, but this organism was recovered from the small intestine of two of the eight patients operated on for acute appendicitis. These findings are not dissimilar to those obtained by earlier workers (Tabaqchali, 1970; Gorbach, 1971) using intestinal intubation in which up to 10^4 organisms/ml were recovered in duodenal aspirates.

Effects of gastric acid secretion

The normal fasting gastric juice contains less than 10^4 organisms/ml which are derived mainly from the oral flora: a mixture of aerobic and anaerobic species usually totalling some 10^6 organisms/ml of mixed saliva. Susceptibility to acid attack is greatest for gram-negative bacilli and least for the sporing anaerobes such as clostridia. *Escherichia coli* strains are killed within seconds of exposure to gastric acid. The effectiveness of gastric acid in killing bacteria will depend on complete mixing of the swallowed material with the gastric acid. Rapid emptying of incompletely acidified stomach contents, following for example the ingestion of a large volume of fluid or as a result of gastric surgery, will lead to a less effective kill of swallowed bacteria. Reduction of gastric acid secretion by vagotomy, atrophic gastritis, or by treatment with histamine H_2 receptor antagonists leads to an increase of the bacterial population of gastric juice (Ruddell et al, 1980; Milton-Thompson et al, 1982). Ruddell and Losowsky (1980) have reported a case of intestinal bacterial overgrowth, with large numbers of enterococci, *Streptococcus viridans*, coliforms and *Bacteroides*, in which the abnormal bacterial population and the diarrhoeal symptoms were reversed without antibiotic treatment when cimetidine was withdrawn.

Effects of motility

It is now well established that the human small intestine has a cyclical pattern of motor activity (Thompson et al, 1980) similar to that described in dogs (Szurszewski, 1969). This cyclical activity may be recorded by myoelectric activity or as changes in intraluminal pressure and comprises a resting phase (I), a phase of irregular activity (II), and a phase of regular rapid spikes of myoelectric activity producing a rise in intraluminal pressure sustained for one to three minutes (III). Phase III activity is a wave of contraction which moves down the small intestine, and in normal fasting humans occurs on average once every two hours. The phase III activity or migrating myoelectric complex is inhibited by ingestion of a meal. The function of the phase III activity is thought to be the cleansing of the fasting intestine and has been dubbed the 'intestinal housekeeper'. Van Trappen et al (1977) have described abnormalities of phase III activity in patients with bacterial overgrowth syndrome. Of 18 patients with bacterial overgrowth, as shown by an abnormal bile acid breath test, five had abnormal or absent phase III activity: two with bacterial overgrowth of obscure aetiology, one with a gastrectomy, one with Crohn's disease, and one with systemic sclerosis. In these patients antibiotic therapy reversed the abnormality in the bile acid breath test and also tended to restore normality to the motility pattern; phase III activity reappearing as the bacterial overgrowth was reversed. These studies have the interesting implication that the presence of an abnormal bacterial flora in the small intestine may in some way further impair intestinal motility. In patients with jejunoileal bypass a similar response of the colonic pseudo-obstruction to antibiotic therapy has been noted (Barry, Chow and Billesdon, 1977). Experimentally, inhibition of normal gut motility by drugs has variable results. Summers and Kent (1970) found that a slowing of gut transit with mecamylamine produced only small changes in the small intestinal flora of the rat (e.g., counts of *E. coli* were increased from $10^{3.9}$ to $10^{5.6}$/ml) with little evidence of functional disturbance to the gut, while Wehmann, Lifshitz and Teichberg (1978), using the same agents, produced bacterial overgrowth with evidence of small intestinal damage seen in the electron microscope. Intraperitoneal quinacrine, which produces extensive damage to the myenteric plexus, led to enormous dilatation of the small intestine, bacterial overgrowth, and steatorrhoea (Keeler, Richardson and Watson, 1966).

In clinical medicine, small bowel bacterial overgrowth is frequently encountered in patients with intestinal pseudo-obstruction due to a variety of causes (Anuras, 1978) (see Table 1). Probably the most prominent identifiable cause is that of systemic sclerosis (Kahn, Jeffries and Sleisenger, 1966). Other causes, such as myxoedema, diabetes mellitus or motility-inhibiting drugs such as phenothiazines, should be sought, but in a small number of patients no cause may be found, and the disease is then termed idiopathic intestinal pseudo-obstruction. This term undoubtedly embraces a wide variety of pathophysiological entities. Some patients have a form of hereditary visceral myopathy (Schuffler and Pope, 1977), while in other patients there are identifiable morphological changes in the myenteric plexus (Barnett and Wall, 1955; Dyer et al, 1969; Shilkin, Gracey and Joske, 1978). Other patients appear to have abnormal endogenous myo-electrical activity with normal myenteric plexus morphology and normal response to exogenous neurohormonal stimulation (Sullivan et al, 1977). In these patients the normal reflex increase in the duodenal motor activity after distention of the lumen was absent, but fasting motor activity increased normally after stimulation with secretin. It is probable that when careful planar longitudinal preparations of the myenteric plexus are examined (Smith, 1972) many more of these patients with motility disturbances will be identified as having morphological abnormalities of the myenteric plexus.

Influence of bile and pancreatic secretion

Bile has an influence on the in vitro growth of a number of bacteria; anaerobic gram-negative bacteria and in particular *Bacteroides* species are inhibited. In normal subjects, ingestion of a mixture of conjugated bile acids altered the flora of the ileum, reducing the proportion of anaerobic bacteria forming the total from 57 to 16 per cent (Williams, Showalter and Kern, 1975). However, this inhibitory effect of conjugated bile acids or of whole human bile was absent in in vitro testing on *Bacteroides fragilis, Clostridium perfringens, Lactobacillus* and *Enterococcus*, and inhibition of growth was seen only on testing with unconjugated bile acids (Floch et al, 1972). It seems possible that bile has little effect in the normal regulation of the bacterial population of the small intestine, but when the contents are stagnant deconjugation of bile acids by anaerobic species is one of the mechanisms by which their number is regulated (Percy-Robb and Collee, 1972).

Immunity and small bowel flora

The role of immune mechanisms in control of small bowel bacterial flora seems small in comparison with that of gastric acid and small bowel motility. Secretory IgA with its glycoprotein secretory piece probably acts by agglutinating bacteria and preventing their adherence to the mucosa (Freter, 1970). Clearly such a mechanism will have a major role in preventing gut infections with cholera or strains of enteropathogenic *Escherichia coli* but seems unlikely to influence the development of bacterial overgrowth in the stagnant bowel. However, severe immuno-deficiency syndromes, and in particular variable acquired immuno-deficiency, may be complicated by bacterial overgrowth in which *Bacteroides* species are prominent (Brown et al, 1972). Hersh et al (1970) and Parkin, McClelland and Moore (1972) found abnormal jejunal bacterial counts only in those hypogammaglobulinaemic subjects who were achlorhydric, but in these patients the counts were comparable to those of achlorhydric subjects with normal circulating levels of immunoglobulins.

Although both the amount (Crabbe et al, 1968) and specificity (McClelland et al, 1972) of secretory IgA seems to be determined by the local flora in the gastrointestinal tract, circulating agglutinins to a variety of gut organisms are present in normal persons, but do not appear to exert any controlling influence on the luminal flora (Freter, 1971).

Cell-mediated immunity is probably of importance in defence against nematode infestation (Ottaway, Rose and Parrott, 1979). Nude mice lacking T lymphocytes do not appear to develop an abnormal gut flora (Brown and Balish, 1970).

Other causes of abnormal bacterial flora

In both coeliac disease (Prizont, Hersh and Floch, 1970) and non-strictured small bowel Crohn's disease (Beeken, 1975) an abnormal small bowel flora has been described, but the significance of this to either the aetiology or the pathophysiology of mucosal damage and malabsorption in these is unknown. Radiation damage to the intestine appears to be followed by the establishment of an abnormal small bowel bacterial population (Kent, Osborne and Wende, 1968; Gorbach and Tabaqchali, 1969). In the acute stage this is associated with necrosis of the intestinal epithelium, but as a chronic effect irradiation leads to fibrosis, altered mucosal blood flow and villus damage.

PATHOPHYSIOLOGY OF MALABSORPTION IN THE BLIND LOOP SYNDROME

It is perhaps not surprising that the complex flora of the stagnant bowel produces intestinal malabsorption through a wide variety of mechanisms. Not all of these absorptive abnormalities will be present in every patient, and it is presumed that the differences in the malabsorptive pattern observed in patients (e.g., gross protein malabsorption predominating in one patient, or B_{12} malabsorption in another) depends upon the types of bacteria present in the lumen.

Altered Luminal Digestion

The observation that the mucosa in the blind loop is usually only mildly abnormal focused attention on the luminal digestion of fat and other nutrients.

Bile acid abnormalities and steatorrhoea

Dawson and Isselbacher (1960) suggested that the cause of steatorrhoea in the blind loop syndrome was bacterial deconjugation of bile acids which lowered the effective luminal concentration of conjugated bile acids to below the critical micellar concentration. Steatorrhoea in dogs with self-filling blind loops could be reversed by feeding cholic acid (Kim et al, 1966), though this did instead produce watery diarrhoea. However, in patients with blind loop syndrome, although the percentage of the secondary bile acid deoxycholate was increased from 15 to 30 per cent, there was no clear increase in the amount of deconjugated bile acids in intestinal aspirates (Mallory et al, 1973). Other workers (Hamilton et al, 1970) have also found the presence of deconjugated bile acids an inconstant finding. The reason for this may be the rapid non-ionic diffusive absorption of the conjugated bile acids in the small intestine. Evidence for this mechanism was produced by Midtvet et al (1974) who demonstrated that between 6 and 18 per cent of an oral dose of 24-cholyl-glycine was still present as the conjugate in bile after 24 hours. However, despite this very extensive bacterial splitting of the conjugated bile acids, there was usually no free bile acid present in the lumen, presumably due to its rapid duodenal absorption. Bile acid deconjugation may, however, play a role in the mucosal dysfunction also seen in blind loop syndrome (Donaldson, 1965), and the process of bacterial deconjugation in the small intestine may be detected by breath test and has been used clinically to demonstrate bacterial overgrowth. Conversely, Hamilton et al (1970) have recorded a patient with blind loop syndrome whose steatorrhoea was completely corrected by antibiotic therapy despite the persistence of a high degree of deconjugation of luminal bile acids.

Vitamin B$_{12}$ malabsorption

Considerable attention has been paid to the mechanism of malabsorption of B$_{12}$ in blind loop syndrome and several mechanisms appear to operate. A wide variety of bacteria appears to possess the capacity to bind vitamin B$_{12}$ (Schonsby and Hofstad, 1975), although the capacity of the aerobic species tested to take up free cobalamin was much more limited than their capacity to bind cobalamin complexed with intrinsic factor. Giannella, Broitman and Zamchek (1971) and Welkos, Toskes and Baer (1981) have examined the binding of B$_{12}$ to anaerobic species and have clearly demonstrated that anaerobic species, especially *Bacteroides*, have a much higher affinity binding to cobalamin and that 72 per cent of intrinsic factor-cobalamin complex was bound to the bacteria (see Figure 2). They demonstrated that in blind loop rats the absorption of cobalamin was improved by anti-anaerobic agents such as metronidazole, while therapy with antibiotics active mainly against aerobic species had no effect on cobalamin absorption. It is likely that the aerobic species, if they have any effect on B$_{12}$ metabolism in man, are probably net contributors of B$_{12}$. Albert, Mathan and Baker (1980) have demonstrated that a number of species of human small intestinal bacteria, particularly *Pseudomonas* and *Klebsiella* species, are able to synthesize significant amounts of vitamin B$_{12}$. The change in bacterial flora in a stagnant bowel towards a dominance of anaerobic species is therefore likely to lead to severe malabsorption of B$_{12}$.

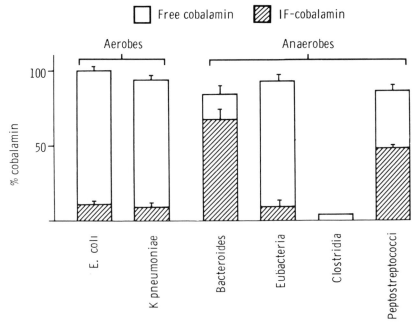

Figure 2. In vitro binding of free- and intrinsic factor (IF)-complexed cobalamin by blind loop flora. Note uniquely high binding of IF-cobalamin by *Bacteroides*. (Adapted from Welkos et al, 1981.)

Cobalamin, whether ingested or synthesized in situ in the intestinal lumen, may be metabolized by *Clostridium, Escherichia coli* and *Propionibacterium* to metabolically inactive substances known as cobamides (Brandt, Bernstein and Wagle, 1977). These may combine with intrinsic factor and block both ileal receptors (Mathan, Babior and Donaldson, 1974) and hepatic receptors to cyanocobalamin. In one patient with jejunal diverticulosis, 11 per cent of an orally administered dose of ^{57}Co B$_{12}$ was converted to 2-methyladeninecyanocobalamin, an inactive cobamide.

The absorption of vitamin B$_{12}$ is also enhanced by the presence in the lumen of a protein secreted by the pancreas. Bacterial degradation of this R protein could also inhibit absorption of cobalamin (Toskes, 1980).

Dietary proteolysis

Hypoalbuminaemia is not uncommon in patients with contaminated small bowel syndrome (Cooke et al, 1963) and is much more frequent than is seen in patients with coeliac disease. These abnormalities have been reviewed by Neale et al (1972). Dietary protein may be deaminated (Jones et al, 1968; Curtis, 1979). In addition, presumably through absorption into the portal blood of some toxic bacterial metabolite, hepatic protein synthesis tends to be impaired (Jones et al, 1968; Yap, Hafkenscheid and van Tongeren, 1974). This impairment of albumin synthesis is probably a non-specific effect of the hepatic damage which is seen in blind loop rats (Aarbakke and Schonsby, 1978) and in jejunoileal bypass (Maxwell, 1980).

Mucosal Damage

Structural abnormalities

In most patients with blind loop syndrome the mucosa is only mildly abnormal, and a finding of villous atrophy strongly suggests the presence of coeliac disease. In rodents the germ-free state is associated with jejunal villus hypoplasia (Abrams, 1977) and the mucosa of jejunal blind loops shows a hyperplastic pattern with increased crypt length, villus height and surface area (Gutschmidt et al, 1982). However, biopsies from within human jejunal diverticula may show villous atrophy (Lee and Toner, 1980). At an ultrastructural level, Ament et al (1972) noted that there was moderate to severe damage to the brush border of jejunal biopsies from patients with bacterial overgrowth. The abnormalities seem to be non-homogeneous within the biopsies, some villi showing greater abnormality than others. In several biopsies a large accumulation of lipid droplets was seen in the apical (supranuclear) portion of the enterocytes. Numerous dilated cytoplasmic vesicles and mitochondrial swellings were present. It was thought that fat transport out of the cell was probably impaired because chylomicrons were seen to be absent from the lateral intercellular spaces of postprandial biopsies. Similar changes have been observed in the mucosa from self-filling jejunal blind loops of rats (Gracey, Papadimitriou and Bower, 1974) (Figure 3). These abnormalities reversed after antibiotic therapy.

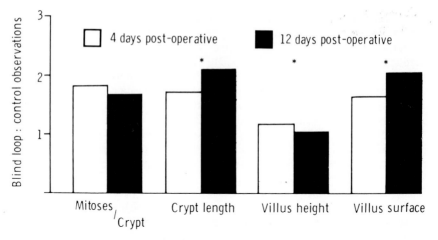

Figure 3. Changes of mucosal morphology in jejunal self-filling blind loops of rats at four days and 12 days after operation, expressed as a ratio to control (sham-operated) animals. Increased crypt mitoses, crypt length, villus height and villus surface at four days are significant ($P<0.01$); differences between observations at four days and 12 days are significant ($P<0.01$) if indicated by an asterisk. (Adapted with permission from Gutschmidt et al, 1982.)

Abnormalities of mucosal enzymes and transport processes

Although structural abnormalities may not be evident in blind loop syndrome, abnormally low levels of brush border enzymes are observed. Giannella, Rout and Toskes (1974) demonstrated depressed levels of maltase, sucrase and lactase in both the blind loop and the segment of jejunum distal to it in rats. Antibiotic treatment corrected the maltase and sucrase levels, but uptake of both 3-O-methylglucose and leucine remained depressed. Such brush border damage was thought to be related to the presence of deconjugated bile acids. Brush border preparations from blind loops also showed reduced levels of disaccharidases and peptidases (Jonas, Flanagan and Forstner, 1977; Mazzacca et al, 1977). Using a dual isotope pulse labelling technique, this loss of enzymes was shown to be due to an abnormally rapid turnover of brush border glycoprotein (see Figure 4) (Jonas and Forstner, 1978). This effect of the luminal bacteria can be attributed to their production of an elastase-like enzyme which degrades glycoproteins (Jonas and Forstner, 1979). Prizont (1981) has demonstrated that the luminal content of rat blind loops contains enzymes capable of degrading blood group substances (also glycoprotein). Levels of α-N-acetyl-galactosaminidase were markedly increased above control levels, and injected ^{14}C-glucosamine was rapidly metabolized by the luminal bacteria to short-chain fatty acids. That this rapid turnover of brush border enzymes was unrelated to the presence of bile acids, whether deconjugated or not, was elegantly demonstrated in further experiments by Jonas and Forstner (1979) in which diversion of the bile distal to the blind loop had no effect on the degree of damage to the brush border enzyme, although the steatorrhoea was greatest in those animals with biliary diversion. Pure bile acids, especially deconjugated bile acids (Gracey et al, 1973) are damaging to the jejunum, altering mucosal disaccharidase levels and impairing the absorption of monosaccharides (Harries and Sladen, 1972), but the presence of lecithin, as found in normal bile, protects the mucosa from bile acid attack (Lamabadasuriya, Quiraldes and Harries, 1975).

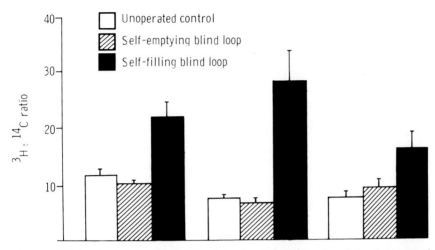

Figure 4. Relative degradation ratios of brush border glycoproteins from jejunal mucosa of non-operated rats and from self-emptying blind loops and self-filling blind loops. The rats were injected with ^{14}C-glucosamine at 19 h and ^{3}H-glucosamine at 3 h before being killed. Left = jejunum proximal to blind loop; centre = blind loop; right = jejunum distal to blind loop. (Adapted from Jonas, Flanagan and Forstner, 1977.)

Malabsorption of other nutrients

Malabsorption deficiencies of water and fat-soluble vitamins have been reported in patients with blind loop syndrome. Vitamin D absorption may be impaired, leading to clinical deficiency (Thompson, 1967). High serum folic acid levels related to an increased synthesis of folic acid by the luminal bacteria have been described, as have patients with clinical evidence of folic deficiency which was corrected by antibiotic therapy (Neale et al, 1972). Severe nicotinic acid deficiency, producing encephalopathy, occurred in one patient with jejunal diverticulosis (Tabaqchali and Pallis, 1970). Iron deficiency has not been reported in uncomplicated blind loop syndrome despite the fact that many gut bacteria have high avidity for ferric iron and possess specific iron binding receptors or siderophores.

SYSTEMIC EFFECTS OF BLIND LOOP SYNDROME

Besides the nutritional deficiencies engendered by malabsorption in the blind loop syndrome, there appears to be a number of other features which are not explained solely by nutritional deficiency. Of these the most serious is the hepatitis and steatosis seen in jejunoileal bypass patients (Fikri and Cassella, 1974). Experimentally, this appears to be related to overgrowth of aerobic organisms in the bypassed segment and can be treated by administration of the appropriate antibiotics (Maxwell, 1980). It may be that this effect is due to absorption into the portal blood of some toxic bacterial metabolite or to the combined effects of malnutrition and bacterial consumption of a hepatotrophic factor such as choline (McGouran et al, 1982).

CLINICAL METHODS IN THE DIAGNOSIS OF BLIND LOOP SYNDROME

The essential features of the blind loop syndrome in clinical medicine are the occurrence of steatorrhoea and B_{12} malabsorption in association with an abnormal small bowel flora. The absorptive defects can be corrected by treatment directed solely to reducing or altering this abnormal flora. In assessing any patient with absorptive defects the clinician should be alerted to the possibility of blind loop syndrome by a previous history of gastric surgery, scleroderma, diabetes, or the long-term use of H_2-antagonists.

Radiology

Demonstration of an anatomical abnormality in the small intestine by means of barium studies is especially valuable, particularly by using barium infusion or enteroclysis techniques (Figure 5). This also directs the investigator to a rational and precise location of a subsequent intestinal intubation and aspiration study from the segment of intestine which is most likely to be the site of bacterial colonization.

Demonstration of bacterial metabolic processes

Indirect clinical tests for the presence of bacterial overgrowth depend on the demonstration of bacterial metabolic processes. Urinary indicans are derived from hepatic metabolism of indoles, products of bacterial metabolism of dietary tryptophan. Variations in urinary indican excretion are likely to occur when the dietary tryptophan is varied, or simply as a result of increased spill of tryptophan into the colon when the small bowel absorption is abnormal, e.g., in coeliac disease (Neale et al, 1972). However, in the absence of severe steatorrhoea, a urinary indican excretion of greater than 200 mg/day is highly suggestive of bacterial overgrowth in the small intestine. Aarbakke and Schonsby (1978) showed that other urinary metabolites, phenol, *p*-cresol and indican, were also valuable indicators. False positive results did not occur with phenol excretion and false negative results were not obtained with urinary indican excretion.

Xylose excretion in the urine after an oral test dose is highly unreliable. The estimation of total serum bile acids may be of some value in the diagnosis of blind loop syndrome particularly if the unconjugated fraction can be shown to be elevated.

Valuable non-invasive aids to the diagnosis of blind loop syndrome have been the various breath tests. These depend upon the detection in the breath

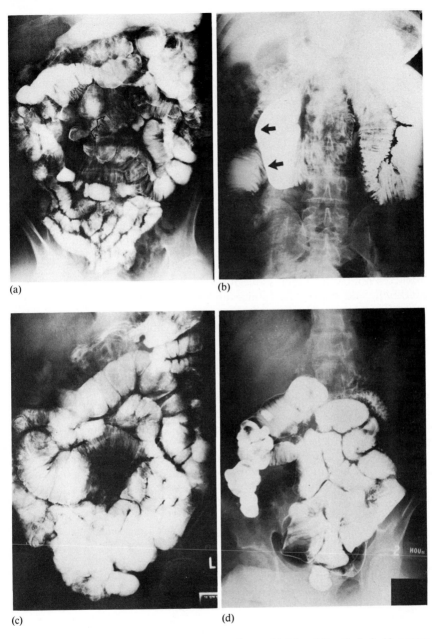

(a)

(b)

(c)

(d)

Figure 5. Small bowel radiology and blind loop syndrome. (a) Jejunal diverticulosis. Numerous diverticula have been demonstrated; the arrows indicate the mouths of two. (b) Scleroderma. Note the featureless duodenum (arrowed) and dilated jejunal loops. (c) Partial jejunal obstruction; in this case the obstruction is due to an intestinal lymphoma. (d) Intestinal pseudo-obstruction. Two hours after ingestion of barium dilated jejunal and ileal loops are visible. (Radiographs courtesy of Dr E. O. L. Hoskins.)

of a peak of hydrogen or $^{14}CO_2$ when an ingested bolus of a bacterial substrate such as xylose passes through the small intestine. The amount of substrate given and its rate of transit through the small intestine will influence the results obtained, as the colonic bacteria will also metabolize unabsorbed substrate. Furthermore, the bacterial flora present in the stagnant small intestine does not always have the ability to deconjugate bile acids, for example, rendering the bile acid breath test less reliable than the use of ^{14}C-xylose as a substrate. (See Chapter 17 for a full discussion of this.)

Quantitative bacteriology of the small intestine

Direct examination of the small bowel contents should ideally be performed in all patients in whom blind loop syndrome is suspected. Samples of intestinal fluid are obtained using a long weighted-tip intestinal tube. The collection and bacteriological quantification of the samples requires meticulous technique in order to obtain reproducible results. It is of particular importance to ensure that the patient has not been treated with antibiotics for at least the preceding two weeks. Patients should be instructed not to clean their teeth or use mouthwash on the morning of the aspiration, and during the intubation procedure they should spit out all saliva. Tubes should be free of all antibacterial chemicals and positioned under fluoroscopic controls as rapidly as possible. A sample should be saved after aspirating a volume of intestinal juice equivalent to that of the dead space within the tube. The fasting normal jejunum usually contains only a little fluid which has a clear and bile-stained appearance. In patients with gross blind loop syndrome large volumes of foul-smelling turbid fluid may be aspirated. The sample should be immediately sent to the laboratory under anaerobic conditions. This is most conveniently done by taking the sample into a disposable syringe, expelling all air, and sealing the syringe with a blind (needleless) hub.

Quantification of a bacterial population in the intestine presents a much greater problem than in other types of clinical specimen. The problem of qualitative bacteriology of the flora of fluid from a blind loop is considerable. The bacteriologist is not attempting to identify a single infecting organism such as occurs in the classic transmitted infections. Instead his task is to give an overall picture of the complex flora which exists in the stagnant bowel and to indicate whether the contamination is of a degree severe enough to produce active abnormalities. Undoubtedly the largest number of bacteria will be cultivated when the rigorous anaerobic techniques laid down in the Virginia Polytechnic Institute guidelines are used (Holdeman and Moore, 1972). These involve the handling of the specimens in an oxygen-free environment or glove box. Most hospitals are not equipped with full anaerobic culture facilities, but usually employ a commercial system for anaerobic culture. Results of cultures are expressed as the number of colony-forming units grown per millilitre of fluid, but clearly one colony can form from a large clump of bacteria and this tends to result in underestimation of the total number. More subtle methods for the detection of anaerobic organisms involves the use of gas-liquid chromatography to demonstrate the short-chain fatty acid production by species such as *Bacteroides* (Gorbach et al, 1976; Phillips, Tearle and Willis, 1976). *Bacteroides fragilis* produces acetic and succinic acids. The demonstration of these acids in fasting jejunal contents is proof of bacterial contamination. Interpretation of quantitative bacteriology of the small intestine can be made only in the light of knowledge of the patient's gastric acid secretory status, as achlorhydric subjects always have larger numbers of bacteria in the small intestine. For each laboratory a range of normal values must be established, but in general a total bacterial count of greater than 10^6 organisms/ml and the presence of more than 10^4 bacteroides/ml are highly significant.

TREATMENT

The first aim of treatment in blind loop syndrome is to reverse the absorptive abnormalities by correcting structural or functional abnormalities leading to the bacterial overgrowth. A surgically remediable lesion such as a stricture should always be sought. If the syndrome is not correctable by surgery then therapy with a wide variety of antibiotics (Banwell, 1981) may be effective. It is not possible to permanently eradicate bacterial contamination from a grossly abnormal bowel such as jejunal diverticulosis, and treatment with antibiotics may be given on an intermittent basis with good effect. Clinical trials comparing antibiotic regimes are not available. Tetracycline is of established value and metronidazole is also highly effective clinically. Relapses of blind loop syndrome may be related to recolonization of the intestine with different serotypes of bacteria, and second courses of antibiotics are often just as effective as the first for this reason. Because there is no single pathogenic species in the blind loop syndrome, the isolation of single organisms and antibiotic sensitivity testing seems to have little to commend it; there is certainly no scientific evidence to support this procedure.

TROPICAL MALABSORPTION AND SMALL BOWEL BACTERIAL CONTAMINATION

This topic has been the subject of recent reviews (Tomkins, 1981; Ross and Mathan, 1981; Klipstein, 1981; Cook, 1980). Tropical sprue has been defined as malabsorption, occurring in the tropics, of two unrelated test substances in a patient in whom other specific infections or non-tropical disease cannot be identified (Tomkins, 1981). In general, the more severe degrees of malabsorption are referred to as tropical sprue. Sprue of acute onset is more frequently identified in expatriates of temperate climates visiting sprue endemic areas, notably India, Central and South America and South-East Asia and the Middle East. The sudden onset of diarrhoea followed by malabsorption is highly suggestive of an infective aetiology, but it has never been possible to isolate a single agent which will produce the disease in normal subjects. Bacterial flora of the upper small intestine differs from that of classical blind loop syndrome in that, although total numbers of bacteria may not be dramatically elevated, the gram-negative aerobic organisms isolated tend to be enterotoxigenic (Klipstein, Engert and Short, 1978). These toxins cause water and electrolyte secretion in the upper intestine. Anaerobic organisms such as *Bacteroides* are also present, probably accounting for the presence of deconjugated bile acids (Cassells et al, 1970). Malabsorption of vitamin B_{12} responds rapidly to antibiotic therapy, but the luminal events may differ from the classic blind loop syndrome in that ingested cobalt-57-labelled vitamin B_{12} was not apparently bound to the luminal bacteria (Kapadia et al, 1975).

The susceptibility of individuals to chronic tropical sprue may possibly be related to achlorhydria, as approximately one-third of Indian subjects with this disease were achlorhydric (Baker and Mathan, 1976). Similarly Nalin et al (1978) have suggested that the susceptibility to cholera of overland travellers to India might be related to cannabis abuse inducing achlorhydria. Adhesion of the enterobacteria to the gut mucosa appears to play a role (Drasar et al, 1980), and it may be that a combination of a large bacterial load, achlorhydria and a gut surface conducive to adhesion of enterobacteria all play a part in the genesis of this condition.

Diagnosis of tropical sprue is really one of exclusion of other identifiable causes for malabsorption in a patient who was resident in an endemic area. Jejunal biopsy usually shows only minor degrees of villous abnormality, but intraepithelial lymphocyte counts tend to be increased in the crypts as well as villi (Ross and Mathan, 1981). The most important differential diagnosis is that of giardiasis which can mimic tropical sprue by its acute onset and severe malabsorption. Giardiasis alone may lead to an abnormal luminal bacterial flora (Tandon, Tandon and Satpathy, 1977). Treatment with anti-bacterial agents may lead to a rapid reversal of absorptive defects (Gorbach et al, 1970; Tomkins, Smith and Wright, 1978) but regaining weight is much more dependent on recovery of appetite (Klipstein and Corcino, 1977).

Although there may not be a systemic folic acid deficiency in these patients, supplements of folic acids are well recognized to be beneficial (O'Brien, 1979; Tomkins, 1981). This may be due to a production by the luminal bacteria of some antifolic agent effectively causing local deficiency (Tomkins, 1981).

Therapy of tropical sprue with tetracycline brings about improvement of absorptive function, jejunal morphology and clinical state in about a month (Klipstein, 1981). Chronic sprue in natives of endemic areas tends to be more resistant and requires up to a year's antibiotic treatment. A standard treatment regime combines folic acid (5 mg daily) and tetracycline (250 mg four times daily) for three months. Attention should also be paid to deficiency of vitamin B_{12}, with parenteral supplementation if serum levels are abnormal at the time of diagnosis.

The prevalence of tropical sprue in the indigenous populations of endemic areas is unknown but could be responsible for an enormous wastage of food. The reduction of the problem probably depends on improvement in public health measures, the best protection for the visitor to endemic areas is in the careful attention to dietary hygiene and prompt investigation and treatment of diarrhoea.

REFERENCES

Aarbakke, J. & Schonsby, H. (1978) Impaired oxidation of antipyrine in stagnant loop rats. *Scandinavian Journal of Gastroenterology,* **12,** 929-935.

Abrams, G. D. (1977) Microbial effects on mucosal structure and function. *American Journal of Clinical Nutrition,* **30,** 1880-1886.

Albert, M. J., Mathan, V. I. & Baker, S. J. (1980) Vitamin B_{12} synthesis by human small intestinal bacteria. *Nature,* **283,** 781-782.

Ament, M. E., Shimoda, S. S., Saunders, D. P. & Ruben, C. E. (1972) Pathogenesis of steatorrhea in three cases of small intestinal stasis syndrome. *Gastroenterology,* **63,** 728-747.

Anuras, S. (1978) Intestinal pseudo-obstruction. *Gastroenterology,* **74,** 1318-1324.

Baker, S. J. M. & Mathan, V. I. (1976) Tropical sprue in Southern India. In *Tropical Sprue and Megaloblastic Anaemia.* pp. 189-260. London: Churchill Livingstone.

Banwell, J. G. (1981) Small intestinal bacterial overgrowth syndrome. *Gastroenterology,* **80,** 834-835.

Barnett, W. O. & Wall, L. (1955) Megaduodenum resulting from absence from the parasympathetic ganglion cells in Auerbach's Plexus: a review of literature and report of a case. *Annals of Surgery,* **141,** 527-535.

Barry, R. E., Chow, A. W. & Billesdon, J. (1977) Role of intestinal microflora in colonic pseudo-obstruction complicating jejunoileal bypass. *Gut,* **18,** 356-359.

Beeken, W. L. (1975) Remediable defects in Crohn's disease. *Archives of Internal Medicine,* **135,** 686-690.

Brandt, L. J., Bernstein, L. H. & Wagle, A. (1977) Production of vitamin B_{12} analogues in patients with small bowel bacterial overgrowth. *Annals of Internal Medicine,* **87,** 546-551.

Brown, J. F. & Balish, E. (1970) Gastrointestinal microecology of BALB/c nude mice. *Applied and Environmental Microbiology,* **36,** 144-159.

Brown, W. R., Savage, D. C., Dubois, R. S. et al (1972) Intestinal microflora of immunoglobulin deficient and normal human subjects. *Gastroenterology,* **62,** 1143-1152.

Cameron, P. G., Watson, G. M. & Witts, L. J. (1949) The experimental production of anaemia by operations on the intestinal tract. *Blood,* **4,** 803-805.

Cassells, J. S., Banwell, J. G., Gorbach, S. C. et al (1970) Tropical sprue and malnutrition in West Bengal. IV. Bile salt deconjugation in tropical sprue. *American Journal of Clinical Nutrition,* **23,** 1579-1581.

Cooke, G. C. (1980) *Tropical Gastroenterology.* Oxford: Oxford University Press.

Cooke, W. T., Cox, E. B., Fone, D. J. & Gaddie, R. (1963) The clinical and metabolic significance of jejunal diverticula. *Gut,* **4,** 115-131.

Crabbe, P. A., Bazin, H., Eyssen, H. & Heremans, J. F. (1968) The normal microbial flora as a major stimulus for proliferation of plasma cells synthesising IgA in the gut. *International Archives of Allergy,* **34,** 362-375.

Curtis, K. J. (1979) Protein digestion and absorption in the blind loop syndrome. *Digestive Diseases and Sciences,* **2** (24), 923-929.

Dawson, A. M. & Isselbacher, K. J. (1960) Studies of lipid metabolism in the small intestine with observations on the role of bile salts. *Journal of Clinical Investigation,* **39,** 730-740.

Donaldson, R. M. (1965) Studies on the pathogenesis of steatorrhea in the blind loop syndrome. *Journal of Clinical Investigation,* **44,** 1815-1825.

Drasar, B. S., Agostini, C., Clarke, D. et al (1980) Adhesion of enteropathogenic bacteria to cells in tissue culture. *Developments in Biological Standards,* **46,** 83-89.

Dyer, N. H., Dawson, A. M., Smith, B. F. & Todd, I. P. (1969) Obstruction of the bowel due to lesion in the myenteric plexus. *British Medical Journal,* **i,** 686-689.

Fikri, E. & Cassella, R. R. (1974) Jejunoileal bypass for massive obesity: results and complications in 52 patients. *Annals of Surgery,* **179,** 460-464.

Floch, M. H., Binder, H. J., Allburn, B. & Gershengoren, W. (1972) The effect of bile acids on intestinal microflora. *American Journal of Clinical Nutrition,* **25,** 1418-1426.

Freter, R. (1970) Mechanism of action of intestinal antibody in experimental cholera. II. Antibody-mediated antibacterial reaction at the mucosal surface. *Infection and Immunity,* **2,** 556-566.

Freter, R. (1971) Locally produced and serum derived antibodies and 'local immunity'. *New England Journal of Medicine,* **28,** 1375-1376.

Giannella, R. A., Broitman, S. A. & Zamchek, N. (1971) Vitamin B_{12} uptake by intestinal microorganisms: mechanisms and relevance to syndromes of intestinal bacterial overgrowth. *Journal of Clinical Investigation,* **50,** 1100-1107.

Giannella, R. A., Broitman, S. A. & Zamchek, N. (1972) Gastric acid barrier to ingested microorganisms in man: studies in vivo and in vitro. *Gut,* **13,** 251-256.

Giannella, R. A., Rout, W. R. & Toskes, P. P. (1974) Jejunal brush border injury and impaired sugar and amino acid uptake in the blind loop syndrome. *Gastroenterology,* **67,** 965-974.

Gorbach, S. L. (1971) Intestinal microflora. *Gastroenterology,* **60,** 1110-1129.

Gorbach, S. L. & Tabaqchali, S. (1969) Bacteria, bile and the small bowel. *Gut,* **10,** 963-972.

Gorbach, S. L., Mayhew, J. W., Bartlett, J. G. et al (1970) Rapid diagnosis of anaerobic infections by direct gas-liquid chromatography of clinical specimens. *Journal of Clinical Investigation,* **57,** 478-484.

Gracey, M. (1979) The contaminated small bowel syndrome: pathogenesis, diagnosis and treatment. *American Journal of Clinical Nutrition,* **32,** 234-243.

Gracey, M., Papadimitriou, J. & Bower, G. (1974) Ultrastructural changes in the small intestines of rats with self-filling blind loops. *Gastroenterology,* **67,** 646-651.

Gracey, M., Papadimitriou, J., Burke, V. et al (1973) Effects on small intestinal function and structure induced by feeding a deconjugated bile salt. *Gut,* **14,** 519-528.

Gutschmidt, S., Sandforth, F., Menge, H. et al (1982) Adaptive response of α- and β-glucosidase kinetics along the villi of rat self-filling jejunal blind loops. *Gut,* **23,** 376-381.

Hamilton, J. D., Dyer, N., Dawson, A. M. et al (1970) Assessment and significance of bacterial overgrowth in the small bowel. *Quarterly Journal of Medicine,* **39,** 265-285.

Harries, J. T. & Sladen, G. E. (1972) The effects of different bile salts on the absorption of fluids, electrolytes and monosaccharides in the small intestine of the rat in vivo. *Gut,* **13,** 596-603.

Hentges, D. J. & Maier, B. M. (1972) Theoretical basis for anaerobic methodology. *American Journal of Clinical Nutrition,* **25,** 1299-1305.

Hersh, T., Floch, M. H., Binder, H. J. et al (1970) Disturbance of the jejunal and colonic bacterial flora in immunoglobulin deficiencies. *American Journal of Clinical Nutrition,* **23,** 1595-1601.

Holdeman, L. V. & Moore, W. E. C. (1972) *Anaerobe Laboratory Manual. Anaerobe Laboratory.* Virginia: Blacksburg.

Holdeman, L. V. & Moore, W. E. C. (1977) Gram-negative anaerobic bacteria. In *Bergey's Manual of Determinative Bacteriology* (Ed.) Buchanan R. E. & Gibbons, N. E. pp. 384-426. Baltimore: Williams & Wilkins.

Jonas, A. & Forstner, G. C. (1978) Pathogenesis of mucosal injury in the blind loop syndrome. *Gastroenterology,* **75,** 791-795.

Jonas, A. & Forstner, C. G. (1979) The effect of biliary diversion on mucosal enzyme activity and brush border glycoprotein degradation in rats with self-filling blind loops. *European Journal of Clinical Investigation,* **9,** 167-173.

Jonas, A., Flanagan, P. R. & Forstner, G. C. (1977) Pathogenesis of mucosal injury in the blind loop syndrome. Brush border enzyme activity and glycoprotein degradation. *Journal of Clinical Investigation,* **60,** 1321-1330.

Jones, E. A., Craigie, A., Tavill, A. S. et al (1968) Protein metabolism in the intestinal stagnant loop syndrome. *Gut,* **9,** 466-469.

Kahn, I. J., Jeffries, J. H. & Sleisenger, M. H. (1966) Malabsorption in intestinal scleroderma and correction by antibiotics. *New England Journal of Medicine,* **274,** 1339-1344.

Kapadia, C. R., Bhat, P., Jacobs, E. & Baker, S. J. (1975) Vitamin B_{12} malabsorption. A study of intraluminal events in control subjects and patients with tropical sprue. *Gut,* **16,** 988-993.

Keeler, R., Richardson, H. & Watson, A. J. (1966) Enteromegaly and steatorrhea in the rat following intraperitoneal quinacrine. *Laboratory Investigation,* **15,** 1253-1262.

Kent, T. H., Osborne, J. W. & Wende, C. M. (1968) Intestinal flora in whole body and intestinal x-irradiated rats. *Radiation Research,* **35,** 635-651.

Kim, Y. S., Spritz, N., Blum, M. et al (1966) The role of altered bile acid metabolism in the steatorrhea of experimental blind loop. *Journal of Clinical Investigation,* **45,** 956-962.

King, C. E. & Toskes, P. P. (1981) Small intestinal bacterial overgrowth syndrome. *Gastroenterology,* **80,** 834-845.

Klipstein, F. A. (1981) Tropical sprue in travellers and ex-patriates living abroad. *Gastroenterology,* **80,** 590-600.

Klipstein, F. A. & Corcino, J. J. (1977) Factors responsible for weight loss in tropical sprue. *American Journal of Clinical Nutrition,* **30,** 1703-1708.

Klipstein, F. A., Engert, R. F. & Short, H. (1978) Enterotoxigenicity of colonising coliform bacteria in tropical sprue and blind loop syndrome. *Lancet,* **ii,** 342-344.

Klipstein, F. A., Holdeman, L. B., Corcino, J. J. & Moore, W. E. C. (1973) Enterotoxingenic bacteria in tropical sprue. *Annals of Internal Medicine,* **79,** 632-645.

Lamabadusuriya, S., Quiraldes, P. & Harries, J. T. (1975) Influence of mixtures of taurocholate, fatty acids and monolein on the toxic effects of deoxycholate on rat jejunum in vivo. *Gastroenterology,* **69,** 463-469.

Lee, F. D. & Toner, P. G. (1980) *Biopsy Pathology of the Small Intestine.* London: Chapman and Hall.

Mallory, A., Savage, B., Kern, F. & Smith, J. G. (1973) Patterns of bile acids and microflora in the human small intestine. II. Microflora. *Gastroenterology,* **64,** 34-42.

Mathan, V. I., Babior, B. M. & Donaldson, R. M. (1974) Kinetics of the attachment of intrinsic factor-bound cobamides to ileal receptors. *Journal of Clinical Investigation,* **54,** 598-608.

Mazzacca, G., Musella, S., Andria, G. et al (1977) Brush border peptidases and arylamidases in the experimental blind loop syndrome of the rat. *Acta Hepatogastroenterologica* (Stuttgart), **24,** 364-367.

Maxwell, J. D. (1980) Intestinal bypass and the liver. In *Surgical Management of Obesity* (Ed.) Maxwell, J. D., Gazet, J. C. & Pilkington, T. pp. 235-255. London: Academic Press.

McClelland, D. B. L., Samson, R. R., Parkin, D. R. & Shearman, D. J. C. (1972) Bacterial agglutination studies with secretory IgA prepared from human gastrointestinal secretions and colostrum. *Gut,* **13,** 450-458.

McGouran, R. C., Rutter, K. P., Ang, L. et al (1982) Role of anaerobic bacteria in weight loss and reduced food intake after jejunoileal bypass in the rat. *International Journal of Obesity,* **6,** 197-204.

Midtvedt, T. (1974) Microbial bile acid transformation. *American Journal of Clinical Nutrition,* **27,** 1341-1347.

Milton-Thompson, G., Lightfood, M. F., Ahmet, Z. et al (1982) Intragastric acidity, bacteria, nitrite and N-nitroso compounds before, during and after cimetidine treatment. *Lancet,* **i,** 1091-1095.

Nalin, D. R., Levine, M. M., Rhead, J. et al (1978) Cannabis, hypochlorhydria and cholera. *Lancet,* **ii,** 859-862.

Neale, G., Gompertz, D., Schjonsby, H. et al (1972) The metabolic and nutritional consequemces of bacterial overgrowth in the small intestine. *American Journal of Clinical Nutrition,* **25,** 1409-1417.

O'Brien, D. (1979) Tropical sprue. *Journal of the Royal Society of Medicine,* **22,** 916-920.

Ottaway, C. A., Rose, M. L. & Parrott, D. M. F. (1979) The gut as an immunological system. *International Review of Physiology* (Ed.) Crane, R. K. pp. 323-356. Baltimore: University Park Press.

Parkin, D. M., McClelland, D. B. L. & O'Moore, R. R. (1972) Intestinal bacterial flora and bile salt studies in hypogammaglobulinaemia. *Gut,* **13,** 182-188.

Percy-Robb, I. W. & Collee, J. G. (1972) Bile acids: a pH-dependent antibacterial system in the gut? *British Medical Journal,* **iii,** 813-815.

Phillips, K. D., Tearle, P. D. & Willis, A. T. (1976) Rapid diagnosis of anaerobic infections by gas-liquid chromatography of clinical material. *Clinical Pathology,* **29,** 428-434.

Prizont, R., Hersh, T. & Floch, M. H. (1970) Jejunal bacterial flora in chronic small bowel disease. I. Celiac disease. II. Regional Enteritis. *American Journal of Clinical Nutrition,* **23,** 1602-1607.

Prizont, R. J. (1981) Glycoprotein degradation in the blind loop syndrome. Identification of glycosidases. *Journal of Clinical Investigation,* **67,** 336-344.

Rolfe, R. D. (1977) Oxygen tolerance of human intestinal anaerobes. *American Journal of Clinical Nutrition,* **30,** 1762-1769.

Ross, I. M. & Mathan, V. I. (1981) Immunological changes in tropical sprue. *Quarterly Journal of Medicine,* **50,** 435-449.

Ruddell, W. S. & Losowsky, M. S. (1980) Severe diarrhoea due to small intestinal bacterial colonisation during cimetidine treatment. *British Medical Journal,* **281,** 273.

Ruddell, W. S. J., Axon, A. G. R., Findlay, J. M. et al (1980) Effects of cimetidine on the gastric bacterial flora. *Lancet,* **i,** 673-674.

Savage, D. C. (1977) Microbial ecology of the gastrointestinal tract. *Annual Review of Microbiology,* **31,** 107-133.

Schonsby, H. & Hofstad, T. (1975) The uptake of vitamin B_{12} by the sediment of jejunal contents in patients with the blind loop syndrome. *Scandinavian Journal of Gastroenterology,* **10,** 305-309.

Schuffler, M. V. & Pope, C. E. (1977) Studies of idiopathic intestinal pseudo-obstruction. (i) Hereditary hollow visceral myopathy: clinical and pathological studies. *Gastroenterology,* **73,** 327-338.

Shilkin, K. B., Gracey, M. & Joske, R. A. (1978) Idiopathic intestinal pseudo-obstruction. *Australian Paediatric Journal,* **14,** 102-106.

Smith, B. H. (1972) *The Neuropathology of the Alimentary Tract.* London: Edward Arnold.

Sullivan, M. A., Snape, W. J., Matarazzo, R. J. et al (1977) Gastrointestinal myoelectrical activity in idiopathic intestinal pseudo-obstruction. *New England Journal of Medicine,* **297,** 233-238.

Summers, R. W. & Kent, P. H. (1970) Effects of altered propulsion on rat small intestinal flora. *Gastroenterology,* **59,** 740-744.

Szurzewski, J. H. (1969) A migrating electric complex of the canine small intestine. *American Journal of Psychology,* **217,** 1737-1750.

Tabaqchali, S. (1970) The pathophysiological role of small intestinal bacterial flora. *Scandinavian Gastroenterology* (Supplement), **6,** 139-163.

Tabaqchali, S. & Pallis, C. (1970) Reversible nicotinamide deficiency encephalopathy in a patient with jejunal diverticulosis. *Gut,* **11,** 1024-1027.

Tandon, B. N., Tandon, R. K. & Satpathy, B. K. (1977) Mechanism of malabsorption in giardiasis: a study of bacterial flora and bile salt deconjugation in the upper jejunum. *Gut,* **18,** 176-181.

Thadepalli, H., Lou, M. A., Bach, V. T. et al (1979) Microflora of the human small intestine. *American Journal of Surgery,* **138,** 845-860.

Thompson, D. G., Wingate, D. L., Archer, L. et al (1980) Normal patterns of human upper small bowel motor activity recorded by prolonged radio-telemetry. *Gut,* **21,** 500-506.

Thompson, G. R. (1967) A case of osteomalacia, osteoporosis and hypercalcaemia. *British Medical Journal,* **1,** 219-225.

Tomkins, A. M. (1981) Tropical malabsorption: recent concepts in pathogenesis and nutritional significance. *Clinical Science,* **60,** 131-137.

Tomkins, A. M., Smith, T. & Wright, S. J. (1978) Assessment of early and delayed responses in vitamin B_{12} absorption during antibiotic therapy in tropical malabsorption. *Clinical Science and Molecular Medicine,* **55,** 533-539.

Toskes, P. P. (1980) Current concepts of cobalamin (vitamin B_{12}) absorption and malabsorption. *Journal of Clinical Gastroenterology,* **2,** 287-297.

Vantrappen, G., Janssens, J., Hellemans, J. & Ghoos, Y. (1977) The interdigestive motor complex of normal subjects and patients with bacterial overgrowth of the small intestine. *Journal of Clinical Investigation,* **59,** 1158-1166.

Wehmann, H. J., Lifshitz, F. & Teichberg, S. (1978) Effects of enteric microbial overgrowth on small intestinal ultrastructure in the rat. *American Journal of Gastroenterology,* **70,** 249-258.

Welkos, S. L., Toskes, P. P. & Baer, H. (1981) Importance of anaerobic bacteria in the cobalamin malabsorption of the experimental rat blind loop syndrome. *Gastroenterology,* **80,** 313-320.

Williams, R. C., Showalter, E. & Kern, H. F. (1975) In vivo effect of bile salt and cholestyramine on intestinal anaerobic bacteria. *Gastroenterology,* **69,** 483-491.

Yap, S. H., Hafkenscheid, J. C. M. & Van Tongeren, J. H. M. (1974) Rate of synthesis of albumin in relation to serum levels of essential amino acids in patients with bacterial overgrowth in the small bowel. *European Journal of Clinical Investigation,* **4,** 279-284.

6

Intestinal Immunity and Malabsorption

WILLIAM F. DOE
ANDREW J. HAPEL

The intestinal mucosa is exposed to sustained antigenic challenge from the wide range of ingested substances and agents which bathe its surface. In common with other mucosae, the intestine has evolved specialized immune mechanisms by which antigen recognition and handling, induction of cellular and humoral responses, memory, regulation of tolerance and recruitment of effector systems are adapted to respond to the constant threat of injury. Since the observations of Besredka (1919) that oral immunization of rabbits using killed *Salmonella* organisms provided solid protection against dysentery irrespective of serum titres of specific antibody, the concept of a secretory immune system and its importance to homeostasis in the intestine has contributed substantially to our understanding of the pathogenesis of many intestinal disorders. In this chapter the physiology of the immune system in the gut and the disorders of its function which may result in widespread mucosal injury and malabsorption will be discussed. Intestinal disorders which cause malabsorption and are associated with disturbances of immunity, such as gluten sensitive enteropathy and Crohn's disease, are discussed in Chapters 10 and 12.

CELLS INVOLVED IN MUCOSAL IMMUNITY

The antigen-reactive cells of the intestinal tract which are present either as focal aggregates, as in Peyer's patches and the appendix, or as scattered lymphocytes and plasma cells in the lamina propria and epithelium (Doe, 1982) have been collectively called gut-associated lymphoid tissue (GALT). Peyer's patches are covered with an epithelium which includes a unique cell type, the membranous cell (M cell), which provides specialized access for antigens (Owen and Jones, 1974). This mechanism for preferential and controlled antigen uptake allows Peyer's patches to play a pivotal role in the induction and regulation of the secretory immune response. The major antibody-producing cells (B cells) of Peyer's patches are committed to secretion of IgA. The thymus-derived lymphocytes (T cells) present in Peyer's patches represent a smaller population which includes both the T cell inducer/helper and the T cell suppressor/cytotoxic subsets which are characterized in part by specific monoclonal antibodies (Lyscom and

0300-5089/83/1202-415 $05.00©1983 W. B. Saunders Company Ltd

Brueton, 1982). Antigen-specific suppressor cells have been found in rat Peyer's patches following oral administration of sheep erythyrocytes (Mattingly and Waksman, 1978). Subsets of suppressor cells specific for IgE and IgG have been described in mouse Peyer's patches (Ngan and Kind, 1978) but Peyer's patches apparently lack natural killer (NK) cells as well as the precursors which could be induced to differentiate into NK cells by immune interferon (IFN-β) (Tagliabue et al, 1981).

Lymphocytes, including NK cells (Tagliabue et al, 1981), are also present in substantial numbers in the gut epithelium, but plasma cells are conspicuously lacking. The intraepithelial lymphocyte population includes T cells, B cells and lymphocytes which do not express either T or B cell markers, the so-called null cells (Bartnik et al, 1980). In human intestinal epithelium, 70 per cent of the T cells react with a monoclonal antibody, designated OKT8, indicating that they are part of the suppressor/cytotoxic subset of lymphocytes involved in dampening the immune response or in acting as cytotoxic effector cells (Selby et al, 1981). Small numbers of eosinophils, mast cells, neutrophils and macrophages (Bartnik et al, 1980; Bienenstock and Befus, 1980) are also found in the epithelial monolayer of the intestine. The epithelial cells of human small intestine display HLA-DR-like antigens which may be involved in antigen processing (Scott et al, 1980), and could potentially act in a manner analogous to the M cells of Peyer's patches. HLA-DR-like antigens are absent from normal colon epithelium, but are expressed in 50 per cent of cancerous colon mucosa (Daar et al, 1982).

A striking feature of lamina propria cells is the predominance of cells containing IgA (Crabbé and Heremans, 1966). These cells greatly outnumber IgM- and IgG-producing cells, and the sparsely represented IgE and IgD cells. The dense population of lymphocytes and plasma cells appears to result from exposure of the neonatal intestine to microorganisms. In animals raised under germ-free conditions, the lamina propria is practically devoid of antibody-containing cells. Following exposure to a normal environment, however, the numbers of mucosal lymphocytes and plasma cells increase within three to four weeks to levels similar to those found in conventional animals (Crabbé et al, 1970). Like the epithelial layer, the lamina propria contains small numbers of eosinophils, mast cells, neutrophils and macrophages, and mast cells have been successfully isolated from rat mucosa (Befus et al, 1982). T cells are also present in the lamina propria where the majority belong to the inducer/helper subset which is detected by the monoclonal antibody designated OKT4, while only 39 per cent express the OKT8[+] phenotype, i.e., belong to the suppressor/cytotoxic subset (Selby et al, 1981). Some T cells in the rabbit lamina propria bind immuno-globulins via Fc receptors for IgA and IgG (ReMine et al, 1981; Stafford, Knight and Fanger, 1982).

Lamina propria lymphocytes are also involved in mitogen-induced cellular cytotoxicity (MICC), spontaneous cell-mediated cytotoxicity (SCMC), and antibody-dependent cellular cytotoxicity (ADCC) (Arnaud-Battandier et al, 1978; Chiba et al, 1981; Falchuk, Barnhard and Machado, 1982). SCMC and ADCC may be important effector mechanisms in elimination of malignant cells. Antibody-dependent (K cell) and NK activity were absent in the lymphocyte population harvested from colon cancers and from adjacent unaffected mucosa. By contrast, MICC was present. The responsiveness of tumour-invasive lymphocytes and lamina propria lymphocytes to mitogens was similar to that found in the peripheral blood of colon cancer patients, although the proportions of T cells differed in the populations tested from these different sites (Bland et al, 1981).

INTESTINAL FLUID IMMUNOGLOBULINS

The relative concentrations of the major immunoglobulin classes — IgA, IgM and IgG — in intestinal juice are in substantial agreement with the distribution of these different classes in the antibody-containing cells of the intestinal mucosa, IgA being the predominant immunoglobulin class (Tomasi, 1970). A specific form of IgA, known as secretory IgA, is characteristic of the IgA found in external secretions (Tomasi and Zigelbaum, 1962). Unlike serum IgA, which is predominantly a 7S monomer (comprising the paired light and heavy chains common to all immunoglobulin structural units), secretory IgA is an 11S dimer (MW 390 000) consisting of two monomers of 7S IgA (Tomasi, 1970) joined by a covalently linked peptide named 'J' for joining (Halpern and Koshland, 1970). The assembly of secretory IgA is completed by the addition of a glycopeptide component called secretory piece which appears to protect IgA from digestion by the proteolytic enzymes bathing the mucosal surface. In addition, secretory piece is involved in the transport of IgA from the lamina propria across the epithelium (Brown, 1978). Both sub-classes of IgA, IgA_1 and IgA_2, are represented in the lamina propria, but a higher proportion of IgA_2 is present in the intestine and in other secretory sites than is found in bone marrow (Andre, Andre and Fargier, 1978). Amongst the other immunoglobulin classes only IgM binds secretory piece and is transported across the epithelium as a secretory immunoglobulin (Brandtzaeg, 1973).

Secretory pathway of intestinal immunoglobulins

The vast majority of the immunoglobulin present in intestinal secretions is synthesized locally by plasma cells in the intestinal mucosa. In addition, J chain is synthesized by IgA- and IgM-producing plasma cells where it joins up the dimer of IgA or the pentamer of IgM (Koshland and Wilde, 1974). Secretory piece, however, is synthesized independently of IgA in the epithelial cells and is displayed on the external surfaces of the lateral and basal membranes of the epithelial cells, particularly the crypt epithelial cells. IgA and IgM bind to secretory piece on the lateral and basal membranes of human intestinal epithelial cells. Pinocytotic vesicles containing IgA or IgM with secretory piece have been observed within the cytoplasm of the epithelial cell and as invaginations of its laterobasal membrane (Brown, 1978). These findings, together with the identical distribution of secretory piece, IgA and IgM, suggest that the secretory pathway for IgA and IgM involves binding to secretory piece on the external surface of the laterobasal membrane of the crypt epithelial cell, uptake by invagination of the plasma membrane to form a pinocytotic vesicle, and then transport of the secretory immunoglobulin to the apical membrane of the epithelial cell where secretion of IgA or IgM into the lumen occurs by reverse pinocytosis.

ANTIGEN HANDLING AND INDUCTION OF MUCOSAL IMMUNITY

The privileged environment of the lamina propria is protected from antigenic challenge by both non-immune and immune mechanisms which may operate within the lumen, at the mucosal surface, or in some cases within the intestinal mucosa. Amongst the non-immune mechanisms which contribute to protection of the mucosa from antigenic assault are gastric acidity, luminal proteases, peristalsis, the commensal microflora and the mucus coat or glycocalyx of the epithelial surface.

Immune responses are generally initiated by antigen-presenting cells which characteristically express membrane structures called Ia (mouse) or HLA-DR (human). These molecules are essential to the presentation of most antigens and to the subsequent induction of an immune response. Macrophages isolated from Peyer's patches present antigen under experimental conditions (Richman, Graeff and Strober, 1981) and macrophages from animals fed antigen will stimulate peripheral lymph node T cells in an antigen-specific manner. Macrophages are also found in the epithelium, the lamina propria of the human intestine (Golder and Doe, 1983), and in the lumen of the rabbit intestine, where they adhere in large numbers near the Peyer's patches and the appendix (Heatley and Bienenstock, 1982). Ia-like (mouse) or HLA-DR-like (human) antigens are also found on epithelial cells of the human small intestinal villi, where they are expressed in a patchy distribution involving the apices of columnar epithelial cells, and in the upper part of the crypt epithelium (Scott et al, 1980). The role, if any, of HLA-DR-positive epithelial cells in antigen presentation at mucosal surfaces is unknown, but it is of interest that the epithelial cells of the small intestine, the M cells of Peyer's patches and the macrophages found in Peyer's patches, intestinal epithelium and lamina propria represent the cells which are the first to encounter the heavy antigen load that bathes the surface of the small intestine.

Recent insights into the role of Peyer's patches in the local intestinal immune response have shed considerable light on the pathways by which orally given antigen results in the local production of specific secretory IgA antibody in the intestinal mucosa and in the predominance of IgA-containing cells in the lamina propria of the gut. Studies using two Thiry-Vella loops in a rabbit — one loop containing Peyer's patches and the other not — showed that only when the Peyer's patch-containing loop was exposed to topical antigen did a specific secretory antibody response occur when it was found in both loops. By contrast if only the intestinal loop free of Peyer's patches was exposed to antigen, little secretory antibody activity was detectable in either loop (Cebra et al, 1977). Thus Peyer's patches appear to be central to the induction of a secretory antibody response to luminal antigens and the mechanisms whereby these events occur are now clearer. Peyer's patches contain the precursors of IgA plasma cells which appear to seed the small intestine. Following injection into recipients, Peyer's patch B cells migrate to the mesenteric nodes which represent the preferential intermediate site for the proliferation and differentiation of Peyer's patch IgA precursor cells into IgA-secreting cells (Roux et al, 1981). These lymphoblasts, which are committed to IgA production, migrate via the lymphatic system into the peripheral blood from which they enter the intestinal mucosa and other exocrine sites to become mature plasma cells (Figure 1). This traffic pattern suggests that the precursors of IgA plasma cells recognize some feature common to that of high endothelial venules in mesenteric nodes, Peyer's patches and the intestinal mucosa. The preferential homing of the large granular T lymphocyte cells found in the epithelium, and the dividing cells from the lamina propria and mesenteric nodes (McDermott, O'Neill and Bienenstock, 1980) may involve a similar homing mechanism. Selective migration of IgA-containing cells appears to result from both antigen-independent and antigen-dependent systems. Homing of gut-derived lymphoblasts occurs in isografts of fetal small

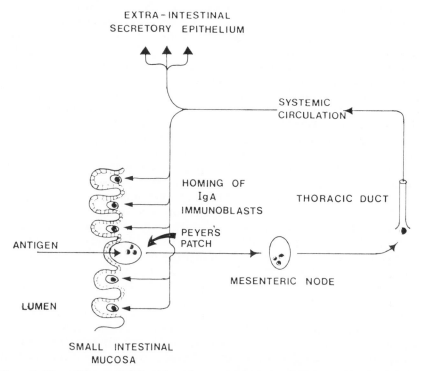

Figure 1. The traffic pattern following antigen exposure for lymphoblasts destined to become lamina propria plasma cells secreting specific IgA antibody. From Doe (1979), with kind permission of the author and the editor of *American Journal of Medicine*.

intestine transplanted under the kidney capsule (Parrott and Ferguson, 1974). Increased localization of IgA-secreting cells occurs at the site of antigen exposure but only after a period of recirculation, suggesting that lymphocyte trapping by specific antigen and subsequent lymphocyte proliferation is superimposed upon a defined traffic pattern which is organ-specific but antigen-independent (Husband and Gowans, 1978).

A novel aspect of mucosal immune responses is the concurrent suppression of systemic immunity to the same antigen. This phenomenon was first observed by Wells in 1911 when guinea pigs, previously fed with ovalbumin, lost the ability to develop an anaphylactic reaction following peripheral inoculation of the antigen. The induction of a systemic state of unresponsiveness to a specific antigen by oral presentation of the antigen was further studied by Chase (1946) who observed antigen-specific suppression of contact sensitization after feeding the allergen.

The mechanism by which such a state of specific immunological unresponsiveness occurs, however, is not fully understood. It is now known that Peyer's patches, mesenteric lymph nodes and spleen contain suppressor cells which block IgM, IgG and IgE responses (Ngan and Kind, 1978; Mattingly and Waksman, 1978; Challacombe and Tomasi, 1980) and depress delayed-type hypersensitivity (DTH) reactions. Tolerance due to oral administration of antigen in rats is similar to classical 'low zone' tolerance in that it is abrogated when normal syngeneic cells are injected into the 'tolerized' animal (Thomas and Parrott, 1974). In immune animals it is clear that the ability to induce tolerance by feeding is under complex genetic control because in LPS-non-responsive C3H/HeJ mice, systemic tolerance does not occur after antigen-feeding and recirculating suppressor cells are not generated in Peyer's patches. These mice instead generate unusually high levels of IgA and have an amplified helper T cell population (Kiyono et al, 1980). Serum antibody can also prevent the intestinal response to cholera toxin (Pierce, 1980). Although much remains to be clarified regarding the interaction of systemic and mucosa-associated lymphoid tissue, elucidation of the regulatory mechanisms that determine immune responses, and their suppression after intestinal exposure to antigen, offer the prospect of understanding mucosal hypersensitivity reactions and their contribution to malabsorption states.

The complex mixture of lymphoid cells found in GALT is probably modulated locally by mediator released from cells present in the gut epithelium and lamina propria. Histamine modulates cell cycle changes in bone marrow-derived stem cells (Byron, 1977) and in regulated T cell responses (Roszkowski, Plant and Lichtenstein, 1977) and is present in GALT as a product of the mucosal mast cells. Histamine may therefore modulate differentiation or maturation of leucocytes in the GALT. Similarly, prostaglandins, released by various cells of the immune system, inhibit development of humoral responses and the proliferative response to mitogens (Leung and Mihich, 1980), and may also be involved in regulation of lymphocyte functions in GALT.

Recent work has defined a group of molecules, collectively termed lymphokines, which are polypeptides that are capable of delivering differentiation and growth signals to lymphocytes and macrophages. Immune interferon (IFN-β), which is released following antigen recognition by T cells, enhances cytotoxic activity of NK and cytotoxic T cells, induces plasminogen activator in human macrophages (Hovi, Saksela and Vaher, 1981), and can suppress antigen-dependent leucocyte migration inhibition (Szigetti et al, 1980). Another lymphokine, interleukin 3 (Ihle et al, 1982), modulates expression of steroid resistance in a variety of leucocyte subsets in the mouse, possibly including NK cells (Djeu et al, 1982), T cells and mast cells. During their development, murine T cells are also variably susceptible to β-adrenergic effects (Singh et al, 1979). Each of these soluble mediators may play a role in differentiation, homing, and in the in vitro effector activity of the GALT.

The function of secretory antibody

Perhaps the most important aspect of immunity of mucosal surfaces is the production and secretion of IgA. Uniquely, secretory IgA activity appears to be largely confined to binding to antigens and does not initiate local hypersensitivity reactions. Among its range of antibody activities against viruses, bacteria, toxins and food antigens, secretory IgA is an effective neutralizing antibody against viruses, as shown by the Sabin oral, live poliovirus vaccine where protection correlates with levels of secretory IgA antibody (Ogra and Karzon, 1969). The dimeric structure of secretory IgA comprises four antigen-combining sites which allow this antibody molecule to function efficiently as an agglutinin. Further antibacterial protection is provided by the capacity of secretory IgA to prevent bacteria from binding to surface epithelial cells, as seen for secretory IgA antibodies to *Vibrio cholerae* (Freter, 1972). Moreover, there is evidence that secretory IgA has bacteriocidal potential in cooperation with lysozyme and complement (Adinolfi et al, 1966).

Compared to IgM or IgG, however, secretory IgA appears unable to recruit the powerful effector systems that are activated in systemic immune responses. The classical complement pathway is resistant to activation by secretory IgA, while alternative pathway complement activation is initiated by chemically aggregated IgA but not by the more physiological secretory IgA-antigen complexes (Colten and Bienenstock, 1974). Moreover, secretory IgA appears unable to opsonize bacteria for phagocytosis by monocytes, neutrophils or alveolar macrophages (Reynolds and Thompson, 1974).

Blocking access for food antigens appears to be a further important role for secretory IgA. Patients suffering from selective IgA deficiency have very high titres of circulating antibody to food antigens (Buckley and Dees, 1969), and antigen absorption across the gut mucosa is reduced by the presence of IgA class antibodies (Walker and Isselbacher, 1977). Secretory IgA may also block reaginic hypersensitivity reactions at the surface of the intestinal epithelium, as reported for nasal epithelium (Turk, Lichtenstein and Norman, 1970). Small amounts of dietary antigen, however, are absorbed in normal subjects and many penetrate systemically to give rise to low zone tolerance (Thomas and Parrott, 1974). The importance of 'blocking' antibodies may therefore lie in preventing immunogenic amounts of antigen gaining access to the lamina propria.

THE IMMUNE SYSTEM AND MALABSORPTION

Malabsorption may result from a number of disturbances of the mucosal immune system; immunodeficiency states, proliferation or malignant expansion of immune-related cells, and hypersensitivity reactions can interfere with the absorptive process.

Immunodeficiency States

Primary immunodeficiency states represent natural experiments which have helped elucidate the role of mucosal immunity in the intestine. Of the many defects classified by the WHO Committee (Fundenberg et al, 1971), selective IgA deficiency, adult onset common variable hypogammaglobu-linaemia, and severe combined immunodeficiency are those principally associated with malabsorption states. Immunodeficiency secondary to other diseases less commonly results in gastrointestinal symptoms.

Selective IgA deficiency

Selective IgA deficiency is the commonest of the primary immunodeficiency states and affects about one in 700 of the population. Relatively few such patients, however, have significant gastrointestinal symptoms. In a large survey, Koistinen reported that 13 per cent of deficient subjects suffered from recurrent or chronic diarrhoea (Koistinen, 1975). Part of the explanation for this finding appears to lie in the fact that IgA deficiency is not a global immunological defect. IgM-producing cells, which are found in greatly increased numbers in the intestinal mucosa and provide high concentrations of secretory IgM at the mucosal surfaces (Savilahti, 1973), appear to compensate for the deficiency of secretory IgA.

Since IgA is the first line of defence in the secretory immune system which protects mucosal surfaces, it is not surprising that the intestinal manifestations of IgA deficiency are mainly those of chronic diarrhoea, steatorrhoea, milk intolerance and possibly infestation by *Gardia lamblia*. The patchy reversible histological abnormality associated with giardiasis varies from superficial epithelial injury to complete destruction of villus architecture. The intestinal conditions that have been associated with IgA deficiency include coeliac disease, nodular lymphoid hyperplasia (NLH), ulcerative colitis, Crohn's disease, and the disaccharidase deficiencies (Horowitz and Hong, 1977). The frequency of IgA deficiency in coeliac disease is about ten times that found in the general population (Asquith, Thompson and Cooke, 1969), and this association has provoked the hypothesis that a relative, or qualitative, lack of IgA in the mucosa contributes to the pathogenesis of the mucosal lesion in coeliac disease (Beale et al, 1971).

Little attention has been given to the dissociation which can occur between the serum and secretory levels of IgA. Patients whose serum IgA levels are normal may be completely deficient in secretory IgA and, conversely, reduced serum levels of IgA may occur in patients whose secretory IgA levels are normal (Horowitz and Hong, 1977). This kind of dissociation emphasizes the importance of correlating secretory IgA production in the intestine with intestinal disease state. Indeed, isolated deficiency of secretory piece has recently been described in a patient suffering from intestinal candidiasis and diarrhoea. No evidence of malabsorption was found, however, and the morphological appearances of the jejunal mucosa were normal. Secretory piece was undetectable in the epithelial cells, and, although serum IgA levels were within normal limits, the secretions were completely deficient in IgA (Strober et al, 1976).

Panhypogammaglobulinaemia

Intestinal symptoms, particularly those related to malabsorption, commonly occur in adults who are hypogammaglobulinaemic. In a review of 50 patients with common variable immunoglobulin deficiency, 60 per cent were found to have chronic or recurrent diarrhoea, of whom two-thirds had malabsorption (Hermans, Diaz-Buxo and Stobo, 1976). Infestation by *Giardia lamblia* is common, and secondary disaccharidase deficiencies may result which are usually reflected clinically in lactose intolerance but maltase and sucrase deficiencies may also occur (Dubois et al, 1970). Profound malabsorption, however, also occurs in hypogammaglobulinaemic patients without giardiasis. The intestinal mucosa may show obliteration of villus architecture, but in some instances steatorrhoea occurs even though the villus structure appears normal. In the latter cases the pathogenesis of the malabsorption state is obscure. In rare instances when the intestinal mucosa is flat, patients respond to a gluten-free diet (Webster, 1976), but in most instances the mucosal lesion is not responsive to withdrawal of gluten from the diet. No firm conclusion about the role of antibody in coeliac disease can be drawn from this observation, however, because many patients suffering from serum hypogammaglobulinaemia nevertheless secrete significant amounts of IgM into the jejunal fluid (Webster et al, 1977). Although overgrowth of bacteria is a common finding in the small intestine, there is no correlation between this finding and the patients' symptoms. The rare condition of ulcerative jejunoileitis may also complicate common variable hypogammaglobulinaemia and be associated with severe malabsorption. Although its pathogenesis is not understood, clinical remissions have been reported following steroid and broad spectrum antibiotic therapy. Malabsorption also occurs due to the development of gastric achlorhydria and intrinsic factor deficiency leading to pernicious anaemia or to the more rare syndrome involving neutropenia and pancreatic exocrine deficiency (Doe and Booth, 1973). In contrast to the frequency of intestinal syptoms in common variable hypogammaglobulinaemia, diarrhoea and steatorrhoea are much less common in patients suffering from X-linked agammaglobulinaemia (Rosen and Janeway, 1966).

Nodular lymphoid hyperplasia (NLH) describes the presence of lymphoid nodules in the lamina propria of the small intestine and is usually found in patients suffering from hypogammaglobulinaemia, although it has been described in patients with normal serum immunoglobulin levels (Kahn and Novis, 1974; Matuchansky et al, 1980) and in association with selective IgA deficiency. NLH does not appear to be a distinct clinical entity but rather represents a variation in the morphological expression of humoral immune deficiency. The nodules probably represent proliferating T and B cells akin to the population found in germinal follicles. In common with other variants of antibody secretion defects, the ability to secrete IgM into the gut is often retained (Webster et al, 1977).

Evidence from large series of patients suffering from congenital (Spector, Perry and Kersey, 1978) and common variable immunoglobulin deficiency (Hermans, Diaz-Buxo and Stobo, 1976) suggests that the incidence of generalized lymphomas is significantly higher than that found in the general population. Whether the incidence of intestinal lymphomas is increased in immunodeficient patients, however, is less certain. Jejunal lymphoma complicating late-onset hypogammaglobulinaemia and nodular lymphoid hyperplasia has been reported (Lamers et al, 1980). In a review of 50 cases of common variable hypogammaglobulinaemia, lymphoma developed in two patients, and in one of these there was a primary lymphoma affecting the rectum and sigmoid in association with nodular lymphoid hyperplasia of the small intestine (Hermans, Diaz-Buxo and Stobo, 1976). Small intestinal lymphoma has also been reported in patients shown to have nodular lymphoid hyperplasia of the small intestine but whose serum immunoglobulin levels were normal (Kahn and Novis, 1974; Matuchansky et al, 1980), raising the question as to whether nodular lymphoid hyper-plasia itself predisposes to malignancy. In one of these cases, both the lymphomatous cells in the jejunum and the lymphocyes present in nearby lymphoid hyperplastic nodules were part of a monoclonal expansion of B lymphocytes of IgM-K type, whereas staining of the lymphoid hyperplastic nodules in the intestinal tissue, far distant from the lymphomatous involve-ment, showed polyclonal B lymphocytes in the germinal centres. This finding suggests that the jejunal lymphoma had arisen as a malignant transformation of the nodular lymphoid hyperplasia (Matuchansky et al, 1980).

In infants suffering from severe combined immunodeficiency, in whom both humoral and cellular immune mechanisms are deficient, diarrhoea and malabsorption are common, but few detailed investigations of the patho-genesis of the malabsorption state have been possible because the outcome is usually fatal unless a successful bone marrow graft is established. Studies of the jejunal mucosa reveal stunting of the villi and marked mucosal oedema together with large numbers of vacuolated macrophages. Treat-ment by bone marrow grafting may cause a graft-versus-host reaction resulting in marked villus shortening and consequent malabsorption. In primary cell-mediated immunodeficiency, intestinal disease is uncommon, but again foamy macrophages are seen in the intestinal mucosa (Horowitz and Hong, 1977).

Although not strictly an immunodeficient state, chronic granulomatous disease, a sex-linked deficiency of bacteriocidal function in phagocytic cells, is also associated with malabsorption. Jejunal biopsies reveal villus stunting and the presence of foamy vacuolated macrophages in the lamina propria (Ament and Ochs, 1973).

Hypersensitivity Reactions and Malabsorption

Hypersensitivity is an abnormally heightened state of reactivity to antigen which, far from being protective, frequently results in tissue injury. A number of hypersensitivity states have been characterized which may damage the intestinal mucosa to cause a malabsorption syndrome.

Immediate-type hypersensitivity reactions involve cross-linking by antigen of specific IgE antibody on the surface of mast cells or basophils, causing release of vasoactive amines and consequent oedema and hyperaemia. In atopic subjects who are predisposed to make excessive IgE responses to particular antigens, immediate hypersensitivity may occur to dietary antigens, resulting in an inflammatory reaction in the intestinal mucosa characterized by oedema, eosinophilia, lymphocyte infiltration and increased intestinal motility (Gray, Harten and Walzer, 1940). The reaction is shortlived, however, and this form of hypersensitivity is unlikely to cause malabsorption unless combined with other tissue injury mechanisms. In milk allergy, for example, both immediate- and immune complex- (Arthus-) type hypersensitivities may be present, but it is the latter reaction which is implicated in the villus shortening and malabsorption seen in some infants suffering from an allergy to cow's milk (Kuitunen et al, 1973).

The Arthus-type of immediate hypersensitivity reaction results from the precipitation of complement-fixing antigen-antibody complexes in tissue following the interaction of diffusing antigen with circulating antibody. Activation of complement by immune complex deposits in vessel walls results in the recruitment of neutrophils, platelet aggregation, fibrin deposition and tissue injury. This reaction appears to be an attractive model for the pathogenesis of intestinal mucosal injury in cow's milk allergy (Mathews and Soothill, 1970), gluten-sensitive enteropathy (Doe, Henry and Booth, 1974), and, possibly, in some cases of selective IgA deficiency. In these disorders the presence of precipitating complement-fixing antibody and evidence for polymorphonuclear accumulation and deposition of IgM and complement four to six hours after antigen challenge suggest that this reaction contributes to the injury mechanism of these malabsorption states (Doe, Henry and Booth, 1974).

The delayed hypersensitivity reaction which is due to interaction between antigen and T lymphocytes results from release of lymphokines from activated lymphocytes causing a local inflammation and recruitment of macrophages over 24 to 48 hours. In the intestine, delayed-type hypersensitivity reactions occur following bone marrow transplant when a graft-versus-host reaction may cause intestinal damage and malabsorption (Meunissen et al, 1971).

Malabsorption States Causing Secondary Immune Deficiency

Lesions of the intestinal mucosa characterized by malabsorption and protein-losing enteropathy, such as coeliac disease, cause increased catabolism of immunoglobulins as part of the non-selective protein loss from the intestinal mucosa. IgG levels are usually depressed, whereas IgA and IgM levels often remain within normal limits, reflecting the much slower synthetic rate of IgG (Waldmann and Strober, 1969). In addition to losing immunoglobulins, profound depletion of lymphocytes may occur in some malabsorption states, particularly intestinal lymphangiectasia, Crohn's disease and Whipple's disease. These secondary immunodeficiencies result in an increased susceptibility to infections and may interfere with cell-mediated immune responses.

Immunoproliferative Small Intestinal Disease

Diffuse intestinal lymphomas are prevalent in developing countries, particularly the Middle East and the Mediterranean basin, and comprise the commonest cause of malabsorption in these regions (Eidelman, Parkins and Rubin, 1966). Clinical studies suggest evolution from a diffuse, premalignant plasmacytoid infiltrate of the small intestine to frank lymphoma involving more primitive immunoblasts. Immunoglobulin fragments comprising incomplete heavy chains of IgA are found in the sera and secretion of the majority of patients. Most, if not all, so-called 'Mediterranean lymphomas' represent the malignant phase of a remarkable disorder of the secretory IgA system called alpha-chain disease (αCD) (Rambaud et al, 1968; Seligmann et al, 1968). αCD results from monoclonal expansion of IgA-containing B lymphoid cells which proliferate in the intestinal mucosa and secrete abnormal IgA fragments similar to the Fc piece and free of light chains. The finding of respiratory variants of αCD (Stoop et al, 1971) and the geographical diversity of the disorder have led to the intestinal condition being re-named immunoproliferative small intestinal disease (IPSID) (WHO Bulletin, 1976).

Young adults who come from underprivileged backgrounds and are in the second and third decades of life develop a progressive malabsorption syndrome over several years. The major symptoms are diarrhoea, with the features of steatorrhoea, generalized colicky abdominal pains and weight loss (Doe et al, 1972; Salem et al, 1977). Ankle swelling and ascites may develop from protein-losing enteropathy. At an advanced stage of the disease when frank lymphoma supervenes, bleeding, intestinal obstruction, perforation or intussusception may be presenting features (Doe, 1975; Lewin, Kahn and Novis, 1976). Wasting, marked finger clubbing and oedema are the predominant physical signs, although in advanced cases abdominal lymphoid masses may be palpable. Tests of intestinal function reveal malabsorption in both jejunum and ileum, together with steatorrhoea, suggesting diffuse involvement of the whole length of the small intestine. A stagnant loop syndrome may contribute to the malabsorption of some IPSID patients. One striking biochemical finding is the marked increase in the alkaline phosphatase level in plasma due to the intestinal isoenzyme of alkaline phosphatase (Ramot and Streifler, 1966).

Histopathology

The small intestinal mucosa presents a characteristic appearance. Villi are shortened and broadened, giving the appearance of total or partial obliteration of villus architecture. The basic abnormality is a diffuse, dense, mononuclear infiltrate of the lamina propria causing wide separation of the crypts of Lieberkuhn and effacement of villus structure without significant impairment of the integrity of the surface epithelium. The cellular infiltrate is predominantly plasma cell in type, but the stage of maturation of plasma cells varies in the biopsies of different patients. Topographically, the infiltrate usually begins in the upper small intestine and is diffuse and extensive, often involving the entire length of the small intestine; the distribution therefore contrasts with the western type intestinal lymphomas which, with the exception of malignant histiocytosis, are typically solitary and show a predilection for the ileum. In early cases of IPSID, the cellular infiltrate is confined to the lamina propria and bears none of the histological stigmata of malignancy — a finding consistent with the view that there is a premalignant stage of the disease. When infiltration beyond the muscularis mucosa occurs, invasion of the sub-mucosa, destruction of mesenteric lymph node architecture and apparent spread to rectum, postnasal space, blood and bone marrow may occur (Bognel et al, 1972; Doe et al, 1972). These findings, together with the abnormal appearances of the invading cells, clearly establish the malignant potential of IPSID.

The relationship between the apparently benign plasma cell infiltrate which characterizes the premalignant phase of IPSID, the secretion of αCD polypeptides by these cells, and the development of frank lymphoma affecting the intestine and mesenteric nodes, is becoming clearer. There is strong evidence that the lymphoma that supervenes in IPSID results from malignant transformation of the same clone of proliferating plasma cells which constituted the premalignant phase. Biosynthetic studies of cells from a lymphoma which developed in the intestine of a patient suffering from IPSID showed that both the benign-appearing plasma cell infiltrate and the lymphoma cells synthesized αCD polypeptide, strongly indicating that the immunoblastic tumour cells arose by dedifferentiation from the same defective clone and not from a separate clone of pathological cells (Ramot et al, 1977; Preud'homme, Brouet and Seligmann, 1979). These findings are supported by immunoelectronmicroscopic studies of lymphoma tissue from IPSID patients which show evidence for the presence of αCD polypeptide in the cytoplasm and on the membranes of the large immunoblasts which constitute the lymphoma (Brouet et al, 1977).

Clinical variants

Two patients presenting with the typical clinicopathological features of IPSID were shown to have complete monoclonal IgA gammopathy (Chantar, Escartin and Plaza, 1974; Tangun et al, 1975) and in a third patient, γ heavy chain protein was demonstrated in serum and in the plasma cells of the intestinal infiltrate (Seligmann, 1975). A non-secretory variant of IPSID has also been discussed. In this case the small intestine was diffusely infiltrated by plasma cells but no αCD polypeptide was detectable in serum, urine or concentrated jejunal fluid. The presence of αCD polypeptide in the cytoplasm of the infiltrating plasma cells was suggested by positive immunofluorescence for α-chains in the absence of staining for light chains (Rambaud, Modigliani and Nguyen Phuoc, 1980).

Protein studies

The aberrant protein, which comprises incomplete α heavy chains of IgA related to the Fc piece and devoid of light chains, is found in the serum, jejunal fluid and urine of the majority of IPSID patients (Figure 2). The molecular weight of the monomeric polypeptide varies between 29 000 and 34 000 daltons (Dorrington, Mihaesco and Seligmann, 1970). The missing portion of the α heavy chain lies in the Fd segment. While the C-terminal sequence is identical to that of normal subclass 1 α heavy chains, N-terminal sequences show marked heterogeneity.

The detection of the diagnostic polypeptide in biological fluids depends upon immunochemical analysis. Serum protein electrophoresis is abnormal in only 50 per cent of cases when it shows an abnormally broad band in the α_2 or β region. The characteristic narrow band of a monoclonal immunoglobulin abnormality is not seen. Where no abnormal electrophoretic band is seen, the only changes present are those of a reduced serum albumin and hypogammaglobulinaemia.

Testing by immunoelectrophoresis using antisera monospecific for IgA usually reveals an abnormal precipitin arc extending from the α_1 to the β_2 region which often has a faster electrophoretic mobility than normal IgA. The inability of αCD polypeptide to precipitate with antisera and light chains can also be used as the basis for a diagnostic test, but the failure of some IgA myeloma proteins to precipitate with anti-light chain antisera may produce false positive results. The most sensitive technique for the detection of αCD polypeptide involves the use of an immunoselection technique in which the test serum is electrophoresed into agarose containing an antiserum which recognizes the conformational specificities of the Fab fragment of IgA (Doe and Spiegelberg, 1979). This step results in the precipitation of normal IgA present in the serum close to the origin. The αCD polypeptide, which lacks Fab α determinants and is therefore unaffected by the presence of anti-Fab antibody in the agarose, migrates unimpeded. The αCD polypeptide can then be detected by an antiserum which is monospecific for IgA (Figure 2) (Doe, Danon and Seligmann, 1979). In most IPSID patients, αCD polypeptide can also be detected at low levels in concentrated urine and jejunal fluid (Seligmann et al, 1968).

Prognosis and therapy

The prognosis of IPSID depends upon the stage of progression of the disease at the diagnosis. Very few staging laparotomies have been performed, however, and the sparse data available are derived from attempts

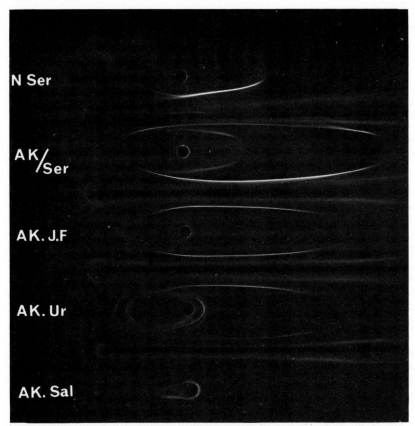

Figure 2. Immunoselection plates identifying free alpha-chain (αCD) polypeptide as a long precipitin arc in serum (Ser), concentrated jejunal fluid (J.F) and concentrated urine (Ur) from a patient (AK) suffering from immunoproliferative small intestinal disease. No αCD polypeptide was detected in the patient's saliva (Sal). The appearances of control normal serum (N Ser) are seen in the upper well which identifies the precipitin arc for normal IgA.

at clinical staging. In the initial 'premalignant' stage, where the plasma cell infiltrate is confined to the lamina propria of the small intestine, remission of the clinical, histological and immunological features has been reported in seven of 17 patients. The remissions, which followed therapy using broad spectrum antibiotics and/or a chemotherapy regime as used for multiple myeloma, comprising prednisone and melphalan or cyclophosphamide, were often sustained for more than five years (reviewed by Galian et al, 1977). In one instance an apparently complete remission in a patient diagnosed in 1971 (Doe et al, 1972) and sustained for two years after cessation of therapy (Manousos et al, 1974), ultimately developed a plasma-cytoma confined to the ileum (Skinner et al, 1976).

In IPSID patients suffering from more advanced disease, no clear therapeutic guidelines are available. When the cellular infiltrate is clearly invading the submucosa but there is no clinical evidence of overt lymphoma, chemotherapy with broad spectrum antibiotics have occasionally induced remission. When the immunoblastoma is clinically evident and confined to the abdomen, radiotherapy has produced prolonged remission in three cases (reviewed by Galian et al, 1977). The use of staging lapotomy as part of the clinical assessment is important to the development of more accurate staging and to reliable assessment of the efficacy of treatment (WHO Bulletin, 1976).

Predisposing factors

The clear predilection of IPSID for underprivileged populations of low socioeconomic status suggests that environmental factors may be implicated in its pathogenesis. Since ingested microorganisms are a powerful proliferative stimulus to the secretory IgA system (Crabbé et al, 1970), the early stage of IPSID could represent an aberrant immune response following sustained antigenic stimulation of the mucosa in populations exposed to an environment of poor hygiene (Seligmann, Mihaesco and Frangione, 1971). Limited bacteriological, parasitic and virological studies have not revealed evidence for a specific agent, but the antigenic stimulation may, of course, have occurred many years before IPSID becomes manifest clinically. The absence of the antigen-combining site from the αCD polypeptide precludes its use for recognition of putative antigenic stimuli.

Several other possible pathogenic mechanisms have been suggested. Cells synthesizing the αCD polypeptide may be present in small numbers in normal subjects and be predisposed to proliferation when there is intense, chronic intestinal exposure to microorganisms. The presence of an oncogenic virus which interferes with IgA synthesis has also been suggested (Rambaud and Matuchansky, 1973).

The importance of genetic predisposition is unknown. Although limited family studies have failed to provide evidence for a heritable trait for IPSID (Novis, Bank and Young, 1973), few data are available on genetic markers, including those represented in the major histocompatibility complex. The finding of the intestinal isoenzyme of alkaline phosphatase in the serum of IPSID patients and their relatives (Ramot and Streifler, 1966; Doe et al, 1972) could form the basis for a prospective study of the natural history of IPSID.

REFERENCES

Adinolfi, M., Glynn, A. A., Lindsay, M. & Milne, C. M. (1966) Serological properties of γ A antibodies to *Escherichia coli* present in human colostrum. *Immunology,* **10**, 517.
Ament, M. E. & Ochs, H. D. (1973) Gastrointestinal manifestations of chronic granulomatous disease. *New England Journal of Medicine,* **288**, 382-387.
Andre, C., Andre, F. & Fargier, M. C. (1978) Distribution of IgA$_1$, IgA$_2$ plasma cells in various normal human tissues and in the jejunum of plasma IgA-deficient patients. *Clinical and Experimental Immunology,* **33**, 327.
Arnaud-Battandier, F., Bundy, B. M., O'Neill, M. et al (1978) Cytotoxic activities of gut mucosal lymphoid cells in guinea pigs. *Journal of Immunology,* **121**, 1059.
Asquith, P., Thompson, R. A. & Cooke, W. T. (1969) Serum immunoglobulins in adult coeliac disease. *Lancet,* **i**, 129-131.

Bartnik, W., ReMine, S. G., Chiba, M. et al (1980) Isolation and characterisation of colonic intraepithelial and lamina proprial lymphocytes. *Gastroenterology,* **78,** 976-985.

Beale, A. J., Parish, W. E., Douglas, A. P. & Hobbs, J. R. (1971) Impaired IgA responses in coeliac disease. *Lancet,* **i,** 1198-1200.

Befus, A. D., Pearce, F. L., Gauldie, J. et al (1982) Mucosal mast cells. I. Isolation and functional characterisation of rat intestinal mast cells. *Journal of Immunology,* **128,** 2475-2480.

Besredka, A (1919) De la vaccination contre les états typhoides par le voie buccale. *Annales de l'Institut Pasteur de Lille,* **33,** 882.

Bienenstock, J. & Befus, A. D. (1980) Mucosal immunity. *Immunology,* **41,** 249-260.

Bland, P. W., Britton, D. D., Richens, E. R. & Pledger, J. V. (1981) Peripheral, mucosal and tumor-infiltrating components of cellular immunity in cancer of the large bowel. *Gut,* **22,** 744-751.

Bognel, J. C., Rambaud, J. C., Modigliani, R. et al (1972) Etude clinique, anatomo-pathologique et immunochimique d'un nouveau cas de maladie des chaines alpha suivi pendant cinq ans. *Revue Européene D'Études Cliniques et Biologiques,* **17,** 362-374.

Brandtzaeg, P. (1973) Structure, synthesis and transfer of mucosal immunoglobulins. *Annual Reviews of Immunology,* **417,** 1246.

Brouet, J. C., Mason, D. Y., Danon, F. et al (1977) Alpha-chain disease: evidence for common clonal origin of intestinal immunoblastic lymphoma and plasmacytic proliferation. *Lancet,* **i,** 861.

Brown, W. R. (1978) Relationships between immunoglobulins and the intestinal epithelium. *Gastroenterology,* **75,** 129.

Buckley, R. H. & Dees, S. C. (1969) Correlation of milk precipitins with IgA deficiency. *New England Journal of Medicine,* **281,** 465.

Bulletin of World Health Organisation (1976) Alpha-chain disease and related small-intestinal lymphoma: a memorandum. **54,** 615-624.

Butcher, E. C., Scollay, R. G. & Weissman, I. L. (1981) Organ specificity of lymphocyte migration: mediation by highly selective lymphocyte interaction with organ-specific determinants on high endothelial venules. *European Journal of Immunology,* **10,** 556-561.

Byron, J. W. (1977) Mechanism for histamine H2-receptor induced cell-cycle changes in bone marrow stem cells. *Agents and Actions,* **7,** 209-213.

Cebra, J. J., Gearhart, P. J., Kamat, R. et al (1977) Origin and differentiation of lymphocytes involved in the secretory IgA response. *Cold Harbor Symposium on Quantitative Biology,* **41,** 201.

Challacombe, S. J. & Tomasi, T. B. Jr (1980) Systemic tolerance and secretory immunity after oral immunisation. *Journal of Experimental Medicine,* **152,** 1459-1472.

Chantar, C., Escartin, P. & Plaza, A. G. (1974) Diffuse plasma cell infiltration of the small intestine with malabsorption associated to IgA monoclonal gammopathy. *Cancer,* **34,** 1620-1630.

Chase, M. W. (1946) Inhibition of experimental dry allergy by prior feeding of the sensitizing agent. *Proceedings of the Society for Experimental Biology and Medicine,* **61,** 257.

Chiba, M., Bartnik, W., ReMine, S. G. et al (1981) Human colonic intraepithelial and lamina proprial lymphocytes: cytotoxicity in vitro, and potential effects of the isolation method on their functional properties. *Gut,* **22,** 177-186.

Colten, H. & Bienenstock, T. (1974) Lack of C3 activation through classical or alternate pathways by human secretory IgA anti-blood group A antibody. In *The Immunoglobulin A System* (Ed.) Mestecky, J. & Lawton, A. R. Volume **45,** p. 305. New York: Plenum Publishing.

Crabbé, A. P. & Heremans, J. F. (1966) Étude immunohistochimique des plasmocytes de la muqueuse intestinale humaine normale. *Revue Francaise Études Cliniques et Biologiques,* **11,** 484.

Crabbé, P. A., Nash, D. R., Bazin, H. et al (1970) Immunohistochemical observations on lymphoid tissues from conventional and germ-free mice. *Laboratory Investigation,* **22,** 448-457.

Daar, A. S., Fuggle, S. V., Ting, A. & Fabre, J. W. (1982) Anomalous expression of HLA-DR antigens on human colorectal cancer cells. *Journal of Immunology,* **129,** 447-449.

Djeu, J. Y., Lanza, E., Hapel, A. J. & Ihle, J. N. (1982) Natural cytotoxic activity of mouse spleen cell cultures maintained with Interleukin-3. In *Natural Cell-Mediated Immunity* (Ed.) Herberman, R. Volume **2**. London: Academic Press.

Doe, W. F. (1975) Alpha chain disease: clinicopathological features and relationship to so-called Mediterranean lymphoma. *British Journal of Cancer,* **31** (Supplement II), 350-355.

Doe, W. F. (1979) An overview of intestinal immunity and malabsorption. *American Journal of Medicine,* **67**, 1077-1084.

Doe, W. F. (1982) Immunology of the gut. In *Clinical Aspects of Immunology* (Gell & Coombs) (Ed.) Luchmann, P. & Peters, D. K. Volume **2**, 985-1010.

Doe, W. F. & Booth, C. C. (1973) Two brothers with congenital pancreatic exocrine insufficiency, neutropenia and depgammaglobulinaemia. *Proceedings of the Royal Society of Medicine,* **66**, 1125.

Doe, W. F. & Spiegelberg, H. L. (1979) Characterization of an antiserum specific for the Fabα fragment. Its use for detection of α-heavy chain disease protein by immuno-selection. *Journal of Immunology,* **122**, 19-23.

Doe, W. F., Danon, F. & Seligmann, M. (1979) Immunodiagnosis of alpha chain disease. *Clinical and Experimental Immunology,* **36**, 189-197.

Doe, W. F., Henry, K. & Booth, C. C. (1974) Complement in coeliac disease. In *Coeliac Disease* (Ed.) Hekkens, W. J. M. & Pena, A. S. p. 189. Leiden: Stenfert Kroese.

Doe, W. F., Henry, K., Hobbs, J. R. et al (1972) Five cases of alpha chain disease. *Gut,* **13**, 947.

Dorrington, K. J., Mihaesco, E. & Seligmann, M. (1970) Molecular size of 3 alpha chain disease proteins. *Biochimica et Biophysica Acta,* **221**, 647-649.

Dubois, R. S., Roy, C. C., Fulginiti, V. A. et al (1970) Disaccharidase deficiency in children with immunologic defects. *Journal of Pediatrics,* **76**, 377-385.

Eidelman, S., Parkins, A. & Rubin, C. (1966) Abdominal lymphoma presenting as malabsorption: a clinico-pathologic study of nine cases in Israel and a review of the literature. *Medicine,* **45**, 111.

Falchuk, Z. M., Barnhard, E. & Machado, I. (1982) Human colonic mononuclear cells; studies of cytotoxic function. *Gut,* **22**, 290-294.

Freter, R. (1972) Parameters affecting the association of vibrios with the intestinal surface in experimental cholera. *Infection and Immunity,* **6**, 134.

Fudenberg, H., Good, R. A., Goodman, H. C. et al (1971) Primary immunodeficiencies. Report of a World Health Organization Committee. *Pediatrics,* **47**, 927.

Galian, F., Lecestre, M. J., Scotto, J. et al (1977) Pathological study of alpha chain disease with special emphasis on evolution. *Cancer,* **39**, 2081-2101.

Golder, J. P. and Doe, W. F. (1983) Isolation and preliminary characterisation of human intestinal macrophages. *Gastroenterology.* (In press.)

Gray, I., Harten, M. & Walzer, M. (1940) Studies in mucous membrane hypersensitiveness. II. The allergic reaction in the passively sensitised mucous membranes of the ileum and colon in humans. *Annals of Internal Medicine,* **13**, 2050.

Halpern, M. S. & Koshland, M. E. (1970) Novel subunit in secretory IgA. *Nature,* **228**, 1276.

Heatley, R. V. & Bienenstock, J. (1982) Luminal lymphoid cells in the rabbit intestine. *Gastroenterology,* **82**, 268-275.

Hermans, P. E., Diaz-Buxo, J. A. & Stobo, J. D. (1976) Idiopathic late-onset immunoglobulin deficiency. *American Journal of Medicine,* **61**, 221-237.

Horowitz, S. D. & Hong, R. (1977) The pathogenesis and treatment of immunodeficiency. In *Monographs in Allergy,* **10**, 27.

Hovi, T., Saksela, O. & Vaher, A. (1981) Increased secretion of plasminogen activator by human macrophages after exposure to leucocyte interferon. *FEBS Letters,* **129**, 233-236.

Husband, A. J. & Gowans, J. L. (1978) The origin and antigen-dependent distribution of IgA-containing cells in the intestine. *Journal of Experimental Medicine,* **148**, 1146-1160.

Ihle, J. M., Rebar, L., Keller, J. et al (1982) Interleukin 3: possible roles in the regulation of lymphocyte differentiation and growth. *Immunological Reviews,* **63**, 1-32.

Kahn, L. B. & Novis, B. H. (1974) Nodular lymphoid hyperplasia of the small bowel associated with primary small bowel reticulum cell lymphoma. *Cancer,* **33**, 837-844.

Kiyono, H., Babb, J. L., Michalek, S. M. & McGhee, J. R. (1980) Cellular basis for elevated IgA responses in C3H/HeJ mice. *Journal of Immunology,* **125**, 732-737.

Kiyono, H., McGhee, J. R., Wannemuehler, M. J. & Michalek, S. M. (1982) Lack of oral tolerance in C3H/HeJ mice. *Journal of Experimental Medicine,* 155, 605-610.

Koistinen, J. (1975) Selective IgA deficiency in blood donors. *Vox Sanguinis* (Basel), 29, 192-202.

Koshland, M. E. & Wilde, C. E. (1974) Mechanism of immunoglobulin polymer assembly. In *The Immunoglobulin A System* (Ed.) Mestecky, J. & Lawton, A. R. Volume 45. p. 129. New York: Plenum Publishing.

Kuitunen, P., Rapola, J., Savilahti, E. & Visakorpi, J. K. (1973) Response of the jejunal mucosa to cow's milk in the malabsorption syndrome with cow's milk intolerance. *Acta Paediatrica Scandinavica,* 62, 585.

Lamers, C. B., Wagener, T., Assmann, K. J. & Van Tongeren, J. H. (1980) Jejunal lymphoma in a patient with primary adult-onset hypogammaglobulinemia and nodular lymphoid hyperplasia of the small intestine. *Digestive Diseases and Sciences,* 25, 553-557.

Leung, K. H. & Mihich, E. (1980) Prostaglandin modulation of development of cell-mediated immunity in culture. *Nature,* 288, 597-600.

Lewin, K. J., Kahn, L. B. & Novis, B. H. (1976) Primary intestinal lymphoma of 'Western' and Mediterranean type, alpha chain disease and massive plasma cell infiltration. *Cancer,* 38, 2511-2528.

Lyscom, N. & Brueton, M. J. (1982) Intraepithelial, lamina propria and Peyer's patch lymphocytes of the rat small intestine; isolation and characterisation in terms of immunoglobulin markers and receptors for monoclonal antibodies. *Immunology,* 45, 775-783.

Manousos, O. N., Economidoou, J. C., Georgiadou, D. E. et al (1974) Complete clinical, histological and immunological recovery in a case of alpha chain disease. *British Medical Journal,* 2, 409.

Matthews, T. D. & Soothill, J. F. (1970) Complement activation after milk feeding in children with cow's milk allergy. *Lancet,* ii, 893.

Mattingly, J. A. & Waksman, B. H. (1978) Immunologic suppression after oral administration of antigen. I. Specific suppressor cells formed in rat Peyer's patches after oral administration of sheep erythrocytes and their systemic migration. *Journal of Immunology,* 121, 1878-1883.

Matuchansky, C., Morichau-Beauchant, M., Touchard, G. et al (1980) Nodular lymphoid hyperplasia of the small bowel associated with primary jejunal malignant lymphoma. Evidence favoring a cytogenetic relationship. *Gastroenterology,* 78, 1587-1592.

McDermott, M. R. & Bienenstock, J. (1979) Evidence for a common mucosal immunologic system. I. Migration of B immunoblasts into intestinal respiratory and genital tissues. *Journal of Immunology,* 122, 1892-1897.

McDermott, M. R., O'Neill, M. J. & Bienenstock, J. (1980) Selective localisation of lymphoblasts prepared from guinea pig intestinal lamina propria. *Cellular Immunology,* 51, 345-348.

Meunissen, H. J., Kersey, J., Pabst, H. et al (1971) Graft versus host reactions in bone marrow transplantation. *Transplantation Proceedings,* 3, 414.

Ngan, J. & Kind, L. S. (1978) Suppressor T cells for IgE and IgG in Peyer's patches of mice made tolerant by oral administration of ovalbumin. *Journal of Immunology,* 120, 861-865.

Novis, B. H., Bank, S. & Young, G. (1973) Alpha chain disease. *Lancet,* ii, 498.

Ogra, P. L. & Karzon, D. T. (1969) Poliovirus antibody response in serum and nasal secretions following intranasal inoculation with inactivated poliovaccine. *Journal of Immunology,* 102, 15.

Owen, R. L. & Jones, A. L. (1974) Epithelial cell specialisation within human Peyer's patches: an ultrastructural study of intestinal lymphoid follicles. *Gastroenterology,* 66, 189.

Parrot, D. M. V. & Ferguson, A. (1974) Selective migration of lymphocytes within the mouse small intestine. *Immunology,* 26, 571.

Pierce, N. F. (1980) Suppression of the intestinal immune response to cholera toxin by specific serum antibody. *Infection and Immunity,* 30, 62-68.

Preud'homme, J. L., Brouet, J. C. & Seligmann, M. (1979) Cellular immunoglobulins in human γ- and α-heavy chain diseases. *Clinical and Experimental Immunology,* 37, 283-291.

Rambaud, J. C. & Matuchansky, C. (1973) Alpha chain disease and relation to Mediterranean lymphoma. *Lancet,* i, 1430-1432.

Rambaud, J. C., Modigliani, R. & Nguyen Phuoc, B. K. (1980) Non-secretory alpha-chain disease in intestinal lymphoma. *New England Journal of Medicine,* **393,** 53.

Rambaud, J. C., Bognel, C., Prost, A. et al (1968) Clinico-pathological study of a patient with 'Mediterranean' type of abdominal lymphoma and a new type of IgA abnormality (α chain disease). *Digestion,* **1,** 321-336.

Ramot, B. & Streifler, C. (1966) Raised serum alkaline phosphatase. *Lancet,* **ii,** 587.

Ramot, B., Levanon, M., Hahn, Y. et al (1977) The mutual clonal origin of the lympho-plasmocytic and lymphoma cell in alpha-heavy chain disease. *Clinical and Experimental Immunology,* **27,** 440-445.

ReMine, S. G., Bartnik, W., Bahn, R. C. & Shorter, R. G. (1981) Further characterisation of lymphocytes from colonic lamina propria; identification of TG cells. *Clinical and Experimental Immunology,* **46,** 294-300.

Reynolds, H. Y. & Thompson, R. E. (1974) Pulmonary host defenses. II. Interaction of respiratory antibodies with *Psuedomonas aeruginosa* and alveolar macrophages. *Journal of Immunology,* **11,** 369.

Richman, L. K., Graeff, A. S. & Strober, W. (1981) Antigen presentation by macrophage-enriched cells from the mouse Peyer's patch. *Cellular Immunology,* **62,** 110-118.

Roux, M. E., McWilliams, M., Phillips-Quagliata, M. J. & Lamm, M. E. (1981) Differen-tiation pathway of Peyer's patch precursors of IgA plasma cells in the secretory immune system. *Cellular Immunology,* **61,** 141-153.

Rosen, F. S. R. & Janeway, C. A. (1966) The gamma globulins. III. The antibody deficiency syndromes. *New England Journal of Medicine,* **275,** 709.

Roszkowski, W., Plant, M. & Lichtenstein, L. M. (1977) Selective display of histamine receptors on lymphocytes. *Science,* **195,** 683.

Salem, P. A., Nassar, V. H., Shahid, M. J. et al (1977) Mediterranean abdominal lymphoma or immunoproliferative small intestinal disease. Part I: clinical aspects. *Cancer,* **40,** 2941-2947.

Savilahti, E. (1973) IgA deficiency in children. Immunoglobulin containing cells in the intestinal mucosa, immunoglobulins in secretions and serum IgA levels. *Clinical and Experimental Immunology,* **13,** 395-406.

Scott, H., Solherm, B. G., Brandtzaeg, P. & Thorsby, E. (1980) HLA-DR-like antigens on the epithelium of the human small intestine. *Scandinavian Journal of Immunology,* **12,** 77-82.

Selby, S., Janossy, G., Goldstein, G. & Jewell, D. P. (1981) T lymphocyte subsets in human intestinal mucosa: the distribution and relationship to MHC-derived antigens. *Clinical and Experimental Immunology,* **44,** 453-458.

Seligmann, M. (1975) Alpha-chain disease. *Journal of Clinical Pathology,* **29** (Supplement 6), 72-76.

Seligmann, M., Mihaesco, E. & Frangione, B. (1971) Studies on α chain disease. *New York Academy of Sciences Annals,* **190,** 487-500.

Seligmann, M., Danon, F., Hurez, D. et al (1968) Alpha chain disease: a new immunoglobulin abnormality. *Science,* **162,** 1396-1398.

Singh, U., Millson, D. S., Smith, P. A. & Owen, J. J. T. (1979) Identification of β-adreno-ceptors during thymocyte ontogeny in mice. *European Journal of Immunology,* **9,** 31-35.

Skinner, J. M., Manousos, O. N., Economidou, J. et al (1976) Alpha-chain disease with localised plasmacytoma of the intestine. *Clinical and Experimental Immunology,* **25,** 112-116.

Spector, B., Perry, G. S. & Kersey, J. H. (1978) Genetically determined immunodeficiency diseases (GDID) and malignancy report from the immunodeficiency-cancer registry. *Clinical Immunology and Immunopathology,* **11,** 12-29.

Stafford, H. A., Knight, K. L. & Fanger, M. W. (1982) Receptors of IgA on rabbit lymphocytes. II. Characterisation of their binding parameters for IgA. *Journal of Immunology,* **128,** 2201-2205.

Stoop, J. W., Ballieux, R. E., Hijmans, W. & Zegers, B. J. M. (1971) Alpha chain disease with involvement of the respiratory tract in a Dutch child. *Clinical and Experimental Immunology,* **9,** 625-635.

Strober, W., Krakauer, R., Klaeveman, H. L. et al (1976) Secretory component deficiency. A disorder of the IgA immune system. *New England Journal of Medicine,* **294,** 351-356.

Szigeti, R., Masucci, M. G., Masucci, G. et al (1980) Interferon suppresses antigen and mitogen induced leucocyte migration inhibition. *Nature,* **288,** 594-596.

Tagliabue, A., Luini, W., Soldateschi, D. & Boraschi, D. (1981) Natural killer activity in gut mucosal lymphoid cells in mice. *European Journal of Immunology,* **11,** 912-922.

Tangun, Y., Saracbasi, Z., Inceman, S. et al (1975) IgA myeloma globulin and Bence-Jones proteinuria in a diffuse plasmacytoma of small intestine. *Annals of Internal Medicine,* **83,** 673.

Thomas, H. C. & Parrott, D. M. V. (1974) The induction of tolerance to a soluble protein antigen by oral administration. *Immunology,* **27,** 631-639.

Tomasi, T. B. Jr (1970) Structure and function of mucosal antibodies. *Annual Review of Medicine,* **21,** 281.

Tomasi, T. B. Jr & Zigelbaum, S. D. (1962) The excretion of gamma globulin in human saliva, colostrum and urine. *Arthritis and Rheumatism,* **5,** 662.

Turk, A., Lichtenstein, L. M. & Normal, P. S. (1970) Nasal secretory antibody to inhalant antigens in allergic and non-allergic patients. *Immunology,* **19,** 85.

Waldman, R. H. & Strober, W. (1969) Metabolism of immunoglobulins. *Progress in Allergy,* **13,** 1.

Walker, W. A. & Isselbacher, K. J. (1977) Intestinal antibodies. *New England Journal of Medicine,* **294.**

Webster, A. D. B., Kenwright, S., Ballard, J. et al (1975) Nodular lymphoid hyperplasia of the bowel in primary hypogammaglobulinaemia: study of in vivo and in vitro lymphocyte function. *Gut,* **18,** 364-372.

Webster, D. (1976) The gut and immunodeficiency disorders. *Clinics in Gastroenterology,* **5** (2), 323.

Wells, H. G. (1911) Studies on the chemistry of anaphylaxis. III. Experiments with isolated proteins, especially those of the hen's eggs. *Journal of Infectious Diseases,* **9,** 147.

7

Importance of Vitamin B_{12} and Folate Metabolism in Malabsorption

N. D. GALLAGHER

Dietary folate and cobalamin are essential for DNA synthesis. Folate is a general term for any member of the folic acid or pteroylmonoglutamic acid family. Folate in food is present mainly in conjugated form, the second and subsequent glutamic acid molecules being linked through γ-carboxyl and amino groups. Cobalamin, formerly called vitamin B_{12}, is present in most animal tissues and products. Progressive depletion of either vitamin leads to the development of megaloblastic anaemia and, in the case of cobalamin, to neurological disturbances. The rapid regeneration of the small intestinal epithelium makes it susceptible to the lack of these cofactors. Thus folate and cobalamin deficiency of any origin may have a malabsorptive component which is due to impaired enterocyte function (Reynolds et al, 1965; Carmel and Herbert, 1967).

MECHANISM OF FOLATE AND COBALAMIN ABSORPTION

As a general rule water-soluble compounds of molecular weight greater than 200 require a specialized transport system to ensure that they are absorbed in adequate amounts. Both folate as the pteroylheptaglutamate (molecular weight 1215) and cobalamin (molecular weight 1335) qualify. Folate undergoes hydrolysis to the pteroylmonoglutamate (molecular weight 441) (Butterworth, Baugh and Krumdieck, 1969) whereas cobalamin binds initially to Castle's intrinsic factor (molecular weight 44 000) before it is absorbed (Donaldson, 1981). Genetic regulation of the absorptive processes is implicit in rare instances of megaloblastic anaemia in which there is an inability to absorb or transport oral cobalamin or folate across the gut (Chanarin, 1982).

Preparative phase of folate and cobalamin absorption

Folate appears to enter the small intestine unchanged and to be avidly taken up by the jejunal epithelium once it has been deconjugated at the microvillous surface. Cobalamin is firmly bound to R protein in the stomach, either as a result of acid pepsin release from dietary protein or by direct transfer (Allen et al, 1978). R proteins are a group of immunologically related proteins found in secretions such as saliva, gastric juice and bile. R protein has a much greater affinity for cobalamin and has the potential to usurp the role of intrinsic factor in transporting the vitamin down the intestine. The threat is short-lived because R protein is readily destroyed by pancreatic proteases (Allen et al, 1978; Marcoullis et al, 1980). The intervention of R protein is unexplained because intrinsic factor has many of the properties of an ideal transport protein.

Mucosal phase of folate and cobalamin absorption

The mechanism of cobalamin absorption is unknown, but a recent study has shown that the intermicrovillous pit of the ileal epithelium is the absorptive locus (Levine, Nakane and Allen, 1982). There are a number of similarities between the absorptive process and receptor-mediated endocytosis which characterizes the internalization of low density lipoprotein cholesterol and other protein carriers by other tissues (Goldstein, Anderston and Brown, 1979). They include the requirement for a specific binding protein, intrinsic factor, calcium-dependent binding of the intrinsic factor-cobalamin complex to high affinity ileal receptors (Hooper et al, 1973), and energy-dependent transfer into the cell (Strauss, Wilson and Hotchkiss, 1960). There is evidence for the participation of lysosomes in the intestinal transport phase (Jenkins et al, 1981), although there is no indication that intrinsic factor is degraded within these organelles. Cobalamin is found in portal blood bound to transcobalamin II after an unaccountable delay of several hours. There is evidence that the transcobalamin II required for the exit phase is provided by the small intestinal epithelium (Chanarin et al, 1978; Katz and Puschalowsky, 1981).

Detailed accounts of folate absorption are provided in the reviews of Halsted (1980) and Rosenberg (1981). The intestinal absorption of folate requires hydrolysis of pteroylpolyglutamate to pteroylmonoglutamate in the lumen of the upper intestine. Uncoupling of the glutamyl peptide bond is due to the action of folate conjugase which is retained in the epithelial microvillous border. The enzyme is believed to provide a shuttle of pteroylmonoglutamate ions. Maximal entry occurs by a saturable process at a pH of 6. There is a second folate conjugase in lysosomes. Its function is unknown. Other enzymes contribute to methylation and reduction with the result that methyl tetrahydrofolate is the principal product of folate metabolism in the intestinal mucosa. While the ability of the jejunal mucosa to take up physiological amounts of monoglutamate is rate limiting, pharmacological doses of folate and also cobalamin are able to gain entry into the intestinal epithelium in therapeutic amounts.

ASSESSMENT OF DIETARY INTAKE

Even when malabsorption is suspected it is essential to review dietary sources (Chanarin, 1979). Intake may be restricted because of anorexia or socioeconomic factors. It has been estimated that folate stores last for up to four months (Herbert, 1962). The recommended daily intake of folate is 400 μg. Rich sources include yeast, offal, dark leafy vegetables and nuts. Levels in beer are higher than in other alcoholic drinks. Cobalamin deficiency, which may take two to five years to develop (Heyssel et al, 1966), is much less likely to arise on a dietary basis. Vegetarians will develop low serum cobalamin levels unless they take milk or eggs. Depletion of cobalamin is delayed because they continue to absorb biliary cobalamin. The recommended daily intake of cobalamin for an adult is 3 μg. Meat, poultry, seafood and milk are good sources. Cobalamin is not present in vegetables unless contaminated by bacteria in the soil or other medium.

Cobalamin malabsorption

Caution has been advised in choosing a method to measure serum cobalamin (Donaldson, 1978). Malabsorption as determined by an impaired ability to absorb radiolabelled cyanocobalamin in the Schilling test is found more frequently than evidence of cobalamin deficiency. Pernicious anaemia is the likely diagnosis when megaloblastic anaemia and cobalamin deficiency are present. The majority of patients with this disorder show improved absorption when intrinsic factor is administered. A small number do not respond in this fashion until they have been treated with parenteral cobalamin (Carmel and Herbert, 1967).

More rigorous testing of cobalamin absorption can be performed by feeding radiolabelled cobalamin bound to chicken serum protein (Streeter et al, 1974). This will define patients who, following gastric surgery, are able to absorb crystalline cobalamin but not serum-bound cobalamin. It will also demonstrate cobalamin malabsorption in patients treated with H$_2$-blocking drugs, but the long-term effects are uncertain (Steinberg, King and Toskes, 1980). Cobalamin malabsorption is usually present in patients with cystic fibrosis or chronic pancreatitis with minimal exocrine secretion (Toskes, 1980). Analysis of the protein-bound form of cobalamin in jejunal fluid indicates that intrinsic factor has exclusive binding rights in normal subjects (Marcoullis et al, 1980). The absence of pancreatic proteases leads to the persistence of R protein-bound cobalamin which is inaccessible to ileal receptors (Brugge et al, 1980; Marcoullis et al, 1980).

Cobalamin malabsorption which is corrected by antibiotics but not by intrinsic factor is a hallmark in bacterial overgrowth syndromes. A number of bacteria are able to divert cobalamin. Impaired cobalamin absorption is almost invariable in patients with a resection of more than 50 cm of distal ileum. Mucosal damage and stricture formation due to Crohn's disease or pelvic irradiation also lead to cobalamin deficiency. When the mucosal lesion of adult coeliac disease extends into the ileum cobalamin malabsorption will result. Involvement of the ileum is a feature of tropical sprue. A detailed discussion of these and other causes of cobalamin malabsorption is to be found in reviews by Donaldson (1975) and Toskes (1980).

Folate malabsorption

Diseases of the jejunal mucosa and drugs account for most instances of folate malabsorption (Halsted, 1980). Folate deficiency is commonplace in coeliac disease and tropical sprue. Jejunal biopsy has a high priority if the diet is adequate and the red cell folate is low. Although the jejunum is the preferred site, distal absorption also occurs because it is unusual to find folate deficiency unless the greater part of the small intestine has been resected. Blind loop syndromes may also cause folate deficiency.

The relationship between alcohol, nutrition and malabsorption is discussed by Green in this volume. Oral contraceptives have been cited as a cause of folate malabsorption but the absorption of the polyglutamate and the activity of jejunal folate conjugase are normal (Stephens et al, 1972). The mechanism of salicylasosulphapyridine (Axulfidine) induced malabsorption is explicable in terms of competitive inhibition of the conjugase (Reisenauer and Halsted, 1981). The activity of the human enzyme is not affected by diphenylhydantoin (Dilantin). Folate malabsorption in patients receiving this drug may be due to a disturbance in the transport phase (Rosenberg, 1981).

SUMMARY

The risk of developing folate deficiency is greatest in patients who have a poor diet and malabsorption secondary to disease of the jejunal mucosa or drugs which interfere with its metabolism. In contrast to cobalamin deficiency, in which body stores delay the onset of major metabolic complications, folate deficiency may develop in a matter of months. It is frequently possible to predict these deficiencies and always possible to reverse them by supplementation.

REFERENCES

Allen, R. H., Seetharam, B., Podell, E. & Alpers, D. H. (1978) Effect of proteolytic enzymes on the binding of cobalamin to R protein and intrinsic factor. In vitro evidence that a failure to partially degrade R protein is responsible for cobalamin malabsorption in pancreatic insufficiency. *Journal of Clinical Investigation,* **61,** 47-54.
Brugge, W. R., Goff, J. S., Allen, N. C. et al (1980) Development of a dual label Schilling test for pancreatic exocrine function based on the differential absorption of cobalamin bound to intrinsic factor and R protein. *Gastroenterology,* **78,** 937-949.
Butterworth, C. E. Jr, Baugh, C. M. & Krumdieck, C. (1969) A study of folate absorption and metabolism in man utilizing carbon-14-labelled polyglutamate synthesized by the solid phase method. *Journal of Clinical Investigation,* **48,** 1131-1142.
Carmel, R. & Herbert, V. (1967) Correctable intestinal defect of vitamin B_{12} absorption in pernicious anaemia. *Annals of Internal Medicine,* **67,** 1201-1207.
Chanarin, I. (1979) *The Megaloblastic Anaemias.* Oxford: Blackwell Scientific Publications.
Chanarin, I. (1982) Disorders of vitamin absorption. *Clinics in Gastroenterology,* **11,** 73-85.
Chanarin, I., Muir, M., Hughes, A. & Hoffrand, A. W. (1978) Evidence for intestinal origin of transcobalamin II during vitamin B_{12} absorption. *British Medical Journal,* **i,** 1453-1455.
Donaldson, R. M. Jr (1975) Mechanisms of malabsorption of cobalamin. In *Cobalamin* (Ed.) Babior, B. pp. 335-368. New York: J. Wiley.
Donaldson, R. M. Jr (1978) Serum B_{12} and the diagnosis of cobalamin deficiency. *New England Journal of Medicine,* **299,** 827-828.
Donaldson, R. M. Jr (1981) Intrinsic factor and the transport of cobalamin. In *Physiology of the Gastrointestinal Tract* (Ed.) Johnson, L. R. pp. 641-658. New York: Raven Press.
Goldstein, J. L., Anderson, R. G. W. & Brown, M. S. (1979) Coated pits, coated vesicles and receptor mediated endocytosis. *Nature,* **279,** 679-685.

Halsted, C. H. (1980) Intestinal absorption and malabsorption of folates. *Annual Review of Medicine,* **31,** 79-87.

Herbert, V. (1962) Experimental folate nutritional deficiency in man. *Transactions of the Association of American Physicians,* **40,** 81-91.

Heyssel, R. M., Bozian, R. C., Darby, J. W. & Bell, M. D. (1966) Vitamin B$_{12}$ turnover in man: the assimilation of vitamin B$_{12}$ from natural foodstuffs by man and estimates of minimal daily dietary requirements. *American Journal of Clinical Nutrition,* **20,** 636-640.

Hooper, D. C., Alpers, D. H., Mehlman, C. S. & Allen, R. H. (1973) Characterisation of ileal vitamin B$_{12}$-binding using homogeneous human and hog intrinsic factors. *Journal of Clinical Investigation,* **52,** 3074-3083.

Jenkins, W. J., Empson, R., Jewell, D. P. & Taylor, K. B. (1981) Subcellular localisation of vitamin B$_{12}$ during absorption in the guinea pig ileum. *Gut,* **22,** 617-622.

Katz, M. & Puschalowsky, W. (1981) Emergence of vitamin B$_{12}$ from cultured guinea pig enterocyte. *Abstract, Americal Society of Hematology,* San Antonio, Texas.

Levine, J. S., Nakane, P. K. & Allen, R. H. (1982) Immunocytochemical localisation of intrinsic factor-cobalamin bound to the guinea pig ileum in vivo. *Gastroenterology,* **82,** 284-290.

Marcoullis, G., Parmentier, Y., Nicolas, J. P. et al (1980) Cobalamin malabsorption due to non degradation of R protein in the human intestine. *Journal of Clinical Investigation,* **66,** 430-440.

Reisenauer, A. M. & Halsted, C. H. (1981) Human jejunal brush border folate conjugase. Characteristics and inhibition by salicylazosulfapyridine. *Biochimica et Biophysica Acta,* **659,** 62-69.

Reynolds, E. H., Hallpike, J. F., Phillips, B. M. & Matthews, D. M. (1965) Reversible absorptive defects in anticonvulsant megaloblastic anaemia. *Journal of Clinical Pathology,* **18,** 593-598.

Rosenberg, I. H. (1981) Intestinal absorption of folate. In *Physiology of the Gastrointestinal Tract* (Ed.) Johnson, L. R. pp. 1221-1230. New York: Raven Press.

Steinberg, W. M., King, C. E. & Toskes, P. P. (1980) Malabsorption of protein bound cobalamin but not unbound cobalamin during cimetidine administration. *Digestive Diseases and Sciences,* **25,** 188-192.

Stephens, M. E. M., Craft, I., Peters, I. J. & Hoffbrand, A. V. (1972) Oral contraceptives and folate metabolism. *Clinical Science,* **42,** 405-414.

Strauss, E. W., Wilson, T. H. & Hotchkiss, A. (1960) Factors controlling B$_{12}$ uptake by intestinal sacs in vitro. *American Journal of Physiology,* **198,** 103-107.

Streeter, A. M., Balasubramaniam, D., Royle, R. et al (1974) Malabsorption of vitamin B$_{12}$ after vagotomy. *Americal Journal of Surgery,* **128,** 340-343.

Toskes, P. P. (1980) Current concepts of cobalamin (vitamin B$_{12}$) absorption and malabsorption. *Journal of Clinical Gastroenterology,* **2,** 287-297.

8

Nutritional Aspects of Malabsorption: Short Gut Adaptation

ELLIOT WESER

Improved techniques in surgery, anaesthesia, and nutritional management have increased recovery and survival after extensive small bowel resection. With this has occurred a better understanding of the pathophysiology of the short gut and its relationship to intestinal adaptation, both of which directly relate to improved treatment of this condition. The metabolic consequences of short gut depend upon a number of factors which influence the absorption of sufficient nutrients to maintain adequate nutrition (Table 1). This review will consider the pathophysiology of short gut and the major determinants of malabsorption with particular emphasis on intestinal adaptation.

EXTENT AND SITE OF RESECTED BOWEL

It is obvious that the amount of small bowel remaining after extensive resection of small intestine is of major importance in determining the mucosal surface area available for nutrient absorption. The transit time of luminal nutrients will also be decreased in a shortened intestine and will thus reduce the contact time between luminal nutrients and pancreatico-biliary secretions. These events may significantly impair normal digestion and absorption and specifically result in malabsorption of fat, carbohydrates, proteins, and other nutrients.

Fortunately, there is a large functional reserve capacity of the small intestine for adequate absorption of nutrients. Forty to fifty per cent of the small bowel may be removed without major metabolic sequelae although, as indicated below, the site of the resection can be extremely important in determining the degree of impaired absorption. The minimum length of small bowel necessary to provide adequate nutrition via oral calorie intake is not known (or absolute), but occasional reports have cited extended survival after near-total resection of small bowel (Anderson, 1965; Winawer et al, 1966). The use of formula defined diets and parenteral nutrition have contributed significantly to the survival of these patients.

Under normal circumstances the digestion and absorption of fat, carbohydrates, protein, minerals and water-soluble vitamins (except vitamin B_{12})

Clinics in Gastroenterology — Vol. 12, No. 2, May 1983
0300-5089/83/1202-443 $05.00©1983 W. B. Saunders Company Ltd

Table 1. *Major factors affecting nutrient absorption after small bowel resection*

Extent and site of resected small bowel
Preservation or removal of ileocaecal junction
Function of remaining small bowel, colon, stomach, liver, pancreas
Adaptive changes in gastrointestinal tract

takes place primarily in the duodenum and jejunum, thereby leaving few nutrients to be absorbed from the ileum. Thus the ileum represents a functional reserve capacity for absorption. After jejunal resection, increased amounts of nutrients enter the ileum and are absorbed from this site. Since cholecystokinin and secretin synthesis and release are associated with the duodenal and jejunal mucosa, extensive loss of proximal small bowel could be accompanied by impaired hormonal stimulation of pancreatico-biliary secretions.

Resection of ileum is generally associated with greater metabolic consequences than resection of equivalent lengths of jejunum. The ileum is the selective site for active reabsorption of conjugated bile salts, the absorption of intrinsic factor-vitamin B_{12} complex, and possibly the reabsorption of metabolites of vitamin D that are excreted in the bile. Increased diffusion of bile salts and vitamin B_{12} across jejunal mucosa after ileal resection may partially compensate for a lost ileal function (Mackinnon et al, 1975; Tilson, Boyer and Wright, 1975; Heubi et al, 1980). There may even be induction of active bile salt transport in the remaining jejunum as well as ileum (Tilson, Boyer and Wright, 1975; Heubi et al, 1980) and limited increases in the hepatic synthesis of bile salts (Ho and Bondi, 1977). Despite these compensatory changes, loss of bile salts because of insufficient ileal reabsorption reduces the size of the circulating bile salt pool and results in decreased bile salt micelle formation in the small bowel lumen. This in turn reduces absorption of water-insoluble 2-monoglycerides, 1-lysophospholipids, fatty acids, and fat-soluble vitamins (A, D, E, K). Increased amounts of unabsorbed fats and conjugated bile acids enter the colon and are acted upon by bacteria with formation of hydroxy-fatty acids and deconjugated bile salts. These substances impede the absorption of water and electrolytes from the colon (Mekhjian, Phillips and Hofmann, 1971; Ammon and Phillips, 1973) and thus contribute to diarrhoea as well as steatorrhoea. Both may also cause secretion of water into the lumen. Removal of less than 100 cm of ileum may cause significant diarrhoea, secondary to the excess of bile salts in the colon, but the steatorrhoea is usually mild (less than 20 g per day). Resection of greater amounts of ileum is associated with more severe steatorrhoea as well as diarrhoea (Hofmann and Poley, 1972).

Significant losses of fat-soluble vitamins may occur with steatorrhoea. Reduced concentrations of serum 25-hydroxy-vitamin D have been found in patients after intestinal resection and attributed to decreased ingestion as well as malabsorption of vitamin D (Compston and Creamer, 1977). Interruption of an enterohepatic circulation of hydroxy-metabolites of vitamin D may play an important role. After the intravenous injection of tritiated 25-hydroxy-vitamin D into experimental animals and normal volunteers significant amounts appear in intestinal aspirates (Arnaud et al, 1975; Kumar et al, 1980).

Extensive ileal resection will also impair absorption of vitamin B_{12}, which over a period of several years may produce clinical evidence of deficient body stores. Vitamin B_{12} deficiency itself may also alter intestinal mucosal cell morphology and transport (Arvanitakis, 1978).

PRESENCE OF ILEOCAECAL JUNCTION

Removal of the ileocaecal junction, as part of the small bowel resection (and usually in addition a partial colectomy), may result in greater diarrhoea than anticipated from the short bowel state alone. Several mechanisms may explain this occurrence. Experimental data have shown that an intact ileocaecal 'valve' prolongs the transit time of luminal contents within the small bowel (Gazet and Kopp, 1964) and may thereby increase mucosal contact time for nutrient absorption. The loss of the ileocaecal junction may also permit increased bacterial colonization of the already shortened small bowel (Isaacs and Kim, 1979; Simon and Gorback, 1982) and further potentiate bacterial deconjugation of bile salts, a reduction in bile salt reabsorption, and increased passage of these bile salts into the colon. Steatorrhoea may thereby be increased. Furthermore, bacterial colonization of the shortened small bowel may further impair absorption of vitamin B_{12} because of bacterial metabolism of this vitamin.

FUNCTION OF REMAINING SMALL BOWEL, COLON, STOMACH, LIVER, PANCREAS

The functional state of residual small bowel and colon is obviously important in determining the course, complications, and long-term survival of the patient with a short bowel. If the residual intestine is diseased or functionally impaired, such as may occur in Crohn's disease, coeliac-sprue, Whipple's disease, radiation enteropathy, or previous gastroenterostomy, nutrient absorption may be further reduced and add to the problems of maintaining adequate nutrition.

After extensive resection, there is initially a significant reduction in mucosal disaccharidase activity in proportion to the amount and (perhaps) location of small bowel removed (Richards, Concon and Mallison, 1971; Bochenck, Narezewska and Gizegieluch, 1973). This usually results in a reduction of disaccharide hydrolysis, and may produce clinical symptoms of carbohydrate malabsorption. Because of its normal relatively low concentration, intestinal lactase is most commonly affected, and thus ingestion of dietary lactose is associated with an increase in small bowel effluent entering the colon. Bacterial hydrolysis and fermentation of unabsorbed lactose to lactic acid and other small short chain acids may produce an osmotic diarrhoea, bloating, and gas, and thus add to the patient's discomfort.

Quantitatively significant absorption of iron, calcium, and magnesium occurs along the entire length of small bowel, even though the rate of mucosal transport of these cations is highest in the duodenum. Therefore deficiencies of these minerals are not unusual after extensive small bowel resection. Metabolites of vitamin D enhance intestinal calcium transport. As indicated above, serum concentrations of 25-hydroxy-vitamin D may be decreased in patients with short bowel (Comston and Creamer, 1977). When steatorrhoea exists, luminal calcium, as well as magnesium, may bind with unabsorbed fat to form insoluble soaps, resulting in further reduction of cation absorption. Negative calcium and magnesium balance as well as bone disease have been reported in these patients (Ladefoged, Nicolaidou and Jarnum, 1980). Deficiencies of zinc and other trace metals may also occur (Atkinson et al, 1978; Ladefoged, Nicolaidou and Jarnum, 1980). Zinc is an essential component of many enzyme systems and is necessary for protein synthesis (Ulmer, 1977). Deficiency of this metal may also lead to altered taste and appetite (Catalonotto, 1978). Fortunately, deficiencies of water-soluble vitamins occur infrequently (except in massive resection with minimal residual bowel), presumably because ileum can adequately absorb these vitamins in the absence of the jejunum.

Patients with a partial or total colectomy, in addition to a short bowel, usually experience greater diarrhoea, dehydration, hypovolaemia, and electrolyte depletion. This emphasizes the importance of the colon as an efficient site of water and electrolyte absorption as well as a storage organ (Mitchel, 1980). In these patients, faecal electrolyte composition is more likely determined by the amount of remaining colon rather than residual ileum (Cummins, James and Wiggins, 1973). In addition, total intestinal transit time is greater in patients with increasing lengths of remaining colon.

The large bowel is also a major site of absorption of oxalate that remains soluble in the lumen of the intestine (Earnest, 1979). Normally, almost all dietary oxalate combines with calcium intraluminally to form calcium oxalate which is insoluble and non-absorbable. In patients with short bowel and steatorrhoea, calcium will preferentially bind with unabsorbed fats and fatty acids, less with oxalate, and thus luminal oxalate is maintained in a soluble state. Therefore, patients with significant and chronic steatorrhoea and an intact colon are prone to absorb increased amounts of dietary oxalate and excrete this substance in the urine (Earnest et al, 1974; Dobbins and Binder, 1977). Persistent hyperoxaluria increases the likelihood of developing calcium oxalate renal stones. In patients with partial or total colectomy the risk of calcium oxalate nephrolithiasis is reduced (Dobbins and Binder, 1977).

Gastric hypersecretion may occur in some patients shortly after extensive small bowel resection (Winawer et al, 1966; Buxton, 1974). An increase in serum gastrin concentrations has been reported in man (Straus, Gerson and Yalow, 1974) and may represent a reduction in gastrin catabolism related to the reduction in small bowel mass (Becker, Reeder and Thompson, 1973). Further, the absence of hormones usually produced in the excised small bowel tissue (i.e., secretin, cholecystokinin, vasoactive intestinal peptide, gastric inhibitory peptide, somatostatin) which could inhibit the action of gastrin, may also account for an increase in gastric secretion. In rhesus monkeys, gastric hypersecretion after small bowel resection can be abolished by removal of the gastric antrum (Hall et al, 1977). This suggests that an alteration in gastrin secretion after resection is an important factor in causing gastric hypersecretion. Fortunately, this hypersecretion diminishes with time after resection (Windsor, Fejfar and Woodward, 1969; Buxton, 1974) and may be related to adaptive changes in the stomach and small bowel. Gastric hypersecretion, when present, can seriously complicate the management of these patients. The excessive volume of gastric juice entering the residual proximal small bowel may dilute pancreatic enzymes, lower the pH of luminal contents, interfere with bile salt micelle formation, and stimulate peristalsis — all contributing to further reductions in fat digestion and absorption. In a manner analogous to Zollinger-Ellison syndrome, patients may have peptic ulceration, breakdown of surgical anastomosis, and fistula formation as additional complications. Improvement in gastric hypersecretion and nutrient absorption may occur by treating these patients with cimetidine (Cortot, Fleming and Malagelada, 1979; Murphy, King and Dubois, 1979).

In patients with severe malnutrition, pancreatic exocrine secretions may be diminished (Pitchumoni, 1973). Furthermore, loss of secretin and cholecystokinin associated with extensive bowel resection, including jejunum, could result in decreased secretagogue stimulation of the pancreas and contribute to functional pancreatic insufficiency. Superimposed on an already shortened intestine, this could further impair digestion and absorption of nutrients. Some patients who have a primary pancreatic insufficiency in addition to a short gut would of course do more poorly. Animal studies have shown transient increase in exocrine pancreatic secretions after extensive small bowel resection (Gelinas, Morin and Morisset, 1982) possibly reflecting adaptive changes in the pancreas, but this has not been described in man. Although an enteropancreatic circulation of pancreatic enzymes has been postulated, its role in regulating pancreatic secretion is uncertain (Toskes, 1980). Experimentally, luminal trypsin and chymotrypsin in the jejunum decrease pancreatic exocrine secretions in the rat, presumably via a feedback inhibition system (Green and Lyman, 1972; Schneeman and Lyman, 1975).

Maldigestion of dietary proteins and subsequent malabsorption of peptides and amino acids may impair hepatic synthesis of albumin within hours (Rothschild, Oratz and Schneiber, 1972). If protein-calorie malabsorption is severe enough a Kwashiorkor-like condition may occur. Impaired liver function may result in a decreased synthesis of bile acids which could contribute to maldigestion and malabsorption. A recent animal study indicated that bile acids may prolong trypsin and chymotrypsin activity in the intestine, which in turn may regulate pancreatic secretion as mentioned above (Green and Nasset, 1980).

INTESTINAL ADAPTATION

Adaptation of the remaining gastrointestinal tract after small bowel resection plays a significant role in nutrient absorption and maintenance of adequate nutrition. Structural, functional, and cytokinetic changes that take place after intestinal resection have been the subject of several recent reviews (Williamson, 1978; Urban and Weser, 1980) and only the more relevant aspects to human short bowel syndrome will be discussed here.

Studies of adaptive changes in man have been relatively few in number and not well controlled. These indicate that some responses may be similar to those found in experimental animals, but overall translation of this data to man cannot be presumed. There are sporadic reports of enlargement and dilatation of remnant bowel and proximal intestinal biopsies have revealed villus hyperplasia (increase in cell numbers) without increases in villus height (Porus, 1965; Weinstein et al, 1969; Dowling and Gleeson, 1973). In patients with jejuno-ileal bypass for obesity, the jejuno-ileum left in continuity with the nutrient stream becomes elongated and the villi in the ileum increase in height (Fenyo, Backman and Hallberg, 1976; Iverson, Selyovsly and Skagen, 1976). The change in villus height is again associated with an increase in cell numbers (hyperplasia) and not an increase in cell size. There is less agreement concerning changes in the bypassed, defunctionalized segment of small bowel. Some studies report atrophy of the jejunum (Dowling and Gleeson, 1973; Fenyo, Backman and Hallberg, 1976; Iverson, Selyovsly and Skagen, 1976) while others reveal little or no decreases in mucosal mass (Dudrick et al, 1977; Tompkins et al, 1977). A few studies in man also document that functional adaptation or improvement occurs with time after intestinal resection. Usually there is a gradual reduction in postoperative diarrhoea or ileostomy output. Improved absorption of nitrogen, fat, carbohydrates, water, electrolytes, and vitamin B_{12} has been reported (Winawer et al, 1966; Dowling and Booth, 1966; Weinstein et al, 1969; MacKinnon et al, 1975).

Intestinal adaptation has been extensively studied in animals using a variety of experimental models, including resection of the small bowel (Robinson, Dowling and Riecker, 1982). These and other studies clearly indicate that after small bowel resection, adaptive changes occur in the remaining stomach, small bowel, colon, and pancreas. Similar to man, gastric hypersecretion and increased serum gastrin concentrations have been reported (Caridis, Roberts and Smith, 1969; Goldman, Durn and Weinberger, 1972; Wickbom, Landor and Bushkin, 1975). There is some correlation between the magnitude of the gastric hypersecretion and extent of small bowel removed. After both proximal and distal small bowel resection, proliferation of the gastric glandular epithelium occurs which persists for many months (Winborn et al, 1974; Seelig, Winborn and Weser, 1977). A trophic effect of gastrin on the gastric mucosa probably contributes to the hypersecretion and is discussed below.

As shown in Figure 1, the remaining small bowel undergoes mucosal hyperplasia, particularly striking in residual ileum (after jejunectomy), provided the animals are fed orally (Nygaard, 1967; Dowling and Booth, 1967; Tilson and Wright, 1970a; Weser and Hernandez, 1971). Adaptive responses occur in the jejunum remaining after ileal resection, but are less dramatic, more variable, and may partly be related to adaptive changes in food intake (Young and Weser, 1974). Although muscle and serosa may also increase in size, these tissues have not been well studied. It is not clear

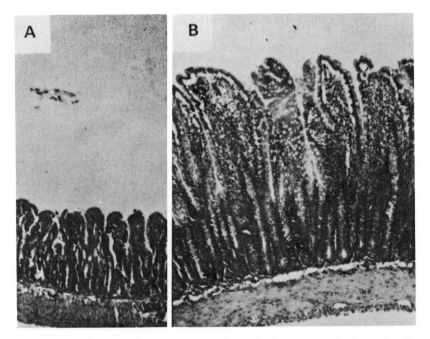

Figure 1. Ileal hyperplasia one month after jejunal resection in a rat maintained on a chow diet. (A) Normal ileum. (B) Ileum after jejunal resection. Haematoxylin and eosin stained, formalin-fixed, sections; magnification × 1400. From Weser (1979), with kind permission of the editor of *American Journal of Medicine.*

whether ultrastructural components of the epithelial cell (brush border, lateral cell membranes) also show adaptive changes (Genyk, 1971; Tilson and Wright, 1972c). The mucosal hyperplasia results from an increase in the rate of cell renewal (which expands the proliferative zone in the crypts) and an increase in the rate of cell migration up the villus (Hanson and Osborne, 1971; McDermott and Roudnew, 1976). It appears that a maximal rate of cell renewal is established by 12 days after small bowel resection and is related to the amount of intestine resected (Hanson, Osborne and Sharp, 1977). The adaptive increase in cell renewal begins as early as two days following surgical resection (Obertop et al, 1977).

Similarly, adaptive hyperplasia of colonic mucosa occurs after both jejunal and ileal resection (Tilson, Michand and Livstone, 1976; Williamson, Bauer and Ross, 1978; Loeschke, Fabritius and Hatz, 1982; Urban, Michel and Weser, 1982) beginning as early as two days after surgery (Nundy et al, 1977). These changes are associated with improved segmental absorption of water and electrolytes (Loeschke, Fabritius and Hatz, 1982; Urban, Michel and Weser, 1982). After extensive resection adaptive hyperplasia occurs in the pancreas as well (Stock et al, 1982). Ileal mucosa may also undergo hyperplasia after colectomy with an associated increase in water absorption (Wright et al, 1969; Woo and Nygaard, 1978).

Functional adaptation in residual small bowel accompanies the morphological changes described above. An increase in nutrient absorption per centimetre of remaining bowel segment has been noted for fat, protein, glucose, galactose, sucrose, maltose, sodium, water, bile acids, vitamin B_{12}, calcium, and zinc (Williamson, 1978; Urban and Weser, 1980; Robinson, Dowling and Riecken, 1982; Urban and Cambell, 1982). Increased absorption may be directly proportional to the increase in mucosal mass (greater number of absorbing epithelial cells), or may be relatively greater, indicating a selective increase in transport by the population of epithelial cells. Transport function by these epithelial cells could also actually be decreased and thus net segmental absorption would depend upon the decreases in cellular transport relative to the total increase in number of absorbing epithelial cells (hyperplasia). These events depend upon the specific substrate as well as the particular location of remnant small bowel (duodenum, jejunum, or ileum).

Numerous metabolic and enzymatic changes accompany morphological adaptation reflecting biochemical alterations consistent with mucosal growth and compensatory function. Specific disaccharidase activity either decreases or changes little (Weser and Hernandez, 1971; Hietanen and Hanninen, 1972; McCarthy and Kim, 1973) whereas peptide hydrolases, entero-kinase, and sodium-potassium-ATPase increase (Tilson and Wright, 1971b; McCarthy and Kim, 1973), probably related to increased absorption of their respective substrates. A reciprocal decrease of adenyl cyclase specific activity has been reported (Oya and Weser, 1974), suggesting an adaptive decrease in electrolyte secretion while absorption is enhanced. There are conflicting reports on whether alkaline phosphatase increases (Hietanen and Hanninen, 1972; Urban, 1977). A reported increase in lipid re-esterifying enzymes of the remnant ileum would correlate with adaptive increases in lipid absorption after jejunal resection (Rodger and Bochenek, 1970). Recently an increase in ornithine decarboxylase specific activity has been noted in ileal mucosa two days after jejunectomy in the rat (Luk and Baylin, 1982). Although the activity of this enzyme returned to normal 14 days after surgery, its association with polyamine synthesis suggests that it may be important in initiating the adaptive hyperplasia response. Polyamines are thought to facilitate DNA, RNA, and protein synthesis and play a key role in cell proliferation. This enzyme is the first and rate-limiting enzyme in polyamine biosynthesis. Other enzymes related to nucleic acid synthesis also increase in remnant small bowel mucosa, reflecting the biochemical equivalent of increased cell proliferation (Nakayama and Weser, 1972, 1975).

Mechanisms of Intestinal Adaptation

In recent years, much has been learned about the various factors influencing intestinal adaptation in animal models. The major and minor factors are listed in Table 2 and have received critical review (Dowling, 1982). No one mechanism can explain all adaptive responses of the gastrointestinal tract, and probably several contribute to the changes in remnant small bowel. All

Table 2. *Factors influencing intestinal adaptation after small bowel resection*

Major factors:
   Luminal nutrition
   Pancreatico-biliary secretions
   Enteric hormones

Minor factors:
   Mucosal blood flow
   Neural effects

would agree that exposure of residual small intestine to intraluminal chyme is required for mucosal hyperplasia to occur after resection. Early studies with transposition of small bowel showed that the location of the segment within the small intestine was important in determining that mucosal morphology conformed to that typical of the region (Altmann and Leblond, 1970; Gronqvist, Engstrom and Grimelius, 1975; Philipson, 1975). An ileal segment transposed to the jejunum increased its mucosal mass and villus height. A jejunal segment transposed to the ileum underwent opposite changes and decreased its mucosal mass. In addition, bypassed segments of small intestine, denied contact with chyme, underwent mucosal atrophy (Gleeson, Cullen and Dowling, 1972; Keren et al, 1975; Rijke et al, 1977). These findings suggested that the intraluminal environment played an important role in intestine adaptation.

Role of luminal nutrition

After intestinal resection, adaptive mucosal hyperplasia of remaining small bowel occurs only if nutrients are present in the intestinal lumen (Feldman et al, 1976; Levine, Deren and Yezdimir, 1976). Animals given isocaloric nourishment via total parenteral nutrition do not develop mucosal hyperplasia despite adequate gain in body weight. Animals with an intact intestine that are fed by total parenteral nutrition develop jejunal atrophy and lose the proximal-distal gradient of mucosal mass (Levine et al, 1974; Eastwood, 1977). Bulk agents have strikingly less or no effect on mucosal morphology in adult rats (Dowling and Booth, 1967). Recent studies have focused on the effect of infusing single, specific nutrients into the bowel on mucosal adaptation while animals were otherwise completely nourished by total parenteral nutrition. Small quantities of long-chain triglycerides produced growth effects equal to complete macromolecular nutrients suggesting that dietary long-chain fat is a potent stimulator of intestinal adaptation (Morin, Grey and Garofalo, 1982). Other substrates which produce mucosal hyperplasia include glucose, galactose, fructose, mannose, 3-O-methylglucose, and a variety of amino acids including α-amino-isobutyric acid (Spector, Levine and Deren, 1977; Spector et al, 1981; Weser, Tawil and Fletcher, 1982; Weser, Vandeventer and Tawil, 1982a,b). These findings indicate that substrates absorbed by active and diffusion processes, which are both metabolized and non-metabolized, can stimulate morphological adaptation. The passage of a substrate into or through the mucosa seems to trigger the hyperplasia response.

Role of pancreatico-biliary secretions

Although nutrients in the lumen of the intestine may stimulate mucosal growth by direct absorption, they may also do so by causing pancreatico-biliary secretions to enter the lumen. This enteric-pancreatico-biliary secretion response is mediated via the release of cholecystokinin, secretin, and possibly other enteric hormones with less clear function. Pancreatico-biliary secretions have been shown to increase villus height and mucosal mass in the ileum in both normal and intestinally resected animals (Altmann, 1971; Weser, Heller and Tawil, 1977). Pancreatic secretions appear to have a more marked effect. Diversion of pancreatico-biliary secretions into the ileum produces ileal mucosal hyperplasia (as well as pancreatic hyperplasia) in rats orally fed chow and defined formula diets, or maintained on total parenteral nutrition (Miazza et al, 1982; Weser, Drummond and Tawil, 1982). Despite differences in experimental methods and absolute results, all studies indicate that the duodeno-jejunal mucosa has greater mucosal mass when pancreatico-biliary secretions are diverted from proximal intestine into ileum compared to biliary diversion alone (Gelinas and Morin, 1980; Miazza et al, 1982; Weser, Drummond and Tawil, 1982). These findings suggest that jejunal mucosal growth is inhibited by pancreatic secretions or that other factors not present in the ileum influence jejunal mucosal growth. It is possible that secretions from the stomach, duodenum, or jejunum account for some of these differences.

The mechanism for stimulation of ileal mucosal growth by pancreatico-biliary secretions is not certain. A direct nutritive effect of these secretions is possible, but some studies suggest additional growth factors (Altmann, 1974; Hughes et al, 1979).

Trophic effects of enteric hormones

There is impelling evidence that nutrient absorption may be associated with release and circulation of enteric hormones that may exert trophic effects on the gastrointestinal mucosa. Proximal small bowel resection causes greater ileal hyperplasia than a comparable bypass of the jejunum (Tilson, Sweeney and Wright, 1975; Williamson, 1978). Studies in parabiotic rats also suggest a circulating trophic hormone (Loran and Carbone, 1968; Williamson, Bucholtz and Malt, 1978). Perhaps most convincing is the fact that the mucosal atrophy of a bypassed segment (from which nutrients and pancreatico-biliary secretions are absent) is partially reversed if the animal is fed enterally rather than by total parenteral nutrition or undergoes partial resection of small bowel remaining in continuity (Dworkin et al, 1976). Amelioration of the mucosal atrophy in the bypassed segment probably results from release of a humoral (hormonal) agent.

Gastrin. Historically, gastrin has received the most attention as a trophic hormone for the gastrointestinal tract and probably plays an important role in producing mucosal hyperplasia of the stomach after experimental small bowel resection. Gastrin stimulates DNA and protein synthesis in gastric, duodenal, and colonic mucosa (Johnson, Ames and Yuen, 1969;

Lichtenberger, Driller and Erwin, 1973; Johnson and Guthrie, 1974; Ryan, Dudrick and Copeland, 1979). Antrectomy results in atrophy of the gastric mucosa (Martin, Macleoud and Sircus, 1970) and hypergastrinaemia associated with Zollinger-Ellison syndrome or short bowel is related to hyperplasia of the gastric mucosa (Isenberg, Walsh and Grossman, 1973; Straus, Gerson and Yalow, 1974).

There is substantial experimental evidence to indicate that gastrin is not important to the small bowel as a trophic hormone after intestinal resection. Confirmed studies show that mucosal hyperplasia in remnant bowel occurs with enteral nutrition despite removal of gastrin-containing tissues and decreases in circulating gastrin (Oscarson et al, 1977; Johnson, 1982). Furthermore, administering pentagastrin parenterally in short bowel rats maintained on total parenteral nutrition did not produce mucosal hyperplasia (Morin and Ling, 1978).

Cholecystokinin and secretin. Several studies suggest that circulating cholecystokinin peptides, perhaps augmented by secretin, stimulate intestinal mucosal growth by either direct trophism, or more likely via pancreaticobiliary secretions. Administration of parenteral cholecystokinin in combination with secretin for six weeks has been shown to completely prevent the intestinal hypoplasia associated with total parenteral nutrition in dogs with an intact intestine (Hughes, Bates and Dowling, 1978). Other studies have shown that continuous intravenous infusion of octapeptide-cholecystokinin for 7 to 14 days in jejunally resected rats supported by total parenteral nutrition partially prevents intestinal hypoplasia compared with animals who do not receive the hormone infusion (Weser, Bell and Tawil, 1981). As recently reviewed, not all studies with cholecystokinin in rats resulted in similar findings (Dowling, 1982).

Enteroglucagon. Ever since villus hyperplasia was associated with an enteroglucagon-secreting tumour of the kidney (Gleeson et al, 1971) there has been intense interest in enteroglucagon as a trophic hormone to small bowel. In three animal models of intestinal adaptation, including intestinal resection, enteroglucagon immunoactivity was found to be increased in fasting plasma and in small bowel tissue (of rats) which developed adaptive mucosal hyperplasia (Jacobs et al, 1982). Enteroglucagon has also been correlated with increases in crypt cell production rate (Al-Mukhtar et al, 1982). Studies in man have revealed selective increases in plasma concentrations of this hormone in human partial small bowel resection and coeliac disease (Bloom and Polak, 1982). The elevated tissue and plasma enteroglucagon concentrations have been related to increased amounts of nutrients entering the ileum. The increased circulating enteroglucagon may in turn 'trigger' the adaptive response. At the present time, the evidence for a trophic action of enteroglucagon is circumstantial, but with the availability of synthetic enteroglucagon its role should become clear.

Earlier studies suggested that pancreatic glucagon was involved in adaptive changes associated with semi-starvation (Rudo, Lawrence and Rosenberg, 1975). However, recent experiments showed that intravenous infusions of pancreatic glucagon did not prevent intestinal hypoplasia associated with total parenteral nutrition (Weser, Bell and Tawail, 1981). It is therefore unlikely that this species of the glucagon family functions as a trophic hormone for small bowel.

Other hormones. A variety of other hormones including corticosteroids, prolactin, anterior pituitary hormones, and epidermal growth factor have been suggested as potential mediators of adaptive responses (Dowling, 1982). Evidence which would assign them a major role is lacking. Overall, it seems unlikely that a circulating hormone alone is responsible for adaptive hyperplasia after intestinal resection. The impressive growth of mucosa exposed to nutrients or chyme, contrasted with the relative or absolute hypoplasia of mucosa not in contact with the nutrient stream, is difficult to explain by trophism of a circulating hormone.

Chalones. It has been suggested that cell division, migration, and differentiation are intrinsic features of intestinal epithelium, genetically controlled, and regulated by sensitive homeostatic mechanisms. There may be a feedback control system in a rapidly dividing tissue such as intestinal epithelium, so that the number of functioning villus cells determines the rate of cell division in the crypts (Galjaard, Van der Meer-Fieggen and Giesen, 1972). Reduction of the villus cell count (by temporary ischaemia or irradiation) stimulates mitosis in the crypt, increases the size of the proliferative zone, and increases crypt cell uptake of tritiated thymidine. This has suggested the existence of an inhibitor (chalone) in the villus epithelial cell acting on the proliferative zone and suppressing cell division. A partially purified villus cell extract has been shown to have strong and specific inhibitory effects on the incorporation of tritiated thymidine into cellular DNA and on cell division, without cytotoxicity (May et al, 1981). It is conceivable that luminal nutrients, pancreatico-biliary secretions, or a 'trophic' hormone, alone or in concert, alter the villus cell inhibitor (chalone) and permit accelerated crypt cell division to take place, resulting in hyperplasia with a new steady state of mucosal turnover.

Mucosal blood flow

At present, there is not sufficient evidence to assign an important role to intestinal blood flow in intestinal adaptation. After mid-gut resection, blood flow in the ileum was shown to increase two days after surgery, returning to normal after two months (Touloukiain and Spencer, 1972). A transient decrease in blood flow has also been reported after adrenergic denervation of remnant small bowel (Touloukiain, Aghajanian and Rothe, 1972). On the other hand, infusion of a vasoconstrictor noradrenaline (norepinephrine) was associated with an increase in crypt cell proliferation (Tutton and Helme, 1974). This conflicting data obscures any role that blood flow may play in intestinal adaptation.

Neural factors

Adrenaline (epinephrine) has been shown to inhibit mucosal mitosis which can be reversed by beta-adrenergic blockade (Tutton and Helme, 1974).

Cellular proliferation has also been inhibited by sympathectomy (Dupont, Biggers and Sprinz, 1965; Tutton and Helme, 1974), and cell division stimulated by cholinergic drugs (Tutton, 1977). In rats and dogs, mucosal hypoplasia of the small intestine, associated with a subsequent increase in epithelial cell turnover, has followed abdominal vagotomy (Ballinger et al, 1964; Silen, Peloso and Jaffe, 1966; Liavag and Vaage, 1972). Cutting the afferent or sensory fibres of the vagus abolished the adaptive changes in residual intestine of the pig after enterectomy (Laplace, 1982). Recently, chemical sympathectomy with 6-hydroxydopamine exaggerated the intestinal mucosal hypoplasia in rats maintained on total parenteral nutrition (Levine, Kotler and Yezdimir, 1982). However, this mucosal atrophy could be prevented by intragastric infusion of luminal nutrients, suggesting the effect of sympathectomy was minor compared to that of luminal nutrients. Although neural and vascular responses seem to be related, their role in intestinal adaptation, particularly after resection, requires more clarification.

The challenge of interrelating the mechanisms that act alone or together in producing the adaptive changes to intestinal resection has attracted the efforts of many investigators. Although much has been learned, many more questions remain and clinical use of these mechanisms to influence gut morphology or function still lies in the future.

REFERENCES

Al-Mukhar, M. Y. T., Sagor, G. B., Ghater, M. A. et al (1982) The relationship between endogenous gastrointestinal hormones and cell proliferation in models of adaptation. In *Falk Symposium 30. Mechanisms of Intestinal Adaptation* (Ed.) Robinson, J. W. L., Dowling, R. H. & Riecken, E. O. pp. 243-254. Lancaster: MTP Press.

Altmann, G. C. (1971) Influence of bile and pancreatic secretions on the size of the intestinal villi in the rat. *American Journal of Anatomy,* 132, 167-178.

Altmann, G. C. (1974) Demonstration of a morphological control mechanism in the small intestine. Role of pancreatic secretions and bile. In *Intestinal Adaptation* (Ed.) Dowling, R. H. & Riecken, E. O. pp. 75-86. Stuttgart: Schattnauer Verlang.

Altmann, G. C. & Leblond, C. F. (1970) Factors influencing villus size in the small intestine of adult rats as revealed by transposition of intestinal segments. *American Journal of Anatomy,* 127, 15-36.

Ammon, H. V. & Phillips, S. F. (1973) Inhibition of colonic water and electrolyte absorption by fatty acids in man. *Gastroenterology,* 65, 744-749.

Anderson, C. (1965) Long term survival with six inches of small intestine. *British Medical Journal,* i, 419-422.

Arnaud, S. B., Goldsmith, R. S., Lambert, P. W. & Go, V. L. W. (1975) Evidence of an enterohepatic circulation in man. *Proceedings of the Society of Experimental Biology and Medicine,* 149, 570-572.

Arvanitakis, C. (1978) Functional and morphologic abnormalities of the small intestinal mucosa in pernicious anemia. *Acta Hepato-Gastroenterologica,* 25, 313-318.

Atkinson, R. L., Dahms, W. T., Bray, G. A. et al (1978) Plasma zinc and copper in obesity and after intestinal bypass. *Annals of Internal Medicine,* 89, 491-493.

Ballinger, W. F. II, Iida, J., Aponte, G. E. et al (1964) Structure and function of the canine small intestine following total abdominal vagotomy. *Surgery, Obstetrics and Gynecology,* 118, 1305-1311.

Becker, H. D., Reeder, D. D. & Thompson, J. D. (1973) Extraction of circulating endogenous gastrin by the small bowel. *Gastroenterology,* 65, 903-906.

Bloom, S. R. & Polak, J. M. (1982) Enteroglucagon and the gut hormone profile of intestinal adaptation. In *Falk Symposium 30. Mechanisms of Intestinal Adaptation* (Ed.) Robinson, J. W. L., Dowling, R. H. & Riecken, E. O. pp. 189-198. Lancaster: MTP Press.

Bochenek, W. T., Narczewska, B. & Gizegieluck, M. (1973) Effect of massive proximal small bowel on intestinal sucrase and lactase activity in the rat. *Digestion,* 9, 224-230.

Buxton, B. (1974) Small bowel resection and gastric hypersecretion. *Gut,* 15, 229-238.

Caridis, D. T., Roberts, M. & Smith, G. (1969) The effect of small bowel resection on gastric acid secretion in the rat. *Surgery,* 65, 292-297.

Catalanotto, F. A. (1978) The trace metal zinc and taste. *American Journal of Clinical Nutrition,* 31, 1098-1103.

Compston, J. E. & Creamer, B. (1977) Plasma levels and intestinal absorption of 25-hydroxy vitamin D in patients with small bowel resection. *Gut,* 18, 171-175.

Cortot, A., Fleming, C. R. & Malagelada, J. R. (1979) Improved nutrient absorption after cimetidine in short bowel syndrome with gastric hypersecretion. *New England Journal of Medicine,* 300, 79-80.

Cummins, J. H., James, W. P. T. & Wiggins, H. S. (1973) Role of the colon in ileal-resection diarrhoea. *Lancet,* i, 344-347.

Dobbins, J. W. & Binder, H. J. (1977) Importance of the colon in enteric hyperoxaluria. *New England Journal of Medicine,* 296, 298-301.

Dowling, R. H. (1982) Small bowel adaptation and its regulation. *Scandinavian Journal of Gastroenterology,* 17 (Supplement 74), 53-74.

Dowling, R. H. & Booth, C. C. (1966) Functional compensation after small bowel resection in man. *Lancet,* ii, 146-147.

Dowling, R. H. & Booth, C. C. (1967) Structural and functional changes following small intestinal resection in the rat. *Clinical Science,* 32, 139-149.

Dowling, R. H. & Gleeson, M. H. (1973) Cell turnover following small bowel resection and bypass. *Digestion,* 8, 176-190.

Dudrick, S. J., Daly, J. M., Castro, G. & Akhtar, M. (1977) Gastrointestinal adaptation following small bowel bypass for obesity. *Annals of Surgery,* 185, 642-648.

Dupont, J. R., Biggers, D. C. & Sprinz, H. (1965) Intestinal renewal and immunosympathectomy. *Archives of Pathology,* 80, 357-362.

Dworkin, L. D., Levine, G. M., Farber, H. J. & Spector, M. H. (1976) Small intestinal mass of the rat is partially determined by indirect effects of intraluminal nutrition. *Gastroenterology,* 71, 626-630.

Earnest, D. L. (1979) Enteric hyperoxaluria. In *Advances in Internal Medicine* (Ed.) Stollerman, G. H. pp. 407-427. Chicago: Year Book Medical Publishers.

Earnest, D. L., Johnson, G., Williams, H. E. & Admirand, M. D. (1974) Hyperoxaluria in patients with ileal resection: an abnormality in dietary oxalate absorption. *Gastroenterology,* 66, 1114-1122.

Eastwood, C. L. (1977) Small bowel morphology and epithelial proliferation in intravenously alimented rabbits. *Surgery,* 82, 613-620.

Feldman, F. T., Dowling, R. H., MacNaughton, J. & Peters, T. J. (1976) Effect of oral versus intravenous nutrition on intestinal adaptation after small bowel resection. *Gastroenterology,* 70, 712-719.

Fenyo, G., Backman, L. & Hallberg, D. (1976) Morphological changes of the small intestine following jejunoileal shunt in obese subjects. *Acta Chirurgica Scandinavica,* 142, 154-159.

Galjaard, N. H., Van der Meer-Fieggen, W. & Giesen, J. (1972) Feedback control by functional villus cells on cell proliferation and maturation in intestinal epithelium. *Experimental Cell Research,* 73, 197-207.

Gazet, J. C. & Kopp, J. (1964) Surgical significance of ileo-cecal junction. *Surgery,* 56, 565-573.

Gelinas, M. D. & Morin, C. L. (1980) Effects of bile and pancreatic secretions on intestinal mucosa after proximal small bowel resection in rats. *Canadian Journal of Physiology and Pharmacology,* 58, 1117-1123.

Gelinas, M. D., Morin, C. L. & Morriset, J. (1982) Exocrine pancreatic function following proximal small bowel resection in rats. *Journal of Physiology,* 322, 71-82.

Genyk, S. N. (1971) Ultrastructure of the apical part of the epithelial cells of the mucous membrane of the small intestine after extensive experimental enterectomy. *Bulletin of Experimental Biology and Medicine,* 72, 964-967.

Gleeson, M. H., Cullen, J. & Dowling, R. H. (1972) Intestinal structure on function after small bowel bypass in the rat. *Clinical Science,* **43,** 731-742.

Gleeson, M. H., Bloom, S. R., Polak, J. M. et al (1971) Endocrine tumor in kidney affecting small bowel structure, motility and absorptive function. *Gut,* **12,** 773-782.

Goldman, L. I., Durn, B. & Weinberger, M. (1972) The small intestine and gastric secretion in the rat. *Archives of Surgery,* **104,** 73-75.

Green, G. M. & Lyman, R. L. (1972) Feedback regulation of pancreatic enzyme secretion as a mechanism for trypsin-inhibitor induced hypersecretion in rats. *Proceedings of the Society for Experimental Biology and Medicine,* **140,** G-12.

Green, G. M. & Nasset, F. S. (1980) Importance of bile in regulation of intraluminal proteolytic enzyme activities in the rat. *Gastroenterology,* **79,** 695-702.

Gronqvist, B., Engstrom, B. & Grimelius, L. (1975) Morphological studies of the rat small intestine after jejuno-ileal transposition. *Acta Chirurgica Scandinavica,* **141,** 208-217.

Hall, A. W., Moossa, A. R., Wood, P. A. B. et al (1977) Effect of antrectomy on gastric hypersecretion induced by distal small bowel resection. *Archives of Surgery,* **186,** 83-87.

Hanson, W. R. & Osborne, J. W. (1971) Epithelial cell kinetics in the small intestine of the rat 60 days after resection of 70 per cent of the ileum and jejunum. *Gastroenterology,* **60,** 1087-1097.

Hanson, W. R., Osborne, J. W. & Sharp, J. G. (1977) Compensation by the residual intestine after intestinal resection in the rat. I. Influence of the amount of tissue removed. II. Influence of postoperative time interval. *Gastroenterology,* **72,** 692-700 and 701-705.

Heubi, J. E., Balistieri, W. F., Partin, J. C. et al (1980) Enterohepatic circulation of bile acids in infants and children with ileal resection. *Journal of Laboratory and Clinical Medicine,* **95,** 231-240.

Hietanen, E. & Hanninen, O. (1972) Effect of chyme on mucosal enzyme levels in small intestine of the rat. *Metabolism,* **21,** 991-1000.

Ho, K. J. & Bondi, J. L. (1977) Cholesterol metabolism in patients with resection of ileum and proximal colon. *American Journal of Clinical Nutrition,* **30,** 151-159.

Hofmann, A. R. & Poley, J. R. (1972) Role of bile acid malabsorption in pathogenesis of diarrhea and steatorrhea in patients with ileal resection. I. Response to cholestyramine or replacement of dietary long chain triglyceride by medium chain triglyceride. *Gastroenterology,* **62,** 918-934.

Hughes, C. A., Bates, T. & Dowling, R. H. (1978) Cholecystokinin and secretin prevent the intestinal mucosal hyperplasia of total parenteral nutrition in the dog. *Gastroenterology,* **75,** 34-41.

Hughes, C. A., Ducker, D. A., Warren, I. F. & McMeish, A. S. (1979) Effect of pancreatico-biliary secretions on mucosal structure and function of self-emptying jejunal blind loops in rats. *Gut,* **20,** A924.

Isenberg, J. I., Walsh, J. H. & Grossman, M. I. (1973) Zollinger-Ellison syndrome. *Gastroenterology,* **65,** 140-165.

Isaacs, P. E. T. & Kim, Y. S. (1979) The contaminated small bowel syndrome. *American Journal of Medicine,* **67,** 1049-1057.

Iversen, B. M., Schonsby, H., Skagen, D. W. & Solhaug, J. H. (1976) Intestinal adaptation after jejuno-ileal bypass operation for massive obesity. *European Journal of Clinical Investigation,* **6,** 355-360.

Jacobs, L. R., Polak, J. M., Bloom, S. R. & Dowling, R. H. (1982) Intestinal mucosal and fasting plasma levels of immunoreactive enteroglucagon in three animal models of intestinal adaptation: resection, hypothermic hyperphagia and lactation in the rat. In *Falk Symposium 30. Mechanisms of Intestinal Adaptation* (Ed.) Robinson, J. W. L., Dowling, R. H. & Riecken, E. O. pp. 231-240. Lancaster: MTP Press.

Johnson, L. R. (1982) Role of gastrointestinal peptide in intestinal adaptation. In *Falk Symposium 30. Mechanisms of Intestinal Adaptation* (Ed.) Robinson, J. W. L., Dowling, R. H. & Riecken, E. O. pp. 201-211. Lancaster: MTP Press.

Johnson, L. R. & Guthrie, P. D. (1974) Mucosal DNA synthesis: a short term index of the trophic action of gastrin. *Gastroenterology,* **67,** 453-459.

Johnson, L. R., Ames, D. & Yuen, L. (1969) Pentagastrin induced stimulation of the in vitro incorporation of ^{14}C-leucine into protein of the gastrointestinal tract. *American Journal of Physiology,* **217,** 251-254.

Keren, D. F., Elliott, H. L., Brown, G. D. & Yardley, J. H. (1975) Atrophy of villi with hypertrophy and hyperplasia of paneth cells in isolated (Thiry-Vella) ileal loops in rabbits. *Gastroenterology,* **68,** 83-93.

Kumar, R., Nagubandi, S., Mattox, V. R. & Londowsky, J. M. (1980) Enterohepatic physiology of 1,25-dihydroxy vitamin D₃. *Journal of Clinical Investigation,* **65,** 277-284.

Ladefoged, K., Nicolaidoa, P. & Jarnum, S. (1980) Calcium, phosphorus, magnesium, zinc, and nitrogen balance in patients with severe short bowel syndrome. *American Journal of Clinical Nutrition,* **33,** 2137-2144.

Laplace, J. P. (1982) Impairment by vagal differentiation of the compensatory hypertrophy after enterectomy, at high and low feeding levels. In *Falk Symposium 30. Mechanisms of Intestinal Adaptation* (Ed.) Robinson, J. W. L., Dowling, R. H. & Riecken, E. O. pp. 321-331. Lancaster: MTP Press.

Levine, G. M., Deren, J. J. & Yezdimir, E. (1976) Small bowel resection. Oral intake is the stimulus for hyperplasia. *American Journal of Digestive Diseases,* **21,** 542-546.

Levine, G. M., Kotler, D. P. & Yezdimir, E. A. (1982) Luminal nutrition obviates sympathectomy-induced intestinal atrophy in the rat. In *Falk Symposium 30. Mechanisms of Intestinal Adaptation* (Ed.) Robinson, J. W. L., Dowling, R. H. & Riecken, E. O. pp. 311-317. Lancaster: MTP Press.

Levine, G. M., Deren, J. J., Steiger, E. & Zinno, R. (1974) Role of oral intake in maintenance of gut mass and disaccharidase activity. *Gastroenterology,* **67,** 975-982.

Liavag, I. & Vaage, S. (1972) The effect of vagotomy and pyloroplasty on the gastrointestinal mucosa of the rat. *Scandinavian Journal of Gastroenterology,* **7,** 23-27.

Lichtenberger, L. M., Driller, L. R. & Erwin, D. N. (1973) The effect of pentagastrin on adult rat duodenal cells in culture. *Gastroenterology,* **65,** 242-251.

Loeschke, K., Fabritus, J. & Hatz, H. (1982) Electrolyte transport of the rat colon following proximal intestinal resection. In *Falk Symposium 30. Mechanisms of Intestinal Adaptation* (Ed.) Robinson, J. W. L., Dowling, R. H. & Riecken, E. O. pp. 521-526. Lancaster: MTP Press.

Loran, M. R. & Carbone, J. V. (1968) The humoral effect of intestinal resection on cellular proliferation and maturation in parabiotic rats. In *Gastrointestinal Radiation Injury* (Ed.) Sullivan, M. F. pp. 127-139. Amsterdam: Excerpta Medica.

Luk, G. D. & Baylin, S. B. (1982) Ornithine decarboxylase in intestinal maturation, recovery, and adaptation. In *Falk Symposium 30. Mechanisms of Intestinal Adaptation* (Ed.) Robinson, J. W. L., Dowling, R. H. & Riecken, E. O. pp. 65-78. Lancaster: MTP Press.

Mackinnon, A. M., Short, M. D., Elias, E. & Dowling, R. H. (1975) Adaptive changes in vitamin B₁₂ absorption in celiac disease and after proximal small bowel resection in man. *American Journal of Digestive Diseases,* **20,** 835-840.

Martin, F., Macleoud, I. F. & Sircus, W. (1970) Effects of antrectomy on the fundic mucosa of the rat. *Gastroenterology,* **59,** 437-444.

May, R. J., Quaroni, A., Kirsch, K. & Isselbacher, K. J. (1981) A villous cell-derived inhibitor of intestinal cell proliferation. *American Journal of Physiology,* **241,** (Gastrointestinal-Liver Physiology, 4), G520-527.

McCarthy, D. M. & Kim, Y. S. (1973) Changes in sucrase enterokinase and peptide hydrolase after intestinal resection. The association of cellular hyperplasia and adaptation. *Journal of Clinical Investigation,* **52,** 942-951.

McDermott, F. T. & Roudnew, B. (1976) Ileal crypt cell population kinetics after 40 per cent small bowel resection. *Gastroenterology,* **70,** 707-711.

Mekhjian, H. S., Phillips, S. F. & Hofmann, A. F. (1971) Colonic secretion of water and electrolytes induced by bile acids: perfusion studies in man. *Journal of Clinical Investigation,* **50,** 1569-1577.

Miazza, B. M., Levan, H., Vaja, S. & Dowling, R. H. (1982) Effect of pancreatico-biliary diversion (PBD) on jejunal and ileal structure and function in the rat. In *Falk Symposium 30. Mechanisms of Intestinal Adaptation* (Ed.) Robinson, J. W. L., Dowling, R. H. & Riecken, E. O. pp. 467-476. Lancaster: MTP Press.

Mitchel, J. E., Brever, R. I., Zucherman, L. et al (1980) The colon influences ileal resection diarrhea. *Digestive Diseases and Sciences,* **25,** 33-41.

Morin, C. L. & Ling, V. (1978) Effect of pentagastrin on the rat small intestine after resection. *Gastroenterology,* **75,** 224-229.

Morin, C. L., Grey, V. L. & Garofalo, C. (1982) Influence of lipids on intestinal adaptation after resection. In *Falk Symposium 30. Mechanisms of Intestinal Adaptation* (Ed.) Robinson, J. W. L., Dowling, R. H. & Riecken, E. O. pp. 175-184. Lancaster: MTP Press.

Murphy, J. P. Jr, King, D. R. & Dubois, A. (1979) Treatment of gastric hypersecretion with cimetidine in short bowel syndrome. *New England Journal of Medicine,* **300,** 80-81.

Nakayama, H. & Weser, E. (1972) Adaptation of small bowel after intestinal resection: increase in the pentose phosphate pathway. *Biochimica et Biophysica Acta,* **279,** 416-423.

Nakayama, H. & Weser, E. (1975) Pyrimidine biosynthetic enzymes in rat intestine after small bowel resection. *Gastroenterology,* **68,** 480-487.

Nundy, S., Malamud, D., Obertop, H. et al (1977) Onset of cell proliferation in the shortened gut. Colonic hyperplase after ileal resection. *Gastroenterology,* **72,** 263-266.

Nygaard, K. (1967) Resection of the small intestine in rats. III. Morphological changes in the intestinal tract. *Acta Chirurgica Scandinavica,* **133,** 233-248.

Obertop, H., Nundy, S., Malamud, D. & Malt, R. A. (1977) Onset of cell proliferation in the shortened gut. Rapid hyperplasia after jejunal resection. *Gastroenterology,* **72,** 267-270.

Oscarson, J. F. A., Veen, H. F., Williamson, R. C. M. et al (1977) Compensatory post-resectional hyperplasia and starvation atrophy in small bowel: dissociation from endogenous gastrin levels. *Gastroenterology,* **72,** 890-895.

Oya, R. & Weser, E. (1974) Reciprocal adaptive changes in intestinal Na^+-K^+-ATPase and adenyl cyclase after small bowel resection in the rat. *Clinical Research,* **22,** 64A.

Philipson, B. (1975) Morphology in the cat ileal mucosa following construction of an ileal reservoir or transposition of patches to different locations. *Scandinavian Journal of Gastroenterology,* **10,** 369-377.

Pitchumoni, C. S. (1973) Pancreas in primary malnutrition disorders. *American Journal of Clinical Nutrition,* **26,** 374-379.

Porus, R. L. (1965) Epithelial hyperplasia following massive small bowel resection. *Gastroenterology,* **48,** 753-757.

Rijke, R. P. C., Plaisier, H. M., de Ruiter, H. & Galjaard, M. D. (1977) Influence of experimental bypass on cellular kinetics and maturation of small intestinal epithelium in the rat. *Gastroenterology,* **72,** 896-901.

Richards, A. J., Concon, J. R. & Mallison, D. M. (1971) Lactose intolerance following extensive intestinal resection. *British Journal of Surgery,* **58,** 493-494.

Robinson, J. W. L., Dowling, R. H. & Riecken, E. O. (Ed.) (1982) *Falk Symposium 30. Mechanisms of Intestinal Adaptation.* Lancaster: MTP Press. 646pp.

Rodger, J. B. & Bochenek, W. (1970) Localization of lipid re-esterifying enzymes of rat small intestine. Effect of jejunal removal on ileal enzyme activities. *Biochimica et Biophysica Acta,* **202,** 426-435.

Rothschild, M. A., Oratz, M. & Schneiber, S. S. (1972) Medical Progress. Albumin synthesis. *New England Journal of Medicine,* **286,** 748-757 and 816-821.

Rudo, N. D., Lawrence, M. D. & Rosenberg, I. H. (1975) Treatment with glucagon-binding antibodies alters the intestinal response to starvation in the rat. *Gastroenterology,* **69,** 1265-1268.

Ryan, G. P., Dudrick, S. J. & Copeland, F. M. (1979) Effects of various diets on colonic growth in rats. *Gastroenterology,* **77,** 658-663.

Schneeman, B. & Lyman, R. L. (1975) Factors involved in the intestinal feedback regulation of pancreatic enzyme secretion in the rat. *Proceedings of the Society for Experimental Biology and Medicine,* **148,** 897-903.

Seelig, L. L., Winborn, W. B. & Weser, E. (1977) Effect of small bowel resection on the gastric mucosa in the rat. *Gastroenterology,* **72,** 421-428.

Silen, W., Peloso, O. & Jaffe, B. F. (1966) Kinetics of intestinal epithelial proliferation: effect of vagotomy. *Surgery,* **60,** 127-135.

Simon, G. L. & Gorbach, S. L. (1982) Intestinal microflora. In *Intestinal Infections* (Ed.) Sodeman, W. A. pp. 563-567. Philadelphia: W. B. Saunders.

Spector, M. H., Levine, G. M. & Deren, J. J. (1977) Direct and indirect effects of dextrose and amino acids on gut mass. *Gastroenterology,* **72,** 706-710.

Spector, M. H., Traylor, J. B., Young, E. A. & Weser, E. (1981) Stimulation of mucosal growth by gastric and ileal infusion of single amino acids in parenterally nourished rats. *Digestion,* **21,** 33-40.

Stock, C., Marescaux, J., Haegel, P. et al (1982) Comparative effects of small bowel bypass and resection on the rat exocrine pancreas and the intestinal enzyme activities. In *Falk Symposium 30. Mechanisms of Intestinal Adaptation* (Ed.) Robinson, J. W. L., Dowling, R. H. & Riecken, E. O. pp. 453-461. Lancaster: MTP Press.

Straus, E., Gerson, C. D. & Yalow, R. S. (1974) Hypersecretion of gastrin associated with the short bowel syndrome. *Gastroenterology,* **66,** 175-180.

Tilson, M. D. & Wright, H. K. (1970) Adaptation of functioning and bypassed segments of ileum during compensatory hypertrophy of the gut. *Surgery,* **64,** 687-693.

Tilson, M. D. & Wright, H. K. (1971) An adaptive change in ileal Na-K-ATPase activity after jejunectomy or jejunal transposition. *Surgery,* **70,** 421-424.

Tilson, M. D. & Wright, H. K. (1972) The effect of resection of the small intestine upon the fine structure of intestinal epithelium. *Surgery, Gynecology and Obstetrics,* **134,** 992-994.

Tilson, D. M., Boyer, J. L. & Wright, H. K. (1975) Jejunal absorption of bile salts after resection of the ileum. *Surgery,* **77,** 231-234.

Tilson, D. M., Michand, J. T. & Livstone, F. M. (1976) Early proliferative activity in the left colon of the rat after partial small bowel resection. *Surgical Forum,* **27,** 445-446.

Tilson, D. M., Sweeney, T. & Wright, H. K. (1975) Compensatory hypertrophy of the ileum after gastro-duodenojejunal exclusion. *Archives of Surgery,* **110,** 309-312.

Tompkins, R. K., Waisman, J., Watt, C. M. H. et al (1977) Absence of mucosal atrophy in human small intestine after prolonged isolation. *Gastroenterology,* **73,** 1406-1409.

Toskes, P. P. (1980) Does a negative feedback system for the control of pancreatic exocrine secretion exist and is it of any clinical significance? *Journal of Laboratory and Clinical Medicine,* **95,** 11-12.

Touloukiain, R. J. & Spencer, R. P. (1972) Ileal blood flow preceding compensatory intestinal hypertrophy. *Annals of Surgery,* **175,** 320-325.

Touloukiain, R. J., Aghajanian, G. K. & Rothe, R. H. (1972) Adrenergic denervation of the hypertrophied gut remnant. *Annals of Surgery,* **176,** 633-637.

Tutton, P. J. M. (1977) Neural and endocrine control systems acting on the population kinetics of the intestinal epithelium. *Medical Biology,* **55,** 201-208.

Tutton, P. J. M. & Helme, R. D. (1974) The influence of adrenoreceptor activity on crypt cell proliferation in the rat jejunum. *Cell and Tissue Kinetics,* **7,** 125-136.

Ulmer, D. D. (1977) Current Concepts. Trace elements. *New England Journal of Medicine,* **297,** 318-321.

Urban, E. (1977) Intestinal brush border alkaline phosphatase in the rat after proximal small bowel resection. *Proceedings of the Society for Experimental Biology and Medicine,* **155,** 99-104.

Urban, E. & Cambell, M. E. (1982) Adaptive responses for zinc transport in vivo by remnant small bowel after intestinal resection in the rat. *Clinical Research* **30,** 769A (Abstract).

Urban, E. & Weser, E. (1980) Intestinal adaptation. In *Advances in Internal Medicine* (Ed.) Stollerman, G. H. Vol. 26, pp. 265-291. Chicago: Year Book Medical Publishers.

Urban, E., Michel, A. M. & Weser, E. (1982) Dissociation of mucosal mass and adaptive changes in electrolyte, water, and sugar transport in rats after intestinal resection. In *Falk Symposium 30. Mechanisms of Intestinal Adaptation* (Ed.) Robinson, J. W. L., Dowling, R. H. & Riecken, E. O. pp. 529-540. Lancaster: MTP Press.

Weinstein, L. D., Shoemaker, C. P., Hersh, T. & Wright, H. K. (1969) Enhanced intestinal absorption after small bowel resection in man. *Archives of Surgery,* **99,** 560-562.

Weser, E. (1979) Nutritional aspects of malabsorption. Short gut adaptation. *American Journal of Medicine,* **67,** 1014-1020.

Weser, E. & Hernandez, M. H. (1971) Studies of small bowel adaptation after intestinal resection in the rat. *Gastroenterology,* **60,** 69-75.

Weser, E., Bell, D. & Tawil, T. (1981) Effects of octapeptide-cholecystokinin, secretin, and glucagon on intestinal mucosal growth in parenterally nourished rats. *Digestive Diseases and Sciences,* **26,** 409-416.

Weser, E., Drummond, A. & Tawil, T. (1982) Effect of diverting bile and pancreatic secretions into the ileum on small bowel mucosa in rats fed a liquid formula diet. *Journal of Parenteral and Enteral Nutrition,* **6,** 39-42.

Weser, E., Heller, R. & Tawil, T. (1977) Stimulation of mucosal growth in the rat ileum by bile and pancreatic secretions after jejunal resection. *Gastroenterology,* **73,** 524-529.

Weser, E., Tawil, T. & Fletcher, J. T. (1982) Stimulation of small bowel mucosal growth by gastric infusion of different sugars in rats maintained on total parenteral nutrition. In *Falk Symposium 30. Mechanisms of Intestinal Adaptation* (Ed.) Robinson, J. W. L., Dowling, R. H. & Riecken, E. O. pp. 141-149. Lancaster: MTP Press.

Weser, E., Vandeventer, A. & Tawil, T. (1982a) Non-hormonal regulation of intestinal adaptation. *Scandinavian Journal of Gastroenterology,* **17** (Supplement 74), 105-113.

Weser, E., Vandeventer, A. & Tawil, T. (1982b) Stimulation of small bowel mucosal growth by mid-gut infusion of different sugars in rats. *Journal of Pediatric Gastroenterology and Nutrition,* **1**, 411-416.

Wickbom, G., Landor, J. H. & Bushkin, F. L. (1975) Changes in canine gastric acid output and serum gastrin levels following massive small bowel resection. *Gastroenterology,* **69**, 448-452.

Williamson, R. C. N. (1978) Medical progress. Intestinal Adaptation. Part 1. Structural, functional, and cytokinetic changes. *New England Journal of Medicine,* **298**, 1383-1402.

Williamson, R. C. N., Bauer, F. L. R. & Ross, J. S. (1978) Proximal enterectomy stimulates distal hyperplasia more than bypass or pancreatico-biliary diversion. *Gastroenterology,* **74**, 16-23.

Williamson, R. C. N., Bucholtz, T. W. & Malt, R. A. (1978) Humoral stimulation of cell proliferation in small bowel after transection and resection. *Gastroenterology,* **75**, 249-254.

Winawar, S. J., Broitman, S. A., Wolochow, D. A. et al (1966) Successful management of massive small bowel resection based on assessment of absorption defects and nutritional needs. *New England Journal of Medicine,* **274**, 72-78.

Winborn, W. B., Seelig, L. L., Nakayama, H. & Weser, E. (1974) Hyperplasia of the gastric glands after small bowel resection in the rat. *Gastroenterology,* **66**, 384-395.

Windsor, C. W. D., Fejfar, J. & Woodward, D. A. K. (1969) Gastric secretion after massive small bowel resection. *Gut,* **10**, 779-786.

Woo, Z. H. & Nygaard, K. (1978) Small bowel adaptation after colectomy in rats. *Scandinavian Journal of Gastroenterology,* **13**, 903-910.

Wright, H. K., Poskitt, T., Cleveland, J. C. & Herskovic, T. J. (1969) The effect of total colectomy on morphology and absorptive capacity of ileum in the rat. *Journal of Surgical Research,* **9**, 301-304.

Young, E. A. & Weser, E. (1974) Nutritional adaptation after small bowel resection in rats. *Journal of Nutrition,* **104**, 994-1001.

9

Nutritional Management of Patients with Malabsorption Syndrome

JOHN A. MORRIS JR
VAL SELIVANOV
GEORGE F. SHELDON

Malabsorption is associated with anatomical or functional loss of gastrointestinal integrity. The clinical consequences of malabsorption are secondary to deficiency of small intestinal function and are malnutrition and diarrhoea (Table 1).

Although it is possible to provide adequate nutrition indefinitely by intravenous feeding, the small intestine will atrophy if intraluminal foodstuffs are absent. For that reason, rational therapy for patients with malabsorption utilizes intravenous feeding to prevent dehydration, and maintain body cell mass. Daily oral intake of food through the gastrointestinal tract is provided as tolerated.

When malabsorption syndrome is suspected, diagnostic efforts are directed at determining if the defect is in absorption or digestion. *Digestion* is the breakdown of complex molecules into simpler, more absorbable forms. It is initiated by acid and pepsin in the stomach, and continued by amylase, lipase, and trypsin, in the small bowel. *Absorption* occurs by active or passive transport of molecules of foodstuff across the mucosal cell membrane. Transport of by-products of digestion against a concentration gradient has been demonstrated for many essential nutrients (Table 2, Figure 1).

DIGESTION OF SPECIFIC NUTRIENTS

Carbohydrate is ingested mainly as complex polysaccharides such as starch which is hydrolysed by salivary and pancreatic amylase to oligosaccharides and absorbed as monosaccharides or disaccharides into the mucosal cell by a sodium-dependent active transport system.

Protein is degraded in the stomach by the action of pepsin, and in the small bowel by pancreatic enzymes: trypsin, chymotrypsin, and carboxypeptidase. Degradation of protein proceeds to dipeptides, which may be further broken down into amino acids, or absorbed. Dipeptides are absorbed more rapidly than amino acids and probably by a different mechanism

Clinics in Gastroenterology — Vol. 12, No. 2, May 1983
0300-5089/83/1202-463 $05.00©1983 W. B. Saunders Company Ltd

Table 1. *Signs and symptoms of malabsorption syndrome*

Protein-calorie malnutrition (PCM)
Diarrhoea
Anaemia
Amenorrhoea
Glossitis
Tetany, paraesthesias and weakness
Oedema

(Mathews, 1975). Groups of amino acids have different transport mechanisms which may explain the overlap in impaired amino acid metabolism in genetically determined amino acid disorders, such as cystinuria and Hartnup's disease.

Fat digestion is initiated by emulsification, and solubilization. Emulsification takes place in the duodenum, and results in dispersion of triglyceride molecules into lipid droplets which facilitates the action of pancreatic lipase. Lipase cleaves triglyceride to form monoglycerides and free fatty acids.

Bile salts solubilize fat as their surface active properties permit the hydrophobic portions of the lipid molecule to aggregate, resulting in solubilization. Absorption occurs when highly structured aggregations of lipid molecules (micelles) are formed. Individual lipid molecules are released from the micelle, cross the glycocalyx, and enter the epithelial cell.

Free fatty acids and monoglycerides are re-esterified into triglycerides within the endoplasmic reticulum of the mucosal cell, and these aggregate with phospholipids, lipoproteins and cholesterol and form chylomicrons. The chylomicron leaves the intestinal cell, enters the central lacteal of the villus, and is transported to the thoracic duct and into the venous system.

Inadequate concentrations of bile salts will prevent the formation of micelles, inhibiting the solubilization of lipid and resulting in significant steatorrhoea. Bile salts are also responsible for shifting the optimum pH of pancreatic lipase from 8.5 to 6.5 which allows fat absorption to take place in the proximal small bowel.

Bile salts are secreted by the liver, stored in the gall-bladder, released by cholecystokinin, and reabsorbed by the ileum. After reabsorption, bile salts enter the portal vein, and are recirculated to the liver (entero-hepatic circulation). In the normal bowel, 90 per cent of conjugated bile salts reaching the ileum are absorbed, and 20 to 30 g of bile salts recirculate daily.

Table 2. *Nutrients transported against a concentration gradient*

Simple sugars	Bile salts
Electrolytes	Cholesterol
Amino acids	Folic acid
Fatty acids	Vitamin B_{12}

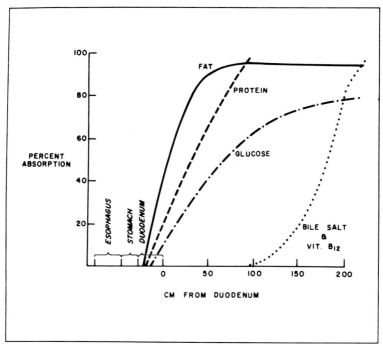

Figure 1. Location of small intestinal absorption. From Borgström et al (1957), with kind permission of the authors and the editor of *Journal of Clinical Investigation.*

An injury to the ileum which results in malabsorption of bile salts will rapidly lead to diarrhoea because of the essential role of bile salts in lipid absorption.

ANATOMY OF THE SMALL INTESTINE

The small intestine provides a large surface area for absorption. Although the human intestine is usually about 18 feet in length, the circular folds, the villi, and the microvilli, increase the absorptive surface area considerably. The circular folds are ridges, from 8 to 10 mm in height, that extend approximately two-thirds of the way around the inner circumference of the intestine.

The villi project into the lumen from the folds in the surrounding mucosal surface, have a density of about 10 to 40 per square mm, and give the mucosa the appearance of velvet to the unaided eye. Their height varies from 0.5 to 1.5 mm. Each villus is covered by epithelium (one cell layer thick) made up of goblet cells which secrete mucus. A continual migration of cells from the crypt of the villus to the tip of the villus occurs. When the migrating cells reach the tip of the villus, they are shed into the lumen, carrying with them whatever digestive enzymes they possess (Moog, 1981).

Each individual epithelial cells is covered by a series of small projections termed microvilli. Microvilli increase the surface area of the intestine by a factor of 20. The membrane of the microvillus is the actual site of admittance of nutrients into the circulation.

THE SHORT BOWEL SYNDROME

Anatomical or functional loss of large segments of the small intestine results in derangements of both digestion and absorption (Table 3). The exact length of small bowel loss compatible with a normal existence is unclear. As a general rule, significant malabsorption results from a 70 per cent loss of small bowel (Tilson, 1980). Residual involvement by diseases of the small intestine in remaining segments obviously influence the absorption of foodstuffs. Isolated case reports are available of long-term survival in patients with 6 to 18 inches of remaining jejunum, ileum and duodenum after resection (Conn, Chavez and Fane, 1972; Strauss et al, 1974; Scheflen et al, 1976). The picture is confused by reports citing the length of intestine remaining after extensive resection which are estimated by measuring the length of resected specimens. A more rational approach to the problem of the small bowel remnant is obtained from intraoperative measurements of the remaining bowel from the ligament of Treitz, or the ileocaecal valve (Chen, 1974).

Table 3. *Classification of malabsorption syndromes*

Inadequate digestion:
  Postgastrectomy syndrome
  Pancreatic insufficiency
  Diminished intraluminal bile salt concentration or availability

Inadequate absorption:
  Loss of absorptive surface area
  Primary mucosal defects
  Inflammatory disease
  Infiltrative disease
  Biochemical or genetic abnormalities

A variety of illnesses result in major loss of the intestine. In infants, necrotizing enterocolitis, volvulus, and intestinal atresias are common reasons for major small intestinal resections. In adults, short bowel syndrome is usually secondary to Crohn's disease, radiation enteritis, cancer, or mesenteric artery occlusion.

Malabsorption syndromes after small bowel resection are dependent on (a) the extent and location of resected bowel, (b) the condition of the remaining bowel and digestive organs, and (c) the ability of the remaining bowel to adapt (Weser, 1976). Anatomical factors which contribute to morbidity following massive small bowel resection include the location of the small bowel remnant, and the presence or absence of the ileocaecal valve and colon. Jejunal resections are better tolerated than ileal resections because the ileum actively transports bile salts and vitamin B_{12}, and has a slower transit time as well as greater potential for adaptation than the jejunum. Resection of less than 100 cm of ileum is defined as a minor resection but may cause watery diarrhoea, as opposed to steatorrhoea, because of incomplete absorption of bile salts. Minor ileal resection usually allows sufficient bile resorption to maintain fat absorption, but incomplete absorption of bile salts irritates the colonic mucosa, resulting in water diarrhoea. Cholestyramine has been recommended to help bind the irritating bile salts (Hoffman and Poley, 1972) in such cases.

Steatorrhoea usually follows a major loss of ileum with depletion of the entero-hepatic pool of bile salts. When bile salts are lost in the stool, after ileal resection, the rate of bile salt synthesis by the liver increases. With massive resection, however, the intraluminal bile salt concentration decreases resulting in diminished solubilization of lipid and malabsorption of both fat and fat-soluble vitamins (Chen, 1974). When the ileocaecal valve is lost by intestinal resection, extensive colonization of the small bowel by coliform bacteria occurs with resultant deconjugation of bile salts and diminished fat absorption (Sheldon, 1979).

Extensive small bowel resection often leaves diseased intestine to perform digestive function. The shortened intestine, particularly if diseased intestine remains, is often inadequate to maintain nutrition. Moreover, protein-calorie malnutrition (PCM) causes malabsorption leading to a 'vicious cycle' of PCM resulting from as well as causing malabsorption (Viteri and Schneider, 1974). PCM is associated with diminution of pancreatic and biliary secretions, which cause lipid malabsorption and deficiency of fat-soluble vitamins (A, D, E, K). As PCM progresses, the intestinal villi atrophy, the mucosal cells become cuboid, absorption is impaired, and diarrhoea occurs. Even when body composition is maintained by hyper-alimentation in patients with malabsorption syndromes, significant atrophy of intestinal villi occurs. The presence of intraluminal foodstuffs is necessary for maintenance of intestinal integrity of mucosa and gut-associated lymphatic tissues.

Surgical procedures and placement of electrodes for control of intestinal mobility have not been effective in the treatment of malabsorption syndromes. However, maintenance of body composition by long-term parenteral nutrition has allowed many patients to lead a relatively normal life. Moreover, approximately 10 to 20 per cent of patients on home hyper-alimentation eventually develop enough intestinal adaptation to live without intravenous feeding (Sheldon, 1979).

Intestinal adaptation by lengthening of the bowel and increasing villus height is well known. However, until the early 1970s, information concerning intestinal adaptation was based on patients who received nutrients orally and were frequently malnourished.

Long-term parenteral feedings are associated with increased acid and pepsin secretion, and a decrease in pancreatic bicarbonate response to secretin. The weight of the protein and DNA contents of enteric mucosa are 20 to 30 per cent lower in rats on trinitrophenol (TPN) for one to three weeks than in controls receiving either normal or elemental diets by mouth (Levine et al, 1974). In addition to causing intestinal hyperplasia, the 'nutrient stream', i.e., gastric, duodenal and pancreatico-biliary secretions (Altmann, 1971), have a trophic effect on the intestinal mucosa, which improves mucosal permeability (Williamson et al, 1978).

The complex process by which intestinal adaptation occurs after extensive bowel resection is incompletely understood. Therapy is broadly directed at minimizing malabsorption and diarrhoea and avoiding malnutrition.

Treatment of Short Bowel Syndrome

Optimal management of the patient with extensive bowel resection or significantly diseased intestine begins intraoperatively. The remaining small intestine is accurately measured with an umbilical tape stretched along the antimesenteric border of the remaining length of intestine from the ligament of Treitz. Hyperalimentation is initiated in the postoperative period with access to the venous system by Hickman or Broviac catheters (Evergreen Medical Supplies) (Figure 2). Standard subclavian catheterization with a polyvinyl catheter is avoided because of its high thrombosis rate (10 to 20 per cent) which will limit future intravenous access.

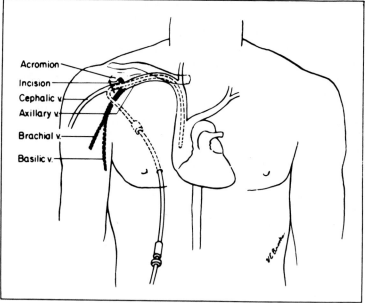

Figure 2. Position of silastic catheter utilized for home hyperalimentation. Note the Dacron® cuff located midway between the two incisions which anchors the catheter and provides a barrier to infection. From Riella and Scribner (1976) with kind permission of the editor of *Surgery, Gynecology and Obstetrics.*

During the postoperative period, the patient is taught to care for the catheter in such a fashion as to avoid mechanical and septic complications of home hyperalimentation. In addition, he is taught to aseptically prepare electrolytes and vitamins based on the minimal quantities necessary to maintain positive nitrogen balance. By learning to use and trouble-shoot an infusion pump the patient can administer his nutrient ration while asleep. Prior to beginning his work day, the infusion rate is decreased in preparation for discontinuing the infusion without developing rebound hypoglycaemia. When the infusion is complete, a heparin lock is placed, and the catheter capped.

Patients usually learn to care for their catheter and nutrient needs within one week. Because the intravenous infusion is in part designed to maintain hydration, patients are taught to monitor their urine osmolarity using a hydrometer. In addition, urine sugars are monitored on a daily basis. Patients on home hyperalimentation are followed weekly as outpatients for the first month after hospital discharge and then at three-monthly intervals. Because many commercial companies will deliver nutrient solutions and supplies to any site of the patients choosing, many have remarkably unrestricted life styles which include camping and fishing vacations in wilderness areas.

In addition to an extensive education programme in intravenous nutrition, patients with malabsorption must learn the fundamentals of nutrition under the instruction of dietitians. They must know the fat content of various foods in order to adhere to a low-fat diet and thus minimize steatorrhoea. During the early period after extensive intestinal resection, when gastric hypersecretion occurs and ingestion of all foodstuffs causes diarrhoea, minimal oral intake is encouraged. We usually allow the patient to eat dry food of his choosing while minimizing the fat content of the food and its propensity for causing diarrhoea. It is emphasized to the patient that intravenous feeding will maintain normal nutrition and that they may eat favourite foods for pleasure if they understand that excess quantities may induce diarrhoea. As intestinal adaptation occurs, more stringent adherence to a low-fat diet makes possible eventual discontinuation of intravenous feeding in some patients. The factors which contribute to diarrhoea associated with malabsorption are treated while nutrition is maintained by home hyperalimentation (Table 4).

Gastric hypersecretion occurs after extensive small bowel resection and may contribute to malabsorption by inactivation of pancreatic enzymes, and acid diarrhoea with fluid and electrolyte losses. Because gastric hypersecretion is associated with elevated levels of serum gastrin, cimetidine is usually administered to patients with short bowel syndrome for the initial three to six months. Because gastric hypersecretion is self-limited, cimetidine therapy need not be maintained indefinitely (Cortat et al, 1979; Murphy et al, 1979).

The osmolality of the ingested solution influences intestinal transit and contact time between the nutrient stream and the absorptive surface. To optimize nutrient-surface contact, fat-free solutions with an osmolality of approximately 230 mOsm/litre are employed in small quantities six times daily to supplement foods selected by the patient. Although some physicians use medium-chain triglyceride oil (MCT) because it is absorbed through the intestinal mucosa without the action of pancreatic lipase, our practice is to prescribe pancreatic enzymes and allow fat in small quantities

Table 4. *Clinical stages of short bowel syndrome*

Stage	Signs	Treatment
Stage I	Diarrhoea exceeds 2.5 l/day	1. Maintain fluid and electrolyte balance 2. Provide adequate TPN 3. Start half-strength Precision LR at 25 to 50 ml/h 4. Small quantities of diet of choice 5. Cimetidine 6. Pancreatic enzymes 7. Codeine
Stage II	Diarrhoea stable at less than 2.5 l/day	1. Continue TPN 2. Continue volume half-strength Precision LR 3. Low fat-free regular diet 4. Discontinue codeine 5. Discontinue cimetidine
Stage III	Stabilization of diarrhoea on low-fat diet.	1. Discontinue TPN if weight hydration maintained 2. Frequent feedings 3. Intermittent use of self-placed silastic naso-gastric tube for nocturnal feeding

to be ingested. MCT oil is a non-essential fat and frequently causes diarrhoea in spite of its ease of absorption.

Specific pharmacological agents such as codeine and belladona-containing compounds are occasionally useful in increasing intestinal transit time and maximizing absorption.

To enhance intestinal adaptation, a nutrient stream should be provided which does not inhibit enteric secretion. Because bile and pancreatic juice play a dominant role in the intestinal hyperplastic response, elemental diets which diminish pancreatic and biliary secretions are seldom indicated (Altmann et al, 1970, 1971). Numerous small feedings, initially of low fat and iso-osmolar solutions, are provided while nutrition is maintained with TPN.

Home hyperalimentation

Standard or special nutritional formulas are tailored to the patient's energy, protein, and micronutrient needs (Table 5). Basal energy requirements are estimated by the Harris-Benedict equations, with energy estimates increased in proportion to stress for females BEE $= 655 + 9.6W \times 1.8H - 4.7A$ and for males BEE $= 66 + 13.7W + 6.8A$; 1 to 2.5 g protein/per kg body weight daily is usually sufficient. The recommended daily allowance (RDA) for vitamins and electrolytes is administered. Fat is intravenously administered at 2 to 4 per cent of daily calories to prevent essential fatty acid deficiency (EFAD). Nitrogen balance is monitored during hospitalization to assess the adequacy of nutrient provided.

A long-term catheter (Hickman or Broviac) is positioned, at the time of initial intestinal resection, by cephalic venotomy with the catheter tip placement in the superior vena cava documented by fluoroscopy. The

Table 5. *Approximate maintenance formulas[a]*

Solutions	1	2	3
Volume	125 ml/h	13 ml/kg/24 h	
	3 l/day	losses	
Protein	18 g	1.0 g	18 g (Amino acids)
	(4.25%)	Amino acids	(4.25%)
Carbohydrate	3000 calories	Dextrose 47%	Dextrose 15%
	(Dextrose 10-47%)	(500-700 ml)	
Fat	500 ml/day	—	500 ml/day (20%)
Na	50 mEq/l	0	50 mEq/l
Cl	50 mEq/l	0	50 mEq/l
K	40 mEq/l	0	40 mEq/l
PO₄	20 mEq/l	0	20 mEq/l
Magnesium	8 mEq/l	0	8 mEq/l
Calcium	10 mEq/l	0	10 mEq/l
Acetate	50 mEq/l	0	50 mEq/l
Zn	5 mg/l	0	5 mg/l
Cu	500 μg/l	0	500 μg/l
Cr	10 μmole/l	0	10 μmole/l
MVI-12	10 ml/day	10 ml/day	10 ml/day
Vitamin K	10 mg IM/wk	10 mg IM/wk	10 mg IM/wk
Folic acid	2 mg/day	2 mg/day	2 mg/day
Vitamin B₁₂	100 μg IM/wk	100 μg IM/wk	100 μg IM/wk

[a]From Kudsk, Stone and Sheldon (1982), with kind permission of the authors and the editor of *Surgical Clinics of North America.*

Examples of daily maintenance solutions for different clinical situations:

If the therapeutic goal is replacement of oral intake, Solution 1 provides a reasonably balanced intravenous diet which can be adjusted based on monitoring panels and nitrogen balance.

Solution 2 is a fluid-restricted, low-nitrogen, high calorie infusion which is used for patients with acute renal failure (ARF). Usually, addition of electrolytes, vitamins and trace metals becomes necessary after several days of use. The role of intravenous fat in ARF is currently unclear. Solution 2 can be modified for use in other situations requiring volume restriction, such as cardiac failure. In patients with heart failure, the base solution is altered to contain K and Zn and limit Na.

Solution 3 is designed for patients with hypercarbic respiratory failure: fat is in part substituted for glucose as the caloric source, to lower the respiratory quotient (R.Q.).

When liver failure occurs, therapy is initiated with a formula comparable to Solution 2 if profound oedema is present, or Solution 1 if absent. Although patients with hepatic insufficiency can tolerate more protein intravenously than enterally, if hepatic encephalopathy is present, protein load is decreased and an intravenous hepatic amine or oral hepaticade solution containing high levels of branched-chain amino acids (BCAA) may be of use.

In most instances, Na:acetate:Cl ratios are maintained at 1:1:1. In all instances, alteration of the base formula should be based on (a) state of nutrition; (b) abnormal losses; and (c) nitrogen balance.

proximal end of the catheter exits the skin through a separate incision near the midline within reach of the patient (see Figure 2). Because venous access is crucial to maintenance of nutrition for the several years necessary for intestinal adaptation, great care of the catheter is required and percutaneous venous access is avoided. Because the life of a 'long-term' catheter is limited by infection or thrombosis (usually two years) it is necessary to plan the home hyperalimentation programme by anticipating the need for future venous access. Patients referred to our unit are evaluated by venograms of the subclavian system performed prior to attempting catheter placement. When subclavian, jugular and superior vena caval access is impossible, we place the catheter directly into the right atrium using a median sternotomy (Figure 3).

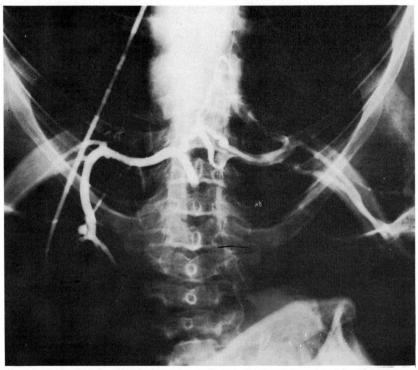

Figure 3. Venogram of patient on home hyperalimentation for eight years. After eight years of combined oral and intravenous feeding, the patient is able to maintain weight and hydration without intravenous supplementation. The venogram illustrates the access problem of long-term intravenous infusion as both subclavian and internal jugular veins and superior vena cava are occluded. For two years, the home intravenous infusions were administered through a catheter placed in the right atrium by thoracotomy. The patient is without oedema, in spite of occlusion of his venous system.

Home hyperalimentation training includes teaching the patient to convert his catheter into a heparin lock, cyclic administration of solutions, and avoidance of mechanical, metabolic and septic complications. The mechanical complications to be most feared are air embolus and venous thrombosis. Air embolism usually occurs from accidental disconnection of intravenous infusion tubing. Patients are provided with catheter repair kits and instructions for repairing broken or leaking catheters external to the skin tunnel.

Septic complications continue to be a problem. The commonest organism recovered from blood and catheter culture is *Staphylococcus epidermidis*. Daily cleansing of the catheter site and application of povidone-iodine paste minimizes but does not totally avoid infectious complications. When positive cultures occur, they are treated with culture-specific antibiotics through the catheter. If the catheter cannot be sterilized, it is removed. An infectious complication rate of nine episodes per 2956 patient days of home parenteral alimentation occurred in 1981 in our unit.

The first metabolic complication which may be encountered after initiation therapy is dehydration. Patients are instructed to measure the specific gravity of their urine with a hydrometer. If urine concentration exceeds 1.020 they call the hyperalimentation unit for adjustments in solution. If glucose is infused at rates greater than 0.5 g/kg/h, hyperglycaemia, hyperosmolar dehydration and coma may occur. Hyperosmolar, non-ketotic coma has a mortality rate exceeding 40 per cent and is an avoidable complication. Lesser degrees of hyperglycaemia are treated by the addition of insulin to the hyperalimentation solution.

The intravenous protein source is synthetic L-amino acids. Since acetate has been substituted for the chloride-amino acid linkage, hyperchloraemic acidosis seldom occurs. Pre-renal azotaemia occurs when the calorie/nitrogen ratio of the infusion is low, or if dehydration is present.

Electrolyte abnormalities occur infrequently in the stable patient receiving home hyperalimentation. However, if the patient is profoundly malnourished when hyperalimentation is initiated, large quantities of electrolytes will be required. Low serum potassium and phosphate values occur during repletion of the starved patient as a result of an ion shift from the extracellular to the intracellular fluid space. Hypokalaemia with cardiac arrhythmias may occur. Haemolytic anaemia, low values of adenosine triphosphate (ATP), and 2,3-diphosphoglycerate (2,3-DPG) accompany hypophosphataemia and are associated with a left-shifted oxy-haemoglobin dissociation curve, elevated cardiac output, and convulsions.

Essential fatty acid deficiency is characterized by flaky erythematous dermatitis, and may be aided by rubbing safflower oil on the skin. As it becomes possible for the patient to ingest some food, fat is gradually added. Essential fatty acid deficiency (EFAD) is prevented by administration of 2 to 4 per cent of the daily calories as fat. Fat emulsions are required (10 per cent soybean or safflower oil) twice weekly until sufficient oral fat can be provided.

Zinc deficiency is the commonest trace element deficiency which occurs during TPN. It will develop rapidly if patients are malnourished or have increased gastrointestinal losses when therapy is initiated. It is characterized by a scaly, dry dermatitis (acrodermatitis, enterohepatic), alopecia, and low serum zinc values. Copper deficiency is the second commonest trace metal deficiency. Copper is essential for normal metabolism of cytochrome C oxidase, ceruloplasmin, and other oxidases. Patients with copper deficiency develop anaemia, leucopenia, and lymphocytosis. Chromium deficiency is uncovered during prolonged (greater than six months) parenteral nutrition.

Chromium combines with insulin to form a ternary complex which acts on cell membrane receptors. Clinically, chromium deficiency presents as glucose intolerance and peripheral neuropathy.

The patient with short bowel syndrome requires considerable emotional support. He should be encouraged to live as independently of the 'medical system' as possible. Proper education in management of intravenous feedings leads to confidence and control of his life. In particular, he should be encouraged to eat and use his gastrointestinal tract in the hope that eventually he will not require intravenous feeding.

ACKNOWLEDGEMENT

Supported by USPHS National Institutes of Health Grants numbers NIGMO 3072 and NIGMS 18470.

REFERENCES

Altmann, G. G. (1971) Influence of bile and pancreatic secretions on the size of intestinal villi in the rat. *American Journal of Anatomy*, **132**, 167.

Altmann, G. G. & Leblond, C. P. (1970) Factors influencing villus size in the small intestine of adult rats as revealed by transposition of intestinal segments. *American Journal of Anatomy*, **127**, 15.

Chen, K. M. (1974) Clinical survey of the patient with massive resection of the small intestine during the last 10 years. *Journal of the Formosan Medical Association*, **73**, 35.

Conn, J. H., Chavez, C. M. & Fane, W. R. (1972) The short bowel syndrome. *Annals of Surgery*, **175**, 803.

Cortat, A., Fleming, R. C. Malagelada, J. R. et al (1979) Improved nutrient absorption after cimetidine in short bowel syndrome with gastric hypersecretion. *New England Journal of Medicine*, **300**, 79.

Hoffman, A. F. & Poley, J. R. (1972) Role of bile acid malabsorption in the pathogenesis of diarrhea and steatorrhea in patients with ileal resection. *Gastroenterology*, **62**, 918.

Kudsk, A. A., Stone, J. M. & Sheldon, J. M. (1982) Nutrition in trauma and burns. *Surgical Clinics of North America*, **62** (1), 183-192.

Levine, G. N., Deren, J. J., Steiger, E. et al (1974) Role of oral intake and maintenance of gut mass and disaccharidase activity. *Gastroenterology*, **67**, 975.

Mathews, D. M. (1975) Intestinal absorption of peptides. *Journal of Physiological Reviews*, **55**, 537.

Moog, F. (1981) The lining of small intestine. *Scientific American*, **245**, 154.

Murphy, J. P., King, D. R., Dubois, A. et al (1979) Treatment of gastric hypersection with cimetidine in short bowel syndrome. *New England Journal of Medicine*, **300**, 80.

Riella, M. C. & Scribner, S. (1976) Right atrial catheter for prolonged parenteral nutrition. *Surgery, Gynecology and Obstetrics*, **43**.

Scheflen, M., Galli, S. J., Perrotto, J. et al (1976) Intestinal adaptation after extensive resection of the small intestine and prolonged administration of parenteral nutrition. *Surgery, Gynecology and Obstetrics*, **143**, 757.

Sheldon, G. F. (1979) Role of parenteral nutrition in patients with short bowel syndrome. *American Journal of Medicine*, **67**, 1021.

Strauss, E., Gerson, C. D., Yalow, R. S. et al (1974) Hypersecretion of gastrin associated with the short bowel syndrome. *Gastroenterology*, **66**, 175.

Tilson, M. D. (1980) Pathophysiology and treatment of the short bowel syndrome. *Surgical Clinics of North America*, **60**, 1273.

Viteri, F. E. & Schneider, R. E. (1974) Gastrointestinal alterations in protein-calorie malnutrition. *Medical Clinics of North America*, **58**, 1487.

Weser, E. (1976) The management of patients after small bowel resection. *Gastroenterology*, **71**, 146-150.

Williamson, R. C., Bauer, F. L., Ross, J. E. et al (1978) Contributions of bile and pancreatic juice to cell proliferation in ileal mucosa. *Surgery*, **83**, 570.

10

Gluten-sensitive Enteropathy

Z. MYRON FALCHUK

Gluten-sensitive enteropathy is a disease of the small intestine in which the presence of a unique sensitivity to dietary gluten results in severe damage to the intestinal epithelial cell, with subsequent flattening of intestinal villi and malabsorption of nutrients. Our knowledge of the clinical and pathogenetic features of this condition has grown considerably during the last 30 years. One of the earliest descriptions of the disease is attributed to Samuel Gee (1888), who wrote that 'there is a chronic indigestion which is not seen in persons of all ages'. He did not appreciate the pathology of the intestine since he could deal only with postmortem tissue riddled with autolytic changes. He went on to add that 'if the patient be cured at all, it must be by means of diet . . . The allowance of farinaceous food must be small'. It is incredible that Gee came to this conclusion without the tools available in more modern times.

It was not until 1950 that investigators would once again come to this independent realization using the scientific armamentaria required to make a definitive statement. Dicke and others (Dicke et al, 1950, 1953; Van de Kamer et al, 1953, 1955), with the insight developed from various epidemiological observations, were able to show a substantial decrease in the wartime incidence of 'coeliac disease' in Holland. (Coeliac disease is a synonymous term for gluten-sensitive enteropathy.) This observation, and the knowledge that wheat was in short supply during the war, suggested that a diminished ingestion of wheat might have contributed to the observed decline in incidence of gluten-sensitive enteropathy. Working with various chemists (Van de Kamer et al, 1953, 1955; Hekkens, 1978), these scientists showed that wheat flour indeed contained the toxic material. Much additional work was required to show that it was gluten and, more precisely, gliadin — the alcohol-soluble glycoprotein in gluten — which was the damaging material. Gliadin is present in wheat, barley, and rye. Originally, oats were also thought to be injurious, but subsequent study did not bear this out.

Gluten is a complex glycoprotein, with sugars and amino acids forming the substance which confers upon dough the sticky, rubbery quality with which all bakers are familiar. Gluten is highly insoluble in water, a feature most investigators found to be a major drawback in studies of the disease.

As little as 3 g per day of gliadin will cause disease in susceptible patients (Van de Kamer, Weijers and Dicke, 1953). Amino acid analysis of gliadin has shown it to be rich in glutamine and proline (Van de Kamer and Weijers, 1955; Hekkens, 1978). Deamidation of the glutamine renders the substance harmless (Van de Kamer and Weijers, 1955). The work of Frazer et al (1959) was a keystone to many subsequent studies. He showed that gluten could be broken down into small fragments (with molecular weights from 2000 to 10 000) (Dissanayake et al, 1974) and still be toxic when fed to patients. The advantage of these small peptic-tryptic digestion products was that they were water-soluble and hence could facilitate a variety of investigations.

CLINICAL FEATURES

The disease typically presents in infancy after weaning and introduction of cereals into the diet. The peak incidence occurs between the ages of nine months and three years, with few cases occurring after the age of ten (Hamilton, Lynch and Reilly, 1969; Barry, Baker and Read, 1974; McNeish and Anderson, 1974). A second peak in incidence occurs in the third decade of life. It is striking to note that the patients in whom clinical disease develops in adult life have frequently been completely asymptomatic until the time of presentation. On the other hand, it is not uncommon for patients with childhood disease to have a clinical remission as adolescents and to tolerate gluten ingestion without symptoms, even though biopsy of the small intestine reveals characteristic pathological changes (Mortimer et al, 1968). The mechanism of these clinical vagaries is not understood.

The typical features of the disease are a diarrhoeal illness with frequent, foul-smelling, bulky stools, weight loss, and irritability (Gee, 1888; Katz and Falchuk, 1975). In children, failure to thrive is common. Secondary lactose intolerance develops as a result of injury to the brush border with decreased activity of all disaccharidase enzymes (Plotkin and Isselbacher, 1964). Oedema secondary to hypoalbuminaemia may appear. Potassium and other electrolytes are actively secreted as a result of an abnormally permeable intestinal mucosa (Fordtran et al, 1967).

All major foods are malabsorbed (protein, carbohydrate, and fat). The D-xylose absorption test is useful in screening for mucosal damage (Rolles et al, 1973). Steatorrhoea is accompanied by loss of fat-soluble vitamins; hence, osteomalacia, rickets (vitamin D), bleeding difficulties (vitamin K), and night blindness (vitamin A) may be encountered. Vitamin D malabsorption can also result in tetany. Of note, if magnesium levels remain normal, endogenous calcium may be mobilized from the skeleton, avoiding difficulties with tetany (Muldowney et al, 1970).

Roentgenological features of gluten-sensitive enteropathy are non-specific and resemble those seen in other malabsorptive disorders. The mucosal folds may become thickened, and the lumen of the bowel is frequently dilated. If non-colloidal barium suspensions are used, flocculation and break-up of the barium column may occur as the column moves down the small intestine. The modern colloidal suspensions of barium do not flocculate.

The disease may be difficult to diagnose since the presenting features may, at times, only obliquely suggest the diagnosis. Thus, constipation rather than diarrhoea (Mann, Brown and Kern, 1970), or osteomalacia (Moss, Waterhouse and Terry, 1965), or pure iron-deficiency anaemia (Mann, Brown and Kern, 1970), or even obesity may be the only manifestation (Mann, Brown and Kern, 1970). It is likely that the paucity of problems at the time of presentation may relate, in some fashion, to involvement of only a limited extent of bowel. The lesion is most severe in the duodenum and proximal jejunum (MacDonald et al, 1964). As one proceeds into the ileum, the lesion tends to become less pronounced and, ultimately, may even disappear. This is due to digestion of the gluten by pancreatic enzymes, causing it to lose its 'toxicity'. That all the small intestine is sensitive to the effects of gluten was shown by direct instillation of gluten into the normal ileum of patients with gluten-sensitive enteropathy. This produced typical lesions of gluten-sensitive enteropathy at the site of gluten infusion. As might be expected, patients with a severe lesion involving the ileum are likely to have vitamin B_{12} malabsorption accompanying the disease.

To establish the diagnosis, it is mandatory, at the outset, to obtain a small intestinal biopsy specimen and to document the characteristic lesion (vide infra). Two subsequent biopsy specimens are required to confirm the diagnosis — one obtained at three months after starting a gluten-free diet, and one obtained after a gluten challenge of at least two weeks (Booth, 1974). The biopsy morphology improves, with decreased inflammation and return of a columnar epithelial cell, only to revert after gluten challenge. If the tissue is normal after a gluten challenge of two weeks, the administration of gluten should be continued for three months. A normal biopsy specimen after such a challenge indicates that the original diagnosis was in error. Since the small intestine in children may become flat in a variety of other diseases, failure to confirm the diagnosis in this manner will result in improper diagnosis in as many as one-third of the patients (Packer et al, 1978).

Treatment requires life-long removal of gluten from the diet. There is no difference in response to gluten restriction between children and adults. Failure to respond adequately to gluten restriction should suggest either unknowing gluten ingestion, or a misdiagnosis. It has been shown more recently that concurrent exocrine pancreatic insufficiency may coexist, either because of abnormal pancreatic function, or because of deficient production of cholecystokinin-pancreozymin (Regan and Dimagno, 1980). Alternative approaches to establishing the diagnosis in a definitive way have been suggested. The approach to be described in more detail below uses organ culture methodology to show in vitro sensitivity to gluten by small intestinal explants (Falchuk et al, 1974). The gluten sensitivity in vitro can be documented by morphological criteria, by measurement of brush border enzyme activity, or by measurement of labelling indices when tissues are cultured with or without gluten peptides (Fluge and Asknes, 1981).

Other tests assess the production of leucocyte migration inhibition factor by lymphocytes from patients with disease when the lymphocytes are exposed in vitro to gluten (Ashkenazi et al, 1978). This test purports to identify 90 per cent of patients, albeit the study was not conducted in a double-blind manner. Finally, there are various tests which measure the permeability of the intestinal mucosa to various macromolecules in an effort to identify the 'leaky' membrane of gluten-sensitive enteropathy. The intestinal membrane in patients with gluten-sensitive enteropathy shows an increase in passive permeability to large polar molecules, including proteins and smaller polysaccharides, using cellobiose, a disaccharide with a molecular radius of 5 Å, and mannitol, a polyhydric alcohol with a radius of 4 Å. Cobden et al (1980) showed that untreated patients absorbed more cellobiose and less mannitol than controls or normals. This was true in 23 of 24 patients. They also showed that in other diseases where the mucosa might be more permeable, such as in Crohn's disease of the proximal intestine, the absorption of these macromolecules would be abnormal.

Except for a few research laboratories, none of the novel approaches described are within reach of the practising physician. Therefore, the final recommendation for establishing the diagnosis of the disease remains as above — three biopsies under appropriate conditions.

There are several complications which may have devastating effects on patients with gluten-sensitive enteropathy. 'Refractory sprue' is a condition which begins as ordinary gluten-sensitive enteropathy, but after some time symptoms and pathology return despite strict adherence to a gluten-free diet (Trier et al, 1978). This condition may respond favourably to treatment with corticosteroids. Ulcerative jejunoileitis (Bayless et al, 1967) may appear as a complication of gluten-sensitive enteropathy. The cause of the condition is unknown. Spontaneous ulceration of the small intestine develops which may perforate, stricture, or bleed. Not all cases of ulcerative jejunoileitis are clearly associated with an antecedent gluten-sensitive entero-pathy. The mortality rate of this complication is very high (60 per cent). Corticosteroids may be useful in its treatment.

Lymphadenopathy in debilitated patients, sometimes associated with lymphocytosis, has been described (Simmonds and Rosenthal, 1981), suggesting the diagnosis of lymphoma. However, the presence of mal-absorption suggests an intestinal lesion, and confirmation of this by small bowel biopsy allows the diagnosis of gluten-sensitive enteropathy. Pro-longed follow up on a gluten-free diet showed resolution of large masses of abdominal, mediastinal, and cervical lymphadenopathy in these patients. The differential diagnosis of unexplained lymphadenopathy should include gluten-sensitive enteropathy.

Certain malignancies of the gastrointesinal tract, including carcinoma and lymphoma (Gough, Read and Naish, 1962), occur more frequently in patients with gluten-sensitive enteropathy. Although the observation appears correct, the precise incidence of malignant transformation in these patients is not entirely clear. Estimates range from incidences as high as 5 to 10 per cent to as low as 1/10 of 1 per cent (Eidelman, Parkins and Rubin, 1966; Harris et al, 1967). In some instances, it is difficult to ascertain whether lymphoma of the small intestine antedates the gluten-sensitive enteropathy, since the biopsy of intestinal lymphoma may be misconstrued to represent gluten-sensitive enteropathy (Eidelman, Parkins and Rubin, 1966). Although suggestive, there are no conclusive data that gluten restriction in these patients will diminish the apparent increased risk of malignancy.

A number of less common associations have been reported with gluten-sensitive enteropathy. Recurrent inflammatory pericarditis (Dawes and Atherton, 1981) was a problem in two men until the diagnosis of gluten-sensitive enteropathy was made. Therapy with a gluten-free diet cured the pericarditis as well as the bowel disease. Another report of cutaneous vasculitis emphasizes the possible importance of immunological features in the disease. Thus, Meyers et al (1981) described a woman with cutaneous leucocytoclastic vasculitis, in whom the skin as well as the intestinal lesions were resolved with institution of a gluten-free diet. Whether circulating immune complexes, present in some patients with gluten-sensitive enteropathy (Doe, Booth and Brown, 1973; Hall et al, 1981), played a role in either the pericarditis or the vasculitis is a matter of conjecture. Finally, alpha-1-antitrypsin activity was reported to be abnormal in patients with gluten-sensitive enteropathy, but more definitive studies do not confirm this (Klasen et al, 1980).

A second disease, dermatitis herpetiformis (DH), has been described in which gluten-sensitive enteropathy is present (Weinstein et al, 1971). DH is an extremely pruritic, papulovesicular eruption of the skin which begins as an erythematous papule, vesicle, or urticarial-like plaque. The lesions tend to occur in groups on the extensor surfaces of the extremities, the back, and the intergluteal folds. The appearance of the lesions can lead to confusion with herpes simplex, erythema multiforme, scabies, and other pruritic skin lesions. The histology of the lesions is typified by collections of neutrophiles and microblisters (Katz et al, 1980). The infiltrate is in marked contrast to the lymphocytes which invade the intestinal wall in gluten-sensitive enteropathy. The diagnosis of DH is established by the clinical presentation, response to treatment with appropriate sulpha compounds, morphology of the lesion, and the presence of IgA deposits along the dermal-epidermal junction of the even normal skin (Cormane, 1967; Seah and Fry, 1975).

The latter point is now considered crucial to establishing unequivocally the diagnosis of DH. In that group of patients, that is, patients with DH documented by all of the above, intestinal biopsy shows a lesion characteristic of gluten-sensitive enteropathy in 80 to 90 per cent (Katz et al, 1980). Both the intestinal and the skin lesions respond favourably to gluten restrictions (Fry et al, 1973; Katz et al, 1980). The relation between the skin and the intestine in these two conditions remains to be established, but the genetic (Katz et al, 1977), immunological (Gebhard et al, 1974), and therapeutic (Fry et al, 1973) similarities suggest the association is not a simple chance occurrence. It is of interest that the intestinal lesion in patients with DH may not be as extensive or as severe as in patients with ordinary gluten-sensitive enteropathy. This probably accounts for the infrequent occurrence of clinical malabsorption in DH: only 5 to 10 per cent of patients.

THE JEJUNAL MUCOSA

The intestinal mucosa is one of the most rapidly proliferating tissues in the body. The normal villus height to crypt-depth ratio is 4:1. The epithelial cells begin in the crypt and ascend the villus in four to five days. The normal epithelial cell is columnar and its nucleus is located in the basal third of the cell. On its ascent out of the crypt, the epithelial cell loses its ability to divide (Trier and Browning, 1970) and acquires a mature brush border, with disaccharidase, peptidase, and alkaline phosphatase enzymes. The most apparent abnormality in the mucosa of patients with gluten-sensitive enteropathy is the loss of the villus architecture. There is a generalized flattening of the mucosa which may range from partial to total absence of villi (Perera, Weinstein and Rubin, 1975). The total thickness of the mucosa, however, may actually be increased since the lamina propria is infiltrated with plasma cells and lymphocytes, and the crypt is markedly hypertrophied (Perera, Weinstein and Rubin, 1975). The surface epithelial cells, rather than being tall and columnar, are cuboidal and become pseudo-stratified. The brush border, normally measuring 1 μm in height and bearing the important disaccharidases (including lactase) and peptidases, is shortened to a mean height of 0.5 μm and becomes sparse in its distribution. The interior of the cell is frequently full of vacuoles. Numerous lysosome-like bodies are present along with free-ribosomes and absent terminal webs (Rubin et al, 1966). The epithelial cell is so damaged as to be incapable of carrying on normal absorption.

In contrast to the villus surface cell, the crypt cell remains normal. The crypt mitotic activity is actually increased several-fold (Wright et al, 1973) and mitotic activity, normally stopping in the lower one-third of the crypt, may continue even to the surface (Trier and Browning, 1970). The migration time of a cell from the crypt to the surface is shortened to one to two days. The intraepithelial lymphocyte population, composed predominantly of T lymphocytes (Ferguson and Parrot, 1972; Arnaud-Battandier et al, 1978), is present in increased numbers in the epithelium of patients with active disease (Ferguson and Murray, 1971). Within three to six days of removing gluten from the diet, the surface epithelial cell is already reverting toward normal. In children maintained on a gluten-free diet, the architecture frequently achieves complete normality with return of villus structure. In adults, this happens less frequently, so that although the surface epithelial cell becomes normal with the return of tall columnar cells, the villus architecture with a villus height to crypt depth ratio of 4:1 rarely returns.

THE PATHOGENESIS OF GLUTEN-SENSITIVE ENTEROPATHY

The precise mechanism by which gluten produces the remarkable changes in the intestinal mucosa of sensitive subjects is not known. In the past 30 years, the data available regarding the pathogenesis of the disease have grown remarkably. The earliest theories regarded gluten-sensitive enteropathy as a disease due to an inborn error of metabolism, in which deficiency of an enzyme necessary for proper metabolism of gliadin allowed accumulation of toxic metabolites (Frazer et al, 1956, 1959; Cornell and Rolles, 1978). Van de Kamer's work (1955) showed that boiling gliadin in normal hydrochloric acid for periods of 45 minutes to two hours abolished the toxic effect of the gluten. Van de Kamer and his associate thought that, since hydrolysis converted glutamine side chains into glutamic acid, glutamine was critical to the toxicity of the gluten. These investigators noted that after the ingestion of gluten, blood glutamine values of patients with gluten-sensitive enteropathy were markedly increased when compared to values of normal children (Weijers and Van de Kamer, 1955), supporting the concept that metabolism of gluten was altered. Numerous investigators have attempted to determine directly whether certain peptidases or other enzymes are missing (Clark and Senior, 1969; Douglas et al, 1969, 1970). To date, no such deficiency has been found in tissues obtained from patients in remission, and enthusiasm for this theory has waned.

Phelan and colleagues (1977) have looked at the possibility that alternative mechanisms are responsible for the toxic effect of gliadin. Thus, they noted the failure of proteolysis of gluten, as performed by Frazer et al (1959), to abolish toxicity of the gluten molecule. They, in turn, postulated that toxicity resides not in a particular sequence of amino acids, but in a side-chain substituent such as a carbohydrate. Using a carbohydrase enzyme, they cleaved the carbohydrate moieties from the gluten and fed this modified gluten to three patients with gluten-sensitive enteropathy. Carbohydrase-treated gliadin did not result in damage to the intestinal mucosa of these three patients. The relevance of the carbohydrate side-chains of gluten to the toxic effects of gluten remains to be shown, and validation of this theory awaits more convincing experiments.

A novel hypothesis has been proposed by Weiser and Douglas (1976) to account for the toxicity of gluten. They postulate a defect of the cell surface membrane which allows gluten to act as a lectin and bind (Douglas, 1976) to the cell surface. As a consequence of this binding, a reaction is initiated which culminates in cell toxicity. However, few data support this concept.

There is an immunological theory regarding the pathogenesis of gluten-sensitive enteropathy. The morphology of the small intestine, with its dense infiltrate of plasma cells and lymphocytes in the lamina propria, as well as the increased number of intraepithelial lymphocytes (Ferguson and Murray, 1971), suggests a role for the immune system. The earliest observations supporting this hypothesis dealt with the presence of circulating antibodies directed at gluten in the bloodstream of patients with disease (Taylor et al, 1961; Alarcon et al, 1964; Katz, Kantor and Hershovic, 1968; Kendrick and Walker-Smith, 1970; Ferguson and Carswell, 1972), as well as the presence of a variety of autoantibodies (Seah et al, 1971; Lancaster-Smith, 1974). Additionally, patients with active disease have elevated levels of serum immunoglobulin A (IgA) (Asquith, Thompson and Cooke, 1969) and diminished levels of serum immunoglobulin M (IgM) (Hobbs and Hepner, 1968). These abnormalities are reversed by a gluten-free diet. Corticosteroids ameliorate the toxic effects of gluten; in patients ingesting a gluten-containing diet, a clinical remission will be achieved if they are given substantial doses of corticosteroids (Lepore, 1958; Wall et al, 1970). Although the mechanism by which glucocorticoids produce this effect is not known, it is known that glucocorticoids interfere with certain immunological functions (Saxon et al, 1978; Wahl, Altman and Rosenstreich, 1975).

Since serum antibodies can arise as a result of an abnormally permeable mucosal barrier which permits protein access to the circulation (Cobden, Rothwell and Axon, 1980), the demonstration of antibody production by the cells of the lamina propria was critical as the first step in providing substantiation that the local immune response participates in the disease process. Indeed, various investigators showed that patients and controls could have circulating antigluten antibody (as well as antibodies to other foods) (Alarcon et al, 1964; Kendrick and Walker-Smith, 1970; Ferguson and Carswell, 1972), indicating the non-specific quality of such serum antibodies in regard to gluten-sensitive enteropathy.

In searching for a more specific basis for implicating the immune response in the pathogenesis of gluten-sensitive enteropathy, Loeb et al (1971) showed that gluten challenge of patients with gluten-sensitive enteropathy in remission results in increased synthesis of IgA and IgM by the intestinal mucosa. Falchuk and Strober (1974), with an affinity chromatography technique (gluten-Sepharose columns), showed that a substantial portion of the increment of IgA and IgM synthesis was antigluten antibody; Brandtzaeg and Baklien (1976) showed that immunoglobulin G (IgG) was also involved. That local immune reactions occur during the ingestion of gluten was further substantiated by showing that gluten challenge results in deposition of immune complexes (of unknown make-up) in the lamina propria (Shiner and Ballard, 1972) and movement of lymphocytes into the intraepithelial location (Ferguson and Murray, 1971).

In support of the concept that antibodies can result in intestinal damage, McCarthy and colleagues described a patient without gluten-sensitive enteropathy in whom villus flattening of the small intestine was associated with an organ-specific anti-epithelial cell antibody in his circulation (McCarthy et al, 1978). The anti-epithelial cell antibody was IgG in class and was quite specific in that it affected only the mature epithelial cell and not the immature crypt cell of the small intestine. This patient was treated with cyclophosphamide immunosuppression, after which his mucosal morphology improved.

Even though IgA is the predominant local mucosal immunoglobulin (Tomasi, 1972), and even though IgA synthesis is markedly increased in the intestinal mucosa of patients with active gluten-sensitive enteropathy (Loeb et al, 1971), it is clear that IgA is not critical to the disease since gluten-sensitive enteropathy does develop in patients with IgA deficiency (Crabbe and Heremans, 1966). Studies by Brandtzaeg et al (1968) have demonstrated that in patients with IgA deficiency, the local immune system compensates for the loss of IgA by increased IgM production. Whatever the role of IgA in mucosal immunity in health and disease, it appears that IgM can replace this immunoglobulin. Patients with IgA deficiency may actually have an increased incidence of gluten-sensitive enteropathy (Crabbe and Heremans,

1966), since IgA may have a role in limiting antigenic absorption of macromolecules (Tomasi, 1972). It is important to emphasize that under no circumstances is gluten-sensitive enteropathy an allergic disease, since the IgE system is not at all abnormal. IgE is the classic antibody in true allergy.

To study the role of the local immune responses cited in the pathogenic process and to determine whether gluten could be directly toxic in intestinal tissue, an in vitro model of gluten-sensitive enteropathy was developed (Falchuk et al, 1974) using organ culture techniques (Browning and Trier, 1969). In the organ culture technique, intestinal biopsy specimens are cultured for periods of 24 to 48 hours. The tissue morphology and the enzyme activity of the brush border serve as markers of tissue condition. In relation to the villus cell, the crypt cell is relatively immature, lacking a fully developed brush border with its full complement of enzymes. In organ culture of normal intestinal tissue, brush border alkaline phosphatase and other enzyme activities increase, indicating occurrence of a general maturation of immature crypt cells. In organ culture of gluten-sensitive enteropathy tissue in gluten-free medium, a similar maturation occurs with a dramatic increase in alkaline phosphatase activity toward normal. These changes are accompanied by development of a tall columnar epithelial cell with a mature brush border. These enzymatic and morphological changes represent an in vitro remission of gluten-sensitive enteropathy tissue. Cultures of tissue in the presence of gluten produce markedly different results in mucosa from normal subjects and mucosa from those with gluten-sensitive enteropathy. Thus, culture of normal tissue in the presence of gluten does not alter either the morphology or the change in alkaline phosphatase activity. In contrast, culture of tissue from patients with gluten-sensitive enteropathy in the presence of gluten results in a drastic inhibition of the increase in alkaline phosphatase activity, and the morphology of the tissue remains unchanged, with numerous intracellular vacuoles, a cuboidal character, and a sparse brush border. This represents an in vitro perpetuation of the diseased state of gluten-sensitive enteropathy tissue.

Thus, the in vitro remission of gluten-sensitive enteropathy tissue in gluten-free medium, and perpetuation of the histological and enzymatic abnormalities of the tissue in a gluten-containing medium, represent an in vitro model of gluten-sensitive enteropathy. Of note, use of other food proteins in culture, for example, casein, does not result in alteration of either the appearance or enzyme activity of intestinal biopsy specimens from patients with gluten-sensitive enteropathy (Falchuk et al, 1974). The lesion is entirely gluten-dependent and is not seen in tissue from normal persons or from patients with other diseases of the small intestine.

The observations in these and other studies indicate that the crypt cell is apparently unharmed by the pathological process in the disease. The toxic effect of gluten occurs at or near the level of the surface, implying that only the more mature cells are at risk. The nature of the cytotoxic event, and the implications of its occurrence exclusively in the more mature cell as it acquires its normal surface components, is discussed further below.

In the organ culture experiments cited previously, it was noted that in contrast to tissue from patients in exacerbation, tissues from patients in remission were not affected by the presence of gluten in the culture medium. This observation suggests that gluten protein is not directly toxic to the epithelial cells of patients with gluten-sensitive enteropathy. Otherwise, during culture, gluten would equally affect tissue from patients with both active and inactive disease. It appears that gluten must first activate an endogenous effector mechanism in vivo which mediates gluten-induced toxicity. The concept that an endogenous effector mechanism is important to the disease was studied further in an experiment in which tissues from patients in remission (remission tissue) and, therefore, not susceptible to injury by gluten in vitro, could be exposed to substances made by tissue from patients in exacerbation (exacerbation tissue). In these studies, the tissue of patients in remission was rendered susceptible to injury by gluten by culturing both tissue specimens together on the same plate. Under these circumstances, exposure of the remission tissue to the medium bathing the exacerbation tissue rendered the remission tissue susceptible to the toxic effects of gluten (Gebhard et al, 1973; Strober et al, 1975). The implication of this observation is that tissue from patients with active disease produces either humoral substances or sensitized cells which can cross the medium and render the remission tissue sensitive to the effect of gluten.

Further support for the relevance of the immune theory in the pathogenesis of gluten-sensitive enteropathy comes from the observation that the inhibitory effect of gluten on both the increase in alkaline phosphatase and recovery of morphology in vitro can be eliminated by adding cortisol to the organ culture medium (Katz et al, 1976). Cortisol has multiple effects on immune phenomena and could interfere with immunoglobulin synthesis (Saxon et al, 1978) or T/B cell function. That sensitized lymphocytes are present under culture conditions and in the intestinal biopsy specimens was shown by Ferguson et al (1975). Macrophage-inhibitory factor is secreted by biopsy specimens cultured in the presence of alpha-gliadin, but not in its absence. The production of magrophage-inhibition factor by such cultures indicates that there is a population of lymphocytes sensitized to gliadin in the intestinal mucosa of patients with untreated gluten-sensitive enteropathy, and supports the theory that local cell-mediated immune reactions to gliadin are taking place in the intestinal mucosa.

In this context, the recent demonstration that intraepithelial lymphocytes (a high proportion of which appear to be T cells) (Ferguson and Parrot, 1972; Arnaud-Battandier et al, 1978) can participate in cellular cytotoxicity reactions of the antibody-dependent, mitogen-induced, and spontaneous variety (Arnaud-Battandier et al, 1978) is noteworthy. Thus, both humoral and cellular cytotoxicity seem to be present in the mucosa of patients with gluten-sensitive enteropathy.

The advent of monoclonal antibodies capable of identifying specific human lymphocyte subsets has allowed additional exploration of the role of lymphocytes in the cytotoxic mechanism of gluten-sensitive enteropathy. Monoclonal antibodies can identify cytotoxic helper and suppressor T lymphocytes (Reinherz and Schlossman, 1980). Theory would predict that in gluten-sensitive enteropathy, the bulk of the intraepithelial lymphocyte populations, that is, those cells in closest contact with the epithelial cells (and therefore the most likely to be involved in the cytotoxic process), would be of the cytotoxic phenotype as identified by the monoclonal reagents. Indeed, preliminary studies showed that the bulk of intraepithelial lymphocytes in patients with active gluten-sensitive enteropathy, but not normals, are cytotoxic T cell marker positive cells (Flores, Winter and Bhan, 1982). If confirmed, the information would go a long way toward conclusively showing the immunological nature of the cytopathic mechanism.

The organ culture technique is potentially useful not only for investigation, but also for establishing the diagnosis of gluten-sensitive enteropathy (Katz and Falchuk, 1978). The flat mucosal lesion of the small intestine results from a number of gastrointestinal disorders, which are particularly prevalent in infants, and include, in addition to gluten-sensitive enteropathy, acute gastroenteritis, chronic diarrhoea of infancy, cow's milk and soy protein allergy, eosinophilic gastroenteritis, immunodeficiency disorders, bacterial overgrowth, tropical sprue and giardiasis (Katz and Falchuk, 1978). As outlined previously, to establish the diagnosis definitively, it is necessary to obtain three biopsy specimens of the small intestine: one at the time of initial presentation, demonstrating the typical pathological lesion; one after adherence to a gluten-free diet to document reversal of the microscopic pathology; and one after a gluten challenge to show return to the disease. Failure to do this will result in an improper diagnosis of gluten-sensitive enteropathy being made in as many as one-third of the patients (Packer et al, 1978) and the condemnation of such patients to lifelong gluten restriction.

We prospectively studied 75 patients who presented with diarrhoea and/or malabsorption, and were able to show that the organ culture model correctly established the presence or absence of gluten-sensitive enteropathy in 70 of them. All 35 patients who had normal intestinal morphology and did not have gluten-sensitive enteropathy were correctly identified. Of the remaining 40 patients with abnormal small bowel biopsy specimens indistinguishable one from the other, 22 of 26 with gluten-sensitive enteropathy and 13 of 14 without it were correctly identified. The false-positive rate was 7 per cent (one of 14) and the false-negative rate was 15 per cent (4 of 26). The false-negative rate could be decreased if the patient's histocompatibility antigen is taken into account, since HLA-B8-negative patients tend not to show gluten sensitivity in vitro (vide infra).

These observations have been generally confirmed by other investigators (Howdle et al, 1981), although there is some outstanding controversy regarding the role of HLA type and in vitro gluten sensitivity (Falchuk, 1981).

GENETIC STUDIES

Gluten-sensitive enteropathy has an increased familial incidence, appearing in as many as 5 to 10 per cent of asymptomatic relatives of patients (McDonald, Dobbins, and Rubin, 1968). A major step forward in our understanding of gluten-sensitive enteropathy came about as a result of observations regarding the histocompatability antigen system. (In the HLA system, the terms gene and antigen are used interchangeably.) Two different HLA antigens appear with great frequency in patients with gluten-sensitive enteropathy. HLA-B8 is found in from 60 to 90 per cent of them (Falchuk, Rogentine and Strober, 1972; Stokes et al, 1972), in contrast to the frequency of 20 to 25 per cent of this antigen in the normal population. Moreover, HLA-DW3, a second HLA antigen, is present in 80 per cent of the patients with gluten-sensitive enteropathy (Keuning et al, 1976), in contrast to the incidence of 20 to 30 per cent in the normal population. Family studies in patients with gluten-sensitive enteropathy indicate that these histocompatibility antigens are, indeed, inherited and not disease-acquired antigen specificities. It should be noted that B8 and DW3 are associated with each other generally as a result of the phenomenon of linkage disequilibrium (i.e., alleles of two loci which do not combine randomly).

The relation of the histocompatibility antigen genes to gluten-sensitive enteropathy may be based on a number of different possibilities which can be gleaned from observations in well-studied animal systems. Thus, in the guinea pig, it has been clearly shown that the ability to mount immune responses to certain antigens is controlled by 'immune-response genes' which, in turn, are closely linked to the histocompatibility genes (McDevitt and Benacerraf, 1969). Animals lacking the appropriate histocompatibility gene cannot mount an immune response. In this regard, it should be pointed out that in gluten-sensitive enteropathy, a specific immune response to gluten which is unique is detected in the intestinal mucosa. It is possible that this represents a response facilitated by an 'immune-response gene' linked to the histocompatibility antigen. Another possibility to account for the increased incidence of HLA genes in a disease is that histocompatibility genes code for production of cell surface proteins which may function as receptors (Vladutiu and Rose, 1974). For example, there are certain viral illnesses in animals in which susceptibility to infection by the virus may be determined by the presence of a receptor for the virus on the cell surface (Lilly, 1970). The receptor, in turn, is coded for by a histocompatibility antigen which by its presence or absence, confers susceptibilty or resistance to infection. In the instance of gluten-sensitive enteropathy, binding of gluten to certain cell surface receptors present on the epithelial cells could facilitate production of immune responses, much as binding of a hapten to a carrier facilitates production of an immune response to the hapten. (Immunofluorescent data generated by Rubin et al (1965) show the presence of gliadin binding to the epithelial cell.)

If HLA-B8 is important to the receptor site for gluten, it might be possible to show differing sensitivity of intestinal biopsy specimens to gluten in vitro between patients with and without the HLA-B8 antigen. Indeed, Falchuk and co-workers showed that biopsies in organ culture from patients who are HLA-B8-positive have an increased susceptibility to the effect of gluten peptides than do tissues from patients who are not HLA-B8-positive (Falchuk et al, 1980). The explanation for this may be the presence of an altered binding site in patients without the HLA-B8 antigen, which can only bind partially degraded gluten. In vivo, such peptides are generated as a result of continued digestion by pancreatic enzymes. In vitro, such peptides are not generated since only a specific form of gluten is placed into the medium, and no additional configurations are generated during the culture. As a result, the in vitro system does not detect a sensitivity even when biopsy specimens from patients with gluten-sensitive enteropathy are cultured, because the gluten cannot bind to the altered site without further digestion.

The study brought into view the more fundamental question as to why the chemical form of gluten protein would influence the amount of toxicity induced in vitro in intestinal tissue obtained from B8-positive as compared to B8-negative patients. While a definitive answer to this question is not possible at this point, one possible hypothesis is based on the current understanding of the relationship of histocompatibility genes to gluten-sensitive enteropathy in particular, and immunologically mediated cytotoxicity in general.

A central feature of the hypothesis regarding the pathogenesis of gluten-sensitive enteropathy is the identification of an appropriate target of cytotoxicity. In this context, it is possible that gastrointestinal epithelial cells in gluten-sensitive enteropathy bear gluten protein-specific receptors and gluten protein binds to such receptors, thus becoming a specific target of local mucosal immunological effector mechanisms. Alternatively, it is possible that gluten protein interacts chemically with the cell surface, and forms an immunologic target in the absence of a specific receptor.

The concept that epithelial cells with bound gluten protein form a target for cytotoxic reactions in gluten-sensitive enteropathy allows one to postulate a role for HLA antigens in the effector mechanisms responsible for tissue injury in this disease. To understand how this may be so, two facts concerning cytotoxicity are pertinent: (1) Stimulation of animals with syngeneic cells which have been chemically or virally modified results in the generation of cytotoxic T cells with specificity for target cells bearing the modifying chemical or viral moiety, as well as the histocompatibility antigen present on the stimulating cells. Thus, if an animal is immunized with chemically modified syngeneic cells, for example cells with surface proteins modified with trinitrophenol (TNP), the animal will form cytotoxic effector cells (T cells) for cell targets bearing both TNP groups and the particular histocompatibility antigens present on the stimulating cells — i.e., histocompatibility antigens already present in the immunized animal. The effector cell either recognizes closely associated but separate modifying antigens and histocompatibility antigens (dual recognition), or recognizes a single, modified histocompatibility antigen (Shearer and Schmitt-Verlhulst, 1977). (2) It has been shown that histocompatibility antigens may determine which modifying antigen will bind to the cell surface. Thus, Bubbers et al (1978) have obtained data that the binding of virus to cell surfaces occurs preferentially at surface sites near particular histocompatibility antigens. In this instance, a histocompatibility antigen may serve as a receptor for a virus.

In view of these facts concerning murine cytotoxicity mechanisms, we can postulate that, in gluten-sensitive enteropathy, the recognition of epithelial cell targets involves concomitant recognition of modifying antigen (in this case, gluten protein) and histocompatibility antigen. Furthermore, the presence of certain histocompatibility antigens determines to some extent the precise nature of the protein bound. In this latter regard, it appears the B8 positivity and B8 negativity impose restrictions on the chemical form of gluten protein interacting with the cell surface: B8-positive individuals form a cytotoxic target with relatively intact protein or with degradation products of gluten protein, whereas B8-negative individuals form cytotoxicity targets only with degraded products of gluten protein.

Thus, the differences between HLA-B8-positive and HLA-B8-negative patients in organ culture studies are consistent with the following: the nature of the HLA antigen present in any given patient places certain restrictions on the chemical form of gluten protein capable of binding to epithelial cells; this, in turn, leads to differences in tissue susceptibility to toxicity in situations where complete degradation of gluten is limited (organ culture). These concepts are compatible with the view that the relevant cyto-toxic mechanism in gluten-sensitive enteropathy is either a T cell-mediated mechanism or a B cell-mediated mechanism. In the former instances, histocompatibility antigens facilitate binding of gliadin or gliadin fragment to epithelial cells and, in addition, form a part of the target on epithelial cells recognized by cytotoxic T cells. In the latter instances, histo-compatibility antigens facilitate binding of gliadin or gliadin fragment to epithelial cells, but do not form part of the epithelial target recognized by cytotoxic antibodies or antibodies, or antibodies cooperating with killer lymphocytes.

The observation that 20 to 30 per cent of normal people without gluten-sensitive enteropathy possess HLA-B8 and/or DW3 suggests that HLA antigens alone are not sufficient to determine disease susceptibility. Genetic analysis of HLA antigens in patients and their families suggested the possible need for a second genetic factor (Falchuk et al, 1978). Such a genetic marker was found by Mann et al, who detected an antigen on the surface of B lymphocytes of patients with gluten-sensitive enteropathy (Mann et al, 1976). This marker is present in 75 to 80 per cent of patients but only in 6 to 18 per cent of normal people. In contrast to the general normal population, the antigen is present in 100 per cent of parents of patients (Pena et al, 1978). Thus, the gene coding for this antigen has a recessive mode of inheritance. Furthermore, it appears that a homozygous condition for this gene, in addition to the HLA antigen, is required for disease manifestation. The role of this B cell-associated gene in gluten-sensitive enteropathy is not clear, but the product of this gene may contribute to the formation of the postulated cell surface receptor.

Data have been developed which suggest that HLA-B8 may be associated with a generalized immune hyperresponsiveness (Vladutiu and Rose, 1974) (or, alternatively, to diminished immunoregulation because of inadequate suppressor mechanisms); for example, HLA-B8 is found in increased incidence in patients with certain diseases of altered immunity or auto-immunity, e.g., myasthenia gravis, juvenile diabetes mellitus, chronic active hepatitis, and Sjogren's syndrome (Vladutiu and Rose, 1974). Individuals with these HLA genes may have a more vigorous immune response to certain antigens. In support of this is the observation of Cunningham-Rundles, in which in vitro lymphocyte transformation to wheat antigens among HLA-B8-positive normal donors was much stronger than among HLA-B8-negative normals (Cunningham-Rundles et al, 1978). Mawhiney showed that oral challenge with polio virus produces a significantly higher antibody response in patients with gluten-sensitive enteropathy than in normals, once again supporting the concept that these patients are hyper-responding to various oral antigens (Mawhiney and Love, 1974). A variety of factors may, therefore, be coinciding to result in gluten-sensitive enteropathy.

Kagnoff (Trefts and Kagnoff, 1981; Kagnoff, 1982) has shown that such complex genetic interactions occur in mice. In that instance, he showed that two genetic loci control the murine response to A-gliadin, the toxic component of gluten. One locus maps to the H-2 region of the mouse, the equivalent of the HLA region in humans, while the other maps to a separate chromosome altogether. The second gene in fact appears linked to genes that code for immunoglobulin heavy chain allotypes. It is alluring to speculate that the two-gene hypotheses for gluten-sensitive enteropathy may have a parallel in the murine species.

A hypothesis regarding the pathogenesis of gluten-sensitive enteropathy can be summarized as follows. Cell surface proteins, which are coded for by histocompatibility antigen genes and the B cell gluten-sensitive enteropathy-associated gene, are present in patients with gluten-sensitive enteropathy. The chance occurrence of the two genes in the same person results in formation of a receptor-complex on the epithelial cell or intestinal lymphocyte, to which gluten can bind. As a result of binding, gluten becomes immunogenic, prompting production of antigluten antibody, sensitized lymphocytes, and probably lymphokines. These various immune products can then return to the epithelial cell and injure it. It is important to note that the epithelial cell of gluten-sensitive enteropathy patients would, in this context, become a specific target for immune lysis by the various effector systems outlined, rendered so by the gluten bound to its surface.

SUMMARY

Gluten-sensitive enteropathy is a disease in which the small intestinal mucosa of susceptible persons is damaged after eating gluten-containing foods. The damaged intestinal mucosa is incapable of normal function, and the affected patients have malabsorption of one or more dietary components. The childhood and adult forms of the disease are identical.

The small intestinal lesion is characterized by villus flattening, cuboidal epithelial cells, and infiltration of the lamina propria with lymphocytes and plasma cells. The diagnosis in all cases must be confirmed by intestinal biopsy before and after treatment with a gluten-free diet, since other conditions may produce a similar lesion. The post-treatment biopsy should disclose reversion toward normal. Treatment with a gluten-free diet is lifelong.

Various theories have been proposed to account for the pathogenesis of the gluten-induced damage. These include the presence of an enzyme deficiency which allows toxic degradation products of gluten to accumulate and kill the epithelial cell, and the presence of surface receptors which allow binding of gluten to the cell surface, with cell death as the result. A third theory states that immune factors are important since antigluten antibodies are made in the mucosa, and cortisone inhibits the lesion in vivo and in vitro. Genetic studies show a familial pattern of the disease and a preponderance of histocompatibility antigens, HLA-B8 and HLA-DW3. The pathogenesis may be related to cell surface receptors, allowing for immunological cytopathic factors to be generated. An in vitro technique of culturing biopsy specimens may be useful in making a diagnosis.

ACKNOWLEDGEMENT

Supported in part by a grant from the United States Public Health Service National Institutes of Health No. AM32054.

REFERENCES

Alarcon, D., Segovia, P., Herskovic, T. et al (1964) Presence of circulating antibodies to gluten and milk fractions in patients with nontropical sprue. *American Journal of Medicine,* **36,** 485.

Arnaud-Battandier, F., Bundy, B. M., O'Neill, M. et al (1978) Cytotoxic activities of gut mucosal lymphoid cells in guinea pigs. *Journal of Immunology,* **121,** 1059.

Ashkenazi, A., Idar, D., Handzel, Z. T. et al (1978) An in vitro immunological assay for diagnosis of coeliac disease. *Lancet,* **i,** 627.

Asquith, P., Thompson, R. A. & Cooke, W. T. (1969) Serum immunoglobulins in adult coeliac disease. *Lancet,* **ii,** 129.

Barry, R. E., Baker, P. & Read, A. E. (1974) Coeliac disease. The clinical presentation. *Clinics in Gastroenterology,* **3,** 55.

Bayless, T. M., Kaplowitz, R. F., Shelley, W. M. et al (1967) Intestinal ulceration as a complication of celiac disease. *New England Journal of Medicine,* **236,** 996.

Booth, C. C. (1974) Definition of adult celiac disease. *Proceedings of the Second Celiac Symposium* (Ed.) Hekkens, W. Th, J. M. & Pena, A. p. 10. Leiden, Holland: H. E. Stenfert Kroese B.V.

Brandtzaeg, P. & Baklien, K. (1976) Immunohistochemical studies of the formation and epithelial transport of immunoglobulins in normal and diseased human intestinal mucosa. *Scandinavian Journal of Gastroenterology,* **11** (Supplement 36), 5.

Brandtzaeg, P., Fjellanger, I. & Gjeruldsen, S. T. (1968) Immunoglobulin synthesis and selective secretion in patients with immunoglobulin A deficiency. *Science,* **160,** 789.

Browning, T. H. & Trier, J. S. (1969) Organ culture of mucosal biopsies of human small intestine. *Journal of Clinical Investigation,* **48,** 1423.

Bubbers, J. E., Chen, S. & Lilly, F. (1978) Non-random inclusions of H-2K and H-2D antigens in Friend virus particles from mice of various strains. *Journal of Experimental Medicine,* **147,** 340.

Clark, M. L. & Senior, J. R. (1969) Small gut mucosal activities of pyrimidine precursor enzymes in celiac disease. *Gastroenterology,* **56,** 887.

Cobden, I., Rothwell, J. & Axon, A. T. R. (1980) Intestinal permeability and screening tests for coeliac disease. *Gut,* **21,** 512.

Cormane, R. H. (1967) Immunofluorescent studies of the skin in lupus erythematosus and other diseases. *Pathologia Europaea,* **2,** 170.

Cornell, H. J. & Rolles, C. J. (1978) Further evidence of a primary mucosal defect in coeliac disease. In vitro mucosal digestion studies in coeliac patients in remission, their relatives, and control subjects. *Gut,* **19,** 253.

Crabbe, P. A. & Heremans, J. F. (1966) Lack of gamma-A immunoglobulin in serum of patients with idiopathic steatorrhea. *Gut,* **7,** 119.

Cunningham-Rundles, S., Cunningham-Rundles, C., Pollack, M. S. et al (1978) Response to wheat antigen in in vitro lymphocyte transformation among HLA-B8-positive normal donors. *Transplantation Proceedings,* **10,** 977.

Dawes, P. T. & Atherton, S. T. (1981) Coeliac disease presenting as recurrent pericarditis. *Lancet,* **i,** 1021.

Dicke, W. K. (1950) Coeliac disease: investigation of harmful effects of certain types of cereal on patients with celiac disease. Thesis. Netherlands University of Utrecht.

Dicke, W. K., Weijers, H. A. & Van de Kamer, J. H. (1953) Coeliac disease. II. The presence in wheat of a factor having a deleterious effect in cases of coeliac disease. *Acta Paediatrica,* **42,** 34.

Dissanayake, A. S., Jerrome, D. W., Offord, R. E. et al (1974) Identifying toxic fractions of wheat gluten and their effect on the jejunal mucosa in coeliac disease. *Gut,* **15,** 931.

Doe, W. F., Booth, C. C. & Brown, D. L. (1973) Evidence for complement-binding immune complexes in adult coeliac disease, Crohn's disease, and ulcerative colitis. *Lancet,* **ii,** 402.

Douglas, A. P. (1976) The binding of a glycopeptide component of wheat to intestinal mucosa of normal and coeliac human subjects. *Clinica et Chimica Acta,* **73,** 357.

Douglas, A. P. & Booth, C. C. (1969) Postprandial plasma-free amino acids in adult coeliac disease after oral gluten and albumin. *Clinical Science,* **37,** 643.

Douglas, A. & Peters, T. J. (1970) Peptide hydrolase activity of human intestinal mucosa in adult coeliac disease. *Gut,* **11,** 15.

Eidelman, S., Parkins, R. A. & Rubin, C. E. (1966) Abdominal lymphoma presenting as malabsorption. A clinicopathological study of nine cases in Israel and a review of the literature. *Medicine* (Baltimore), **45,** 11.

Falchuk, Z. M. (1981) In vitro gluten sensitivity. *Gastroenterology,* **81,** 978.

Falchuk, Z. M. & Strober, W. (1974) Gluten-sensitive enteropathy. Synthesis of antigliadin antibody in vitro. *Gut,* **15,** 947.

Falchuk, Z. M., Rogentine, G. N. & Strober, W. (1972) Predominance of histocompatibility antigen HLA-8 in patients with gluten-sensitive enteropathy. *Journal of Clinical Investigation,* **51,** 1601.

Falchuk, Z. M., Gebhard, R. L., Sessoms, C. et al (1974) An in vitro model of gluten sensitive enteropathy. *Journal of Clinical Investigation,* **53,** 487.

Falchuk, Z. M., Katz, A. J., Shwachman, H. et al (1978) Gluten-sensitive enteropathy: genetic analysis and organ culture study in 35 families. *Scandinavian Journal of Gastroenterology,* **13,** 839.

Falchuk, Z. M., Nelson, D. L., Katz, A. J. et al (1980) Gluten-sensitive enteropathy: influence of histocompatibility type on gluten sensitivity in vitro. *Journal of Clinical Investigation,* **66,** 277.

Ferguson, A. & Carswell, F. (1972) Precipitins to dietary proteins in serum and upper intestinal secretions of coeliac children. *British Medical Journal,* **i,** 75.

Ferguson, A. & Murray, D. (1971) Quantitation of intraepithelial lymphocytes in human jejunum. *Gut,* **12,** 988.

Ferguson, A. & Parrot, D. M. V. (1972) The effect of antigen deprivation on thymus dependent and thymus independent lymphocytes in the small intestine of the mouse. *Clinical and Experimental Immunology,* **12,** 477.

Ferguson, A., MacDonald, T. T., McClure, J. P. et al (1975) Cell-mediated immunity to gliadin within the small intestinal mucosa in coeliac disease. *Lancet,* **i,** 895.

Flores, A. F., Winter, H. S. & Bhan, A. K. (1982) In vitro model to assess immunoregulatory T lymphocyte subpopulations in gluten-sensitive enteropathy. *Gastroenterology,* **82,** 1058.

Fluge, G. & Asknes, L. (1981) Labelling indices of ^{3}H-thymidine incorporation during organ culture of duodenal mucosa in coeliac disease. *Scandinavian Journal of Gastroenterology,* **16,** 921.

Fordtran, J. S., Rector, F. C., Locklear, T. W. et al (1967) Water and solute movement in the small intestine of patients with sprue. *Journal of Clinical Investivation,* **46,** 287.

Frazer, A. C. (1956) Discussion on some problems of steatorrhea and reduced stature. *Proceedings of the Royal Society of Medicine,* **49,** 1009.

Frazer, A. C., Fletcher, R. F., Ross, C. A. C. et al (1959) Gluten induced enteropathy. The effect of partially digested gluten. *Lancet,* **ii,** 252.

Fry, L., Seah, P. P., Riches, D. J. et al (1973) Clearance of skin lesions in dermatitis herpetiformis after gluten withdrawal. *Lancet*, **i**, 288.

Gebhard, R. L., Falchuk, Z. M., Sessoms, C. S. & Strober, W. (1973) Demonstration of gliadin toxicity in vitro. Evidence for an endogenous effector mechanism in gluten sensitive enteropathy. *Journal of Clinical Investigation*, **52**, 32a.

Gebhard, R. L., Falchuk, Z. M., Katz, S. I. et al (1974) Dermatitis herpetiformis: immunologic concomitants of small intestinal disease and relationship to histocompatibility antigen HL-A8. *Journal of Clinical Investigation*, **54**, 98.

Gee, S. (1888) On the coeliac affliction. *St Bartholomews Hospital Reports*, **24**, 17.

Gough, K. R., Read, A. E. & Naish, J. M. (1962) Intestinal reticulosis as a complication of steatorrhea. *Gut*, **3**, 232.

Hall, R. P., Strober, W., Katz, S. I. et al (1981) IgA-containing circulating immune complexes in gluten sensitive enteropathy. *Clinical and Experimental Immunology*, **45**, 234.

Hamilton, J. R., Lynch, M. J. & Reilly, B. J. (1969) Active celiac disease in childhood. *Quarterly Journal of Medicine*, **38**, 135.

Harris, O. D., Cooke, W. T., Thompson, H. et al (1967) Malignancy in adult celiac disease and idiopathic steathorrhea. *American Journal of Medicine*, **42**, 899.

Hekkens, W. Th. & J. M. (1978) The toxicity of gliadin, a review. *Perspectives in Coeliac Disease* (Ed.) McNicholl, B., McCarthy, C. F. & Fottrell, P. F. p. 3. Lancaster: MTP Press.

Hobbs, J. R. & Hepner, G. W. (1968) Deficiency of IgM in coeliac disease. *Lancet*, **i**, 217.

Howdle, P. D., Corazza, G. R., Bullen, A. W., et al. (1981) Gluten sensitivity of small intestinal mucosa in vitro: quantitative assessment of histologic change. *Gastroenterology*, **80**, 442.

Kagnoff, M. F. (1982) Two genetic loci control the murine immune response to A-gliadin, a wheat germ protein that activates coeliac sprue. *Nature*, **296**, 158.

Katz, A. J. & Falchuk, Z. M. (1975) Current concepts in gluten sensitive enteropathy (celiac sprue). *Pediatric Clinics of North America*, **22**, 767.

Katz, A. & Falchuk, Z. M. (1978) The definitive diagnosis of gluten-sensitive enteropathy: use of an in vitro organ culture model. *Gastroenterology*, **75**, 695.

Katz, J., Kantor, F. S. & Hershovic, T. (1968) Intestinal antibodies to wheat fractions in celiac disease. *Annals of Internal Medicine*, **69**, 1149.

Katz, A., Falchuk, Z. M., Strober, W. et al (1976) Gluten-sensitive enteropathy. Inhibition by cortisol on the effect of gluten protein in vitro. *New England Journal of Medicine*, **295**, 131.

Katz, S. I., Hertz, K. C., Rogentine, G. N. et al (1977) HLA-B8 and dermatitis herpetiformis in patients with IgA deposits in skin. *Archives of Dermatology*, **113**, 155.

Katz, S. I., Hall, R. P., Lawley, T. J. et al. (1980) Dermatitis herpetiformis: the skin and the gut. *Annals of Gut Medicine*, **93**, 857.

Kendrick, K. G. & Walker-Smith, A. J. (1970) Immunoglobulins and dietary protein antibodies in childhood coeliac disease. *Gut*, **11**, 635.

Keuning, J. J., Pena, A. S., Van Leeuwen, A. et al (1976) HLA-DW3 associated with coeliac disease. *Lancet*, **i**, 506.

Klasen, E. C., Polanco, I., Biemond, I. et al (1980) α_1-Antitrypsin and coeliac disease in Spain. *Gut*, **21**, 948.

Lancaster-Smith, M. J., Perrin, J., Swarbrick, E. T. et al (1974) Coeliac disease and autoimmunity. *Postgraduate Medical Journal*, **50**, 45.

Lepore, M. J. (1958) Long term maintenance of adrenal steroid therapy in non-tropical sprue. *American Journal of Medicine*, **25**, 381.

Lilly, F. (1970) FV-2, identification and location of a second gene governing the spleen focus response to Friend leukemia virus in mice. *Journal of the National Cancer Institute*, **45**, 163.

Loeb, P. M., Strober, W., Falchuk, Z. M. et al (1971) Incorporation of leucine-^{14}C into immunoglobulins by jejunal biopsies of the patients with celiac sprue and other gastrointestinal disease. *Journal of Clinical Investigation*, **50**, 559.

MacDonald, W. C., Dobbins, W. O. & Rubin, C. E. (1968) Studies on the familial nature of celiac sprue using biopsy of the small intestine. *New England Journal of Medicine*, **272**, 448.

MacDonald, W. C., Brandborg, L. L., Flick, A. L. et al (1964) Studies of celiac sprue. IV. The response of the whole length of the small bowel to a gluten-free diet. *Gastroenterology,* **47,** 573.

Mann, J. G., Brown, W. R. & Kern, F. (1970) The subtle and variable clinical expressions of gluten induced enteropathy. *American Journal of Medicine,* **48,** 357.

Mann, D. L., Katz, S. I., Nelson, D. L. et al (1976) Specific B cell antigens associated with gluten sensitive enteropathy and dermatitis herpetiformis. *Lancet,* **i,** 110.

Mawhiney, H. & Love, A. H. G. (1975) The immunoglobulin class responses to oral polio vaccine in coeliac disease. *Clinical and Experimental Immunology,* **22,** 47.

McCarthy, D. M., Katz, S. I., Gazze, L. et al (1978) Selective IgA deficiency associated with total villous atrophy of the small intestine and an organ-specific anti-epithelial cell antibody. *Journal of Immunology,* **120,** 932.

McDevitt, H. O. & Benacerraf, B. (1969) Genetic control of specific immune responses. *Advances in Immunology,* **11,** 31.

McNeish, A. S. & Anderson, C. M. (1974) Coeliac disease. The disorder in childhood. *Clinics in Gastroenterology,* **3,** 127.

Meyers, S., Dikman, S., Spiera, H. et al (1981) Cutaneous vasculitis complicating coeliac disease. *Gut,* **22,** 61.

Mortimer, P. E., Stewart, J. S., Norman, A. P. et al (1968) Follow-up study of coeliac disease. *British Medical Journal,* **iii,** 7.

Moss, A. J., Waterhouse, C. & Terry, R. (1965) Gluten sensitive enteropathy with osteomalacia but without steatorrhea. *New England Journal of Medicine,* **272,** 825.

Muldowney, E. P., McKenna, T. J., Kyle, L. H. et al (1970) Parathormone-like effect of magnesium replenishment in steatorrhea. *New England Journal of Medicine,* **281,** 61.

Packer, S. M., Charlton, V., Keeling, J. W. et al (1978) Gluten challenge in treated coeliac disease. *Archives of Diseases in Childhood,* **53,** 449.

Pena, A. S., Mann, D. L., Hague, N. E. et al (1978) Genetic basis of gluten sensitive enteropathy. *Gastroenterology,* **75,** 230.

Perera, D. R., Weinstein, W. M. & Rubin, C. E. (1975) Small intestinal biopsy. *Human Pathology,* **6,** 157.

Phelan, J. J., Stevens, F. M., McNicholl, B. et al (1977) Coeliac disease: the abolition of gliadin toxicity by enzymes from *Aspergillus niger. Clinical Science and Molecular Medicine,* **53,** 35.

Plotkin, G. R. & Isselbacher, K. J. (1964) Secondary disaccharide deficiency in adult celiac disease and other malabsorption states. *New England Journal of Medicine,* **271,** 1033.

Regan, P. T. & Dimagno, E. P. (1980) Exocrine pancreatic insufficiency in celiac sprue: a cause of treatment failure. *Gastroenterology,* **78,** 484.

Reinherz, E. L. & Schlossman, S. F. (1980) The differentiation and function of human T lymphocytes. *Cell,* **19,** 821.

Rolles, C. J., Kendall, M. J., Nutter, S. et al (1973) One hour blood xylose screening test for coeliac disease in infants and young children. *Lancet,* **ii,** 1043.

Rubin, W., Fauci, A. S., Sleisinger, M. H. et al (1965) Immunofluorescent studies in adult celiac disease. *Journal of Clinical Investigation,* **44,** 475.

Rubin, W., Ross, L. L., Sleisenger, M. H. et al (1966) An electron microscopic study of adult celiac disease. *Laboratory Investigations,* **15,** 1720.

Saxon, A., Stevens, R. H., Ramer, S. J. et al (1978) Glucocorticoids administered in vivo inhibit human suppressor T lymphocytes function and diminish B lymphocytes responsiveness in in vitro immunoglobulin synthesis. *Journal of Clinical Investigations,* **61,** 922.

Seah, P. P. & Fry, L. (1975) Immunoglobulins in the skin in dermatitis herpetiformis and their relevance in diagnosis. *British Journal of Dermatology,* **92,** 157.

Seah, P. P., Fry, L., Hoffbrand, A. V. et al (1971) Tissue antibodies in dermatitis herpetiformis and adult coeliac disease. *Lancet,* **i,** 834.

Shearer, G. M. & Schmitt-Verlhulst, A. M. (1977) Major histocompatibility complex restricted cell-mediated immunity. *Advances in Immunology,* **25,** 55.

Shiner, M., & Ballard, J. (1972) Antigen-antibody reactions in jejunal mucosa in childhood coeliac disease after gluten challenge. *Lancet,* **i,** 1202.

Simmonds, J. P. & Rosenthal, F. D. (1981) Lymphadenopathy in coeliac disease. *Gut,* **22,** 756.

Stokes, P. L., Asquith, P., Holmes, G. K. T. et al (1972) Histocompatibility antigens associated with adult coeliac disease. *Lancet,* **ii,** 162.

Strober, W., Falchuk, Z. M., Rogentine, G. N. et al (1975) The pathogenesis of gluten-sensitive enteropathy. *Annals of Internal Medicine,* **83,** 242.

Taylor, K. B., Truelove, S. C., Thompson, D. L. et al (1961) An immunological study of coeliac disease and idiopathic steatorrhoea. Serological reactions to gluten and milk products. *British Medical Journal,* **ii,** 1727.

Trefts, P. E., Kagnoff, M. F. (1981) Gluten sensitive enteropathy. I. The T-dependent anti-A-gliadin antibody response maps to the murine major histocompatibility locus. *Journal of Immunology,* **126,** 2249.

Trier, J. S. & Browning, T. H. (1970) Epithelial cell renewal in cultured duodenal biopsies in celiac sprue. *New England Journal of Medicine,* **283,** 1245.

Trier, J. S., Falchuk, Z. M., Carey, M. C. et al (1978) Celiac sprue and refractory sprue. *Gastroenterology,* **75,** 307.

Tomasi, T. B. (1972) Secretory immunoglobulins. *New England Journal of Medicine,* **287,** 500.

Van de Kamer, H. & Weijers, H. A. (1955) Coeliac disease. V. Some experiments on the cause of the harmful effects of wheat gliadin. *Acta Paediatrica,* **44,** 465.

Van de Kamer, H., Weijers, H. A. & Dicke, W. K. (1953) Coeliac disease. IV. An investigation into the injurious constituents of wheat in connection with the action on patients with coeliac disease. *Acta Paediatrica,* **42,** 223.

Vladutiu, A. & Rose, N. (1974) HLA antigens. Association with disease. *Immunogenetics,* **1,** 305.

Wahl, S. M., Altman, L. C. & Rosenstreich, D. (1975) Inhibition of in vitro lymphokine synthesis by glucocorticosteroids. *Journal of Immunology,* **115,** 476.

Wall, A. J., Douglas, A. P., Booth, C. C. et al (1970) Response of the jejunal mucosa in adult celiac disease to oral prednisolone. *Gut,* **11,** 7.

Weijers, H. A. & Van de Kamer, H. (1955) Coeliac disease. VI. A rapid method to test wheat sensitivity. *Acta Paediatrica,* **44,** 536.

Weinstein, W. M., Brow, J. R., Parker, F. et al. (1971) The small intestinal mucosa in dermatitis herpetiformis. II. Relationship of the small intestinal lesion to gluten. *Gastroenterology,* **60,** 362.

Weiser, M. M. & Douglas, A. P. (1976) An alternative mechanism for gluten toxicity in coeliac disease. *Lancet,* **i,** 567.

Wright, N., Watson, A., Morley, A. et al (1973) The cell cycle time in the flat (avillous) mucosa of the human small intestine. *Gut,* **14,** 603.

11

Parasites and Malabsorption

THOMAS A. BRASITUS

Intestinal parasitic infections in man have a worldwide distribution. These infections have become increasingly more prevalent in the United States as foreign travel has increased. It is not generally appreciated that a number of parasites, in addition to causing diarrhoeal illnesses, may result in significant malabsorption of nutrients.

As discussed elsewhere (Brasitus, 1979), reviewing malabsorption due to intestinal parasites gives rise to a number of problems. Since multiple parasitic infections are common, ascribing malabsorption to a single parasite may be difficult. The lack of appropriate socioeconomic and age-matched control populations, as well as the coexistence of malnutrition in infected patients, makes it difficult to determine the true incidence of malabsorption secondary to these parasites. In certain areas many apparently healthy patients have small intestinal mucosal histology which is considered abnormal by North American standards (Klipstein et al, 1968; Brandborg, 1971). Despite these limitations, it is clear that a growing number of parasites may cause malabsorption.

Intestinal parasites can be classified into two major groups: the Protozoa and the Helminths. The latter can be further subdivided into tapeworms, roundworms and flatworms. This paper will review their association with malabsorption.

PROTOZOA

Giardiasis

Giardia lamblia (Figure 1) was first described in 1681 (Dobell, 1920). It has a worldwide distribution with a prevalence rate varying from 2 to 50 per cent (Brandborg et al, 1967; Yardley and Bayless, 1967; Mears and Zinneman, 1969; Kerlin et al, 1978). Giardiasis is both endemic in and imported to the United States, with an overall prevalence of 7.4 per cent (Levine, 1973). In recent years, there have been a number of food- and water-borne epidemics (Brady and Wolfe, 1974; Center for Disease Control, 1974; Shaw et al, 1977). Over a four-year period, 23 per cent of American travellers to Leningrad, Russia developed giardiasis (Mahmoud and Warren, 1975). In Vietnam, 36 per cent of servicemen hospitalized for chronic diarrhoea, were shown to harbour this parasite (Butler et al, 1973).

Clinics in Gastroenterology — Vol. 12, No. 2, May 1983

0300-5089/83/1202-495 $05.00©1983 W. B. Saunders Company Ltd

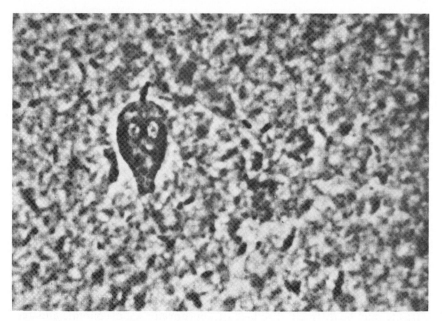

Figure 1. Trophozoite of *Giardia lamblia* in diarrhoeal stool. (Courtesy of Dr Dickson D. Despommier; reprinted with permission from *American Journal of Medicine*, 1979, **67**, 1058-1065.)

G. lamblia resides in the proximal small intestine in man. It has two forms, trophozoite and cyst. The infective cyst form of this parasite is present in formed stools, whereas the trophozoite (Figure 1) is more commonly seen in diarrhoeal stools. The cyst is quite resistant to chlorination (Moore et al, 1969; Brady and Wolfe, 1974) and is usually transmitted by faecally contaminated food or water (Mears and Zinneman, 1969; Brady and Wolfe, 1974; Shaw et al, 1977) and by close interpersonal contact (Petersen, 1972). If the stools are negative for this parasite, the diagnosis is best made by examining a duodenal aspirate and obtaining a small bowel biopsy (Table 1).

There is an increased prevalence of giardiasis in young children (Yardley and Bayliss, 1967; Myers and Zinneman, 1969), in patients with hypo- or achlorhydria (Giannella, Broitman and Zamcheck, 1973), and in certain immunodeficiency states, especially acquired dysgammaglobulinaemia (Hermans et al, 1965; Haskins et al, 1967; Ament and Rubin, 1972) and, rarely, X-linked agammaglobulinaemia (Ochs, Ament and Davis, 1972).

While most patients with giardiasis are asymptomatic, acute diarrhoea, chronic diarrhoea and malabsorption can result from infection with this parasite. The latter can be severe enough to mimic coeliac sprue (Vehelyli, 1939; Cortner, 1959). Faecal fat and nitrogen, D-xylose absorption, serum folate and serum carotene are frequently abnormal (Brandborg et al, 1967; Haskins et al, 1967; Yardley and Bayless, 1967; Mahmoud and Warren,

Table 1. *Diagnosis and treatment of those parasitic diseases which cause malabsorption*

Disease	Diagnosis	Treatment for adults
Giardiasis	Fresh stools for trophozoites or cysts	Quinacrine (Atabrine) hydrochloride 100 mg orally three times a day for seven days
		or
	Small intestinal biopsy with aspiration of intestinal fluid	Metronidazole (Flagyl) 250 mg orally three times a day for seven to ten days (Wolfe, 1975)
Coccidiosis	Allow stool to sit at room temperature for one to two days and check for oocysts.	Furazolidone, 100 mg orally four times a day for ten days (The Medical Letter, 1982)
		or
	Small intestinal biopsy	Trimethoprim-sulphamethoxazole: 160 mg trimethoprim and 800 mg sulphamethoxazole orally four times a day for 10 days and then twice a day for three weeks (The Medical Letter, 1982)
Cryptosporidiosis	Examine stool for oocysts Small intestinal or rectal biopsy Examination of air-dried specimens of small intestine	unknown
P. falciparum malaria	Thin and thick smears of blood	Complex (see The Medical Letter, 1982, for details)
D. latum	Fresh stools for operculated ova	Niclosamide, four 500 mg tablets taken orally at one time and chewed thoroughly (The Medical Letter, 1982)
Capillariasis	Fresh stool for ova Small bowel biopsy	Thiabendazole 25 mg/kg/day orally for several weeks (Whalen et al, 1969)
Strongyloidiasis	Fresh stool for larvae, duodenal aspirate	Thiabendazole 25 mg/kg orally twice a day for three days (Filho, 1978)
Ascariasis	Fresh stool for ova	Mebendazole 100 mg orally twice a day for three days (The Medical Letter, 1982)

1975). Vitamin B_{12} levels may be normal but have been reported to be low in both normal (Cowen and Campbell, 1973) and immunodeficient patients (Ament and Rubin, 1972). The immunodeficient state, bacterial overgrowth, or the parasite itself may contribute to the low vitamin B_{12} levels (Ament and Rubin, 1972). Abnormal Schilling tests in these patients have been attributed to competition between the host and parasite for this vitamin (Cowen and Campbell, 1973).

Roentgenograms may demonstrate thickening and distortion of mucosal folds suggestive of malabsorption (Mahmoud and Warren, 1975). Small bowel biopsy findings have varied from normal to complete villous atrophy (Levinson and Nastro, 1978). In immunodeficient (Cowen and Campbell, 1973) and normal patients (Levinson and Nastro, 1978) with giardiasis, a marked reversal of serum villus abnormalities have been demonstrated after metronidazole (Flagyl) therapy.

Light microscopic studies, using special stains, have demonstrated mucosal invasion by this parasite (Brandborg et al, 1967; Saha and Ghosh, 1977). Morecki and Parker (1967) have shown giardia within mucosal cells by electron microscopy. While it appears that giardia is capable of mucosal invasion, the majority of biopsy specimens do not appear sufficiently abnormal to adequately explain the malabsorption seen with this parasite. A recent study (Hartong, Gourley and Arvanitakis, 1979), however, has demonstrated a significant reduction in several brush border enzyme activities in patients with giardiasis, even when small intestinal biopsies were normal, suggesting that brush border damage may play a role in the malabsorption seen in giardiasis.

A number of other factors may be responsible for malabsorption by this parasite. Erlandsen and Chase (1974), using electron microscopy, have demonstrated direct attachment of the *G. muris* adhesive disc to the rodent microvillus membrane. Others (Poley and Rosenfield, 1981) have demonstrated in man an increased secretory activity by crypt cells harbouring this parasite, with deposition of mucus on top of microvilli. Both studies, therefore, suggest that giardia may create a mechanical barrier to absorption. It may also directly compete with the host for nutrients (Yardley et al, 1967; Cowen and Campbell, 1973) or alter intestinal molitity (Castro et al, 1976). Bacterial overgrowth may coexist with giardiasis and be partially responsible for the associated steatorrhoea (Yardley, Takano and Hendrix, 1965; Tandon et al, 1977; Tomkins et al, 1978; Rogers, 1979). It has been demonstrated that giardial infections may be associated with high luminal free bile acid levels, even when not accompanied by bacterial overgrowth, suggesting that this parasite may be capable of bile salt deconjugation in vivo (Tandon et al, 1973).

Treatment of patients with giardia with Atabrine or metronidazole (Flagyl) (Wolfe, 1975) has usually successfully cured their malabsorption (Table 1). In immunologically deficient patients, higher doses for several weeks may be necessary to eradicate the parasite. In patients in which the parasite seems to have been eradicated and yet malabsorption persists, broad-spectrum antibiotics may be useful (Rogers, 1979).

Coccidiosis

Coccidia are ubiquitous intracytoplasmic parasites which are invariably found in every animal examined, including man (Belding, 1965; Brandborg, Goldberg and Bridenbach, 1970). They belong to the family Eimeriidae (Nime et al, 1976). The *Isospora* species *belli, hominis* and *nateleneis* are found in man. The former two may be the same organism (Zaman, 1968). Despite being endemic in many parts of the world, these parasites have rarely been recognized as pathogens in man (Barksdale and Routh, 1948; Smitskamp and Oey-muller, 1966). Their life cycle is characterized by asexual (schizogony) and sexual (gametogony) phases. The latter phase results in a non-sporulated oocyst which is eliminated in the faeces and is infectious if ingested (Smitskamp and Oey-muller, 1966). Oocysts may be hard to find, making diagnosis by stool examination difficult (Brandborg, Goldberg and Bridenbach, 1970). Faecal specimen are best examined after one to two days at room temperature, which allows the oocysts to mature. Small bowel biopsy with serial sections and examination of intestinal fluids may detect additional cases (Table 1).

Steatorrhoea has been demonstrated in patients infected with this parasite (Barksdale and Routh, 1948; French, Whitby and Whitfield, 1964). Brandborg, Goldberg and Bridenbach (1970) have demonstrated abnormal faecal fat, D-xylose absorption, and low serum carotene levels in several patients. Abnormalities on small bowel biopsies ranged from mild clubbing to a flat mucosa. Almost every stage of this parasite's life cycle was demonstrated within the small intestinal epithelium.

Trier, Moxey and Schimmel (1974) have described a patient with chronic coccidial infection with intermittent diarrhoea for 20 years. This patient appeared to have malabsorption for more than seven years and coccidial infection for at least ten months. The intestinal mucosa showed shortened villi, hypertrophied crypts and cellular infiltration of the lamina propria which reverted to normal after treatment with pyrimethamine and sulpha-diazine. Furazolidone appears to be the drug of choice in the treatment of coccidiosis (The Medical Letter, 1982; Table 1). The malabsorption seen with this parasite is probably secondary to small intestinal mucosal damage (Brandborg, Goldberg and Bridenbach, 1970).

Cryptosporidiosis

Cryptosporidium is also considered to be a member of the coccidia (Jarvis, Merrill and Sprinz, 1966; Meuten, van Kruiningen and Lein, 1974; Pohlenz et al, 1978). It belongs to the family Cryptosporidiae but, unlike *Isospora* species, may be extracellular (Pohlenz et al, 1978) and may not be species specific (Tzipori et al, 1980a, 1982). The life cycle of *C. wrairi* has been recently elucidated in guinea pigs (Vetterling, Takevchi and Madden, 1971). To date, with few exceptions (Nime et al, 1976; Tzipori et al, 1980b; Weinstein et al, 1981), all patients infected with this parasite have been immunosuppressed (Meisel et al, 1976; Lasser, Lewin and Tyning, 1979; Weisberger et al, 1979; Stemmerman et al, 1980; Sloper et al, 1982). Earlier reports failed to document malabsorption with this parasite (Meisel et al, 1976; Nime et al, 1976), but in the last few years several patients have clearly had malabsorption. Abnormal faecal fat, D-xylose tests, and low serum carotene levels have been documented in a number of these patients (Stemmerman et al, 1980; Tzipori et al, 1980b; Sloper et al, 1982). This organism has been shown to produce mild to severe mucosal lesions in the small intestine and colon (Meisel et al, 1976; Nime et al, 1976; Lasser, Lewin and Tyning, 1979; Weisberger et al, 1979; Stemmerman et al, 1980; Sloper et al, 1982). It appears reasonable to ascribe the malabsorption seen with this parasite to small intestinal damage.

The diagnosis of cryptosporidiosis can be difficult. Oocysts can occasion-ally be found in the stools (Tzipori et al, 1980b). The diagnosis may be made by small bowel or rectal biopsy, but the organisms are often hard to find even with special stains (Meisel et al, 1976; Nime et al, 1976) (Table 1). Examination of air-dried specimens of small intestine may also be useful (Weisburger et al, 1979).

Patients on immunosuppressive therapy should, if possible, have these agents stopped (Meisel et al, 1976). To date, despite a myriad of treatments (Meisel et al, 1976; Lasser, Lewin and Tyning, 1979; Weisburger et al, 1979; Stemmerman et al, 1980; Sloper et al, 1982), successful eradication of this parasite has not been shown — unfortunately, since fatal cases have been described (Stemmerman et al, 1980; Weinstein et al, 1981).

Malaria

Gastrointestinal symptoms, including nausea, vomiting and diarrhoea, may be important manifestations of falciparum malaria (Brooks et al, 1967). *Plasmodium knowlesi*-infected monkeys appear to have a decreased amino acid absorption (Migasena and Maegraith, 1969). While there have been reports of steatorrhoea (Karney and Tong, 1972), abnormalities in D-xylose absorption (Olsson and Johnson, 1969; Areekul, Boonyanata and Matrakul, 1972; Karney and Tong, 1972; Cook, 1975), lactose absorption (Olsson and Johnson, 1969; Cook, 1975), and low serum vitamin B_{12} levels (Karney and Tong, 1972; Cook, 1974), many of these studies suffer from technical difficulties. Low folate levels are often seen but may reflect inadequte dietary folate, increased utilization secondary to fever or haemolysis, or inhibition of folate metabolism by the antimalarial drugs (Strickland and Kostinas, 1970). Small intestinal biopsies have revealed congestion and oedema of the lamina propria and even parasitized erythrocytes in capillaries (Olsson and Johnston, 1969; Cook, 1975) (Figure 2). These studies suggest that malaria

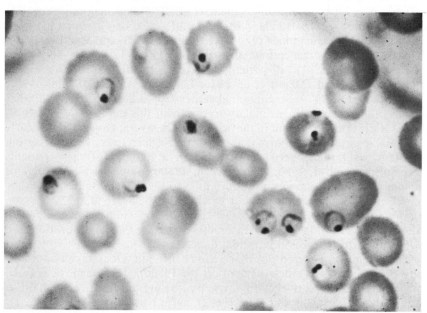

Figure 2. Ring stage of *Plasmodium falciparum* in blood. (Courtesy of Dr Dickson D. Despommier.)

may interfere with absorption by affecting the small intestinal micro-circulation (Olsson and Johnston, 1969; Cook, 1975). Overall, it appears that malaria may be associated with the malabsorption of certain nutrients, including fat, certain disaccharides, and vitamin B_{12} (Olsson and Johnston, 1969). Further studies are clearly needed to elucidate the mechanisms involved in producing malabsorption by this parasite.

HELMINTHS

Tapeworms

Diphylobothrium latum

Adult tapeworms are anchored to the host's intestine by a scolex and have egg-producing units called proglottides. This worm does not possess an intestinal tract but appears to absorb nutrients through its integument (Brandborg, 1978).

Infection results from ingestion of raw infected fish (Strickland and Kostinas, 1970). Although this tapeworm is more commonly seen in Baltic countries, Scandinavia and parts of the USSR, it is also endemic in the northern United States and parts of Canada. While most patients are asymptomatic, vitamin B_{12} deficiency can occur — so-called 'tapeworm pernicious anaemia' (Brandborg, 1978). The mechanisms for this vitamin malabsorption is not entirely clear (Toskes and Doren, 1973), but *D. latum* may take up free vitamin B_{12} (Brante and Ernberg, 1957). It may also absorb vitamin B_{12} complexed to intrinsic factor but at a much slower rate (Brante and Ernberg, 1957). This parasite may secrete a 'releasing' factor capable of freeing the vitamin from intrinsic factor (Nyberg, 1960; Mettrick and Podesta, 1974). Additional studies have shown that *D. latum* depresses gastric intrinsic factor secretion (Toskes and Doren, 1973), although there is no evidence that intrinsic factor is increased after eradication of the worm (Toskes and Doren, 1973).

The diagnosis of this tapeworm rests on finding the characteristic operculated eggs in the stool. The drug of choice for treating *D. latum* appears to be Niclosamide (The Medical Letter, 1982) (Table 1).

Round Worms

Strongyloidiasis

Strongyloides stercoralis (Figure 3) is the species which produces disease in man. This roundworm, while the least common of the intestinal nematodes, deserves particular attention because it may produce overwhelming fatal infections (Cruz, Rebouchaj and Rocha, 1966; Amir-Ahmandi et al, 1968; Civantos and Robinson, 1969; Blumenthal, 1977). It has a worldwide distribution (Filho, 1978) and in the United States is endemic in the rural south, although occasional autochthonous cases have been reported in northern cities (Blumenthal, 1977). It is particularly prevalent in Vietnam veterans (Filho, 1978), in patients confined to institutions for the mentally retarded (Blumenthal, 1977), and in immunosuppressed patients (Filho, 1978).

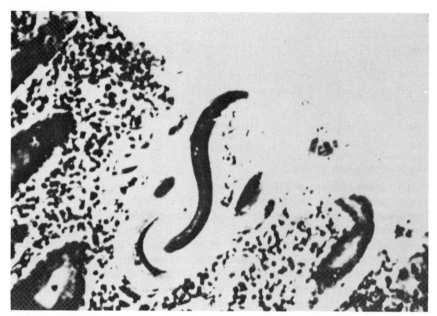

Figure 3. Adult *Strongyloides stercoralis* present in the small intestinal mucosa. (Courtesy of Dr Dickson D. Despommier; reprinted with permission from *American Journal of Medicine*, 1979, **67**, 1058-1065.)

In the host's intestine, eggs are hatched and rhabditiform larvae are passed in the stool. These larvae may become free-living adults that reproduce in the soil, or they may change into infectious filariform larvae and penetrate the host's skin. They then migrate through the venous system to the lungs, then to be coughed up and swallowed to finally reach the small intestine (Blumenthal, 1977; Filho, 1978). Rhabditiform larvae may transform into filariform larvae within the distal small intestine or colon (internal autoinfection) or in the perianal area (external autoinfection) and repeat the cycle of infection (Blumenthal, 1977; Filho, 1978). Occasionally this process can result in an overwhelming fatal 'hyperinfective syndrome' (Blumenthal, 1977; Filho, 1978).

Although the majority of patients harbouring this parasite are asymptomatic, patients with high parasite burdens may have steatorrhoea, abnormal D-xylose absorption and low serum levels of folate and vitamin B_{12} (Toh and Chow, 1969; Filho, 1978). Occasional patients have a severe hypoalbuminaemia, which cannot be adequately explained on a nutritional basis alone, suggesting that it may be secondary to protein-losing enteropathy. Roentgenograms of the gastrointestinal tract may show nonspecific changes compatible with malabsorption or, in severe cases, may show 'pipe-stemming' of the proximal intestine mimicking atypical lymphoma, regional enteritis or intestinal tuberculosis (Johnson and Johnson, 1967; Toh and Chow, 1969; Berkmen and Rabinowitz, 1972; Brasitus et al, 1980). After appropriate treatment (Table 1) this pattern may revert to normal (Toh and Chow, 1969). In one study (Garcia et al, 1977), patients with this severe pattern on x-ray did not have malabsorption, suggesting that the remaining bowel was able to compensate for this relatively small area of diseased mucosa.

This parasitic infection has often been mistaken for tropical sprue. Small bowel biopsy specimens may demonstrate loss of villus height, dilated lacteals, and increase in inflammatory cells (particularly eosinophils) and even microulcerations (Filho, 1978). In patients with negative stool examinations suspected of harbouring this parasite, duodenal aspiration is usually helpful (approximately 90 per cent positive). Small bowel biopsy alone, however, is rarely useful (Filho, 1978).

Even asymptomatic patients harbouring this parasite should be treated since they are always at risk of developing the 'hyperinfective syndrome' (Filho, 1978). Thiabendazole, 25 mg/kg orally twice a day for three days, has been shown to be highly effective in eradicating this parasite in normal hosts. In immunosuppressed patients a longer course may be necessary. In severe cases this agent appears to be less efficacious and fatalities are not uncommon (Filho, 1978).

Ancylostomiasis

The two species of intestinal hookworm that infect humans are *Necator americanus* and *Ancylostoma duodenale* (Tandon et al, 1969; Brandborg, 1978). Their life cycles are similar to strongyloides but antoinfection does not occur (Brandborg, 1978). As much as 0.67 ml of blood per worm may be removed from a host by these hookworms each day (Brandborg, 1978).

There is considerable controversy as to whether hookworm infection can result in malabsorption. A number of studies purport to show steatorrhoea, abnormal D-xylose absorption, abnormal small bowel biopsies and low serum vitamin levels secondary to infection with this parasite (Sheehy et al, 1962; Blackman et al, 1965; Guha and Rashmi, 1968; Pitchumoni and Folch, 1969; Burman, Sengal and Chakravarti, 1970; Nath et al, 1971). However, most studies show poor correlations between worm burden and malabsorption (Banwell et al, 1967; Guha and Rashmi, 1968; Tandon et al, 1969; Saraya and Tandon, 1971; Falaiye, Oladapo and Wall, 1974). Furthermore, malabsorption and even intestinal pathology in these malnourished patients have been reversed solely by a nutritious diet (Mayoral et al, 1966). The results, to date, therefore suggest that hookworm does not cause malabsorption in man (Banwell et al, 1967; Nath et al, 1971; Brandborg, 1978).

Capillariasis

Capillaria philipopinensis, is found only in the Philippines (Whalen et al, 1969). Man appears to be its only host and its mode of transmission is unknown (Whalen et al, 1969). Consumption of uncooked intestine has been suggested to be epidemiologically important (Lindenbaum, 1969). In one large epidemic of capillariasis (Whalen et al, 1969), patients demonstrated a severe sprue-like illness with diarrhoea and malabsorption. Significant steatorrhoea and protein loss into the stools were documented in many of these patients. Small bowel biopsies were equally abnormal in controls and patients, although the worm was present only in infected patients. Thiabendazole, 25 mg/kg/day, rapidly eliminated this parasite from the stools, resulted in clinical improvement, and gradually reversed the abnormal laboratory values (Table 1).

Watten et al (1972) have suggested that these patients may not only have a decrease in conjugated bile acid levels in their intestinal contents but also may have impaired fat digestion as well as fat malabsorption. The reasons for the severe malabsorption seen in these patients remains unclear. It may be a secondary to competition for nutrients by the parasite, elaboration of a toxin, a decrease in bile acid conjugates, or a deficiency in digestive enzyme activities (Watten et al, 1972). Further studies are necessary in this area.

Ascariasis

Ascaris lumbricoides (Figure 4), the largest intestinal nematode, is also known as the 'giant intestinal round worm' (Warren and Mahmoud, 1977). It is distributed worldwide and a recent review estimated that in the United States four million people may harbour this parasite (Warren, 1974). Ascariasis is usually transmitted by ingestion of faecally contaminated raw vegetables and fruits, although pica may explain its high incidence in children. Its life cycle once ingested is similar to that previously described for other nematodes (Warren and Mahmoud, 1977). While most patients are asymptomatic, severe diarrhoea, intestinal obstruction, perforation,

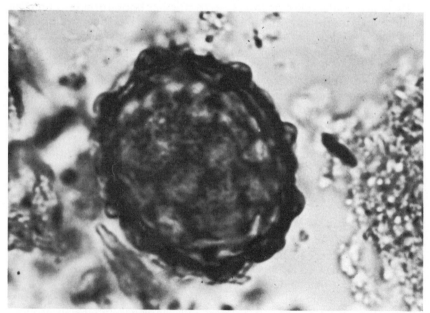

Figure 4. *Ascaris lumbricoides* ovum in diarrhoeal stool. (Courtesy of Dr Dickson D. Despommier.)

appendicitis, pancreatitis and obstructive jaundice have been reported (Brandborg, 1978). It is not clear whether ascariasis can cause widespread malabsorption of nutrients (Tripathy et al, 1971, 1972). It appears, however, that this parasite can interfere with the absorption of vitamin A in children and adults (Siukumar and Reddy, 1975; Mahalanabis et al, 1976), although little correlation has been shown between absorption of vitamin A and stool egg counts. The mechanism for vitamin A malabsorption remains speculative. It does not appear to be caused by either mucosal damage or by ingestion of the vitamin by the worm (Mahalanabis et al, 1976).

Flatworms

Schistosomiasis

Three major species of this flatworm infect man. They include *S. haematobium, S. mansoni* (Figure 5), and *S. japonicum.* Each produces its own characteristic disease. Since the egg-laying female of *S. japonicum* resides in the superior mesenteric venous system, it affects the small intestine to a greater degree than *S. mansoni* which resides in the inferior mesenteric system. The adult female worm of *S. haematobium* usually resides in pelvic veins and less commonly affects the intestine in man (Brandborg, 1978).

The parasitic ova appear to cause overt disease resulting in a granulomatous reaction by the host (Brandborg, 1978). This reaction may

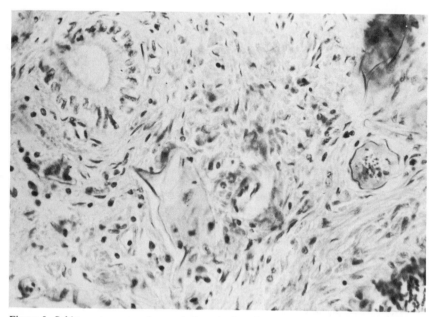

Figure 5. *Schistosoma mansoni* ovum in intestinal section. Note characteristic lateral spine. (Courtesy of Dr Dickson D. Despommier.)

eventually result in polypoid lesions, fibrosis and even stenosis of the intestine (Brandborg, 1978). Despite these complications, there is little data to suggest that schistosomiasis results in malabsorption (Domingo and Warren, 1969; Brandborg, 1978). Experimentally in mice, *S. mansoni* failed to interfere with nutrient absorption, apparently because the absorptive surface of the small intestine was spared (Domingo and Warren, 1969).

While the hypoalbuminaemia often seen in schistosomiasis has been attributed to malnutrition or liver disease, polyposis of the colon secondary to this parasite may cause a protein-losing enteropathy (Brandborg, 1978). El-Saardani et al (1968) have shown a correlation between excess protein loss into the gut lumen with increased portal hypertension. Others (El-Rooby, 1967) also demonstrated intestinal lymphangiectasia in advanced disease. It thus appears that this parasite may cause hypoalbuminaemia for a number of reasons, but that malabsorption does not occur.

SUMMARY

In summary, it appears that giardiasis, coccidiosis, cryptosporidiosis, strongyloidiasis, capillariasis and perhaps *P. falciparum* malaria are the only parasitic diseases which cause malabsorption of many nutrients. *D. latum* and *A. lumbricoides* interfere with vitamin B_{12} and vitamin A absorption, respectively. In view of the increasing use of immunosuppressive therapy, it is likely that malabsorption caused by intestinal parasites may become even more evident in the future.

REFERENCES

Ament, M. E. & Rubin, C. E. (1972) Relation of giardiasis to abnormal intestinal structure and function in gastrointestinal immunodeficiency syndromes. *Gastroenterology, 62*, 216.
Amir-Ahmandi, H., Braun, P., Neva, F. A. et al (1968) Strongyloidiasis at the Boston City Hospital. *American Journal of Digestive Diseases, 13*, 959.
Areekul, S., Boonyanata, C. & Matrakul, D. (1972) Serum vitamin B_{12} and vitamin B_{12} absorption in patients with *Plasmodium falciparum* malaria. *Southeast Asian Journal of Tropical Medicine and Public Health, 3*, 419.
Banwell, J. G., Marsden, P. D., Blackman, V. et al (1967) Hookworm infection and intestinal absorption amongst Africans in Uganda. *American Journal of Tropical Medicine and Hygiene, 16*, 304.
Barksdale, W. L. & Routh, C. F. (1948) *Isospora hominis* infections among American personnel in the southwest Pacific. *American Journal of Tropical Medicine, 28*, 639.
Belding, D. L. (1965) The sporozoa: classification of genera *Sarcocystis* and *Isospora*. In *Textbook of Parasitology*. p. 232. New York: Appleton Century Crofts.
Berkmen, Y. M. & Rabinowitz, J. (1972) Gastrointestinal manifestations of strongyloidiasis. *American Journal of Roentgenology, Radium Therapy and Nuclear Medicine, 115*, 306.
Blackman, V., Marsden, P. D., Banwell, J. et al (1965) Albumin metabolism in hookworm anaemias. *Transactions of the Royal Society of Tropical Medicine and Hygiene, 59*, 472.
Blumenthal, D. S. (1977) Intestinal nematodes in the United States. *New England Journal of Medicine, 297*, 1437.
Brady, P. G. & Wolfe, J. (1974) Water-borne giardiasis. *Annals of Internal Medicine, 81*, 498.
Brandborg, L. L. (1971) Structure and function of the small intestine in some parasite diseases. *American Journal of Clinical Nutrition, 24*, 124.
Brandborg, L. L. (1978) Parasitic disease. In *Gastrointestinal Disease* (Ed.) Sleisenger, M. H. & Fortran, J. S. Chapter 69. Philadelphia: W. B. Saunders.

Brandborg, L. L., Goldberg, S. B. & Bridenbach, W. C. (1970) Human coccidiosis — a possible cause of malabsorption. *New England Journal of Medicine,* **283,** 1306.

Brandborg, L. L., Tankersley, C. B., Gottlieb, S. et al (1967) Histological demonstration of mucosal invasion by *Giardia lamblia* in man. *Gastroenterology,* **52,** 143.

Brante, G. & Ernberg, T. (1957) The in vitro uptake of vitamin B$_{12}$ by *Diphyllobothrium latum* and its blockage by intrinsic factor. *Scandinavian Journal of Clinical and Laboratory Investigation,* **9,** 313.

Brasitus, T. A. (1979) Parasites and malabsorption. *American Journal of Medicine,* **67,** 1058-1065.

Brasitus, T. A., Gold, R. P., Kay, R. M. et al (1980) Intestinal strongyloidiasis. *American Journal of Digestive Diseases,* **73,** 65-69.

Brooks, M., Malloy, J. P., Bartelloni, P. J. et al (1967) Pathophysiology of acute falciparum malaria. *American Journal of Medicine,* **43,** 735.

Burman, N. N., Sengal, A. K. & Chakravarti, R. N. (1970) Morphological and absorption studies of small intestine in hookworm infestation (ankylostomiasis). *Indian Journal of Medical Research,* **58,** 317.

Butler, T., Middleton, F. G., Ernest, D. L. et al (1973) Chronic and recurrent diarrhea in American servicemen in Vietnam. *Archives of Internal Medicine,* **132,** 373.

Castro, G. A. Badial-Aceves, F., Smith, J. W. et al (1976) Altered small bowel propulsion associated with parasitism. *Gastroenterology,* **71,** 620.

Center for Disease Control (1974) *Morbidity and Mortality Weekly Report,* **23** (78), 397.

Civantos, F. & Robinson, M. J. (1969) Fatal strongyloidiasis following corticosteroid therapy. *American Journal of Digestive Diseases,* **14,** 643.

Cook, G. C. (1974) Some factors influencing absorption rates of the digestion products of protein and carbohydrate from the proximal jejunum of man and their possible nutritional implications. *Gut,* **15,** 239.

Cook, G. C. (1975) Relation between malaria, serum globulin concentration and the D-xylose absorption test. *Transactions of the Royal Society of Tropical Medicine and Hygiene,* **69,** 143.

Cortner, J. A. (1959) Giardiasis, a cause of celiac syndrome. *Americal Journal of Diseases of Children,* **98,** 53.

Cowen, A. E. & Campbell, C. B. (1973) Giardiasis — a cause of vitamin B$_{12}$ malabsorption. *American Journal of Digestive Diseases,* **18,** 384.

Cruz, T., Rebouchaj, G. & Rocha, H. (1966) Fatal strongyloidiasis in patients receiving corticosteroids. *New England Journal of Medicine,* **275,** 1093.

Dobell, C. (1920) Discovery of intestinal protozoa in man. *Proceedings of the Royal Society of Medicine,* **13,** 1.

Domingo, E. O. & Warren, K. S. (1969) Pathology and pathophysiology of the small intestine in murine *Schistosomiasis mansoni,* including a review of the literature. *Gastroenterology,* **56,** 231.

El-Rooby, A. A. (1967) Intestinal lymphangiectasis in liver cirrhosis. *Journal of the Egyptian Medical Association,* **50,** 644.

El-Saadani, A. M., El-Sany, A. M., Habib, M. et al (1968) Albumin turnover in schistosomal liver cirrhosis. *American Journal of Tropical Medicine and Hygiene,* **17,** 844.

Erlandsen, S. & Chase, D. G. (1974) Morphological alterations in the microvillous border of villous epithelial cells produced by intestinal microorganisms. *American Journal of Clinical Nutrition,* **27,** 1277.

Falaiye, M. J., Oladapo, J. M. & Wall, J. J. (1974) Hookworm enteropathy. *Journal of Tropical Medicine and Hygiene,* **77,** 211.

Filho, E. C. (1978) Strongyloidiasis. *Clinics in Gastroenterology,* **7** (1), 179.

French, J. M., Whitby, J. L. & Whitfield, A. G. W. (1964) Steatorrhea in man infected with coccidiosis *(Isospora belli). Gastroenterology,* **47,** 642.

Garcia, F. T., Sessions, J. T., Strum, W. B. et al (1977) Intestinal function and morphology in strongyloidiasis. *American Journal of Tropical Medicine and Hygiene,* **26,** 859-865.

Giannella, R. A., Broitman, S. A. & Zamcheck, N. (1973) Influence of gastric acidity on bacterial and parasitic enteric infections. *Annals of Internal Medicine,* **78,** 271.

Guha, D. K. & Rashmi, A. (1968) The D-xylose test in normal microcytic hypochromic anemia and hookworm disease in children. *Indian Journal of Medical Research,* **56,** 1028.

Hartong, W. A., Gourley, W. K. & Arvanitakis, C. (1979) Giardiasis: clinical spectrum and functional-structural abnormalities of the small intestinal mucosa. *Gastroenterology,* 77, 61-69.

Haskins, L. C., Winawar, S. J., Broitman, S. A. et al (1967) Clinical giardiasis and intestinal malabsorption. *Gastroenterology,* 53, 265.

Hermans, P. E., Huizenga, K. A., Hoffman, H. D. et al (1965) Dysgammaglobulinemia associated with nodular lymphoid hyperplasia of the small intestine. *American Journal of Medicine,* 40, 78.

Jarvis, H. R., Merrill, T. G. & Sprinz, H. (1966) Coccidiosis in the guinea pig small intestine due to a cryptosporidium. *American Journal of Veterinary Research,* 27, 408-414.

Johnson, S. & Johnson, C. (1967) A preliminary study of strongyloides infestation. *Journal of Association of Physicians in India,* 15, 513.

Karney, W. W. & Tong, M. J. (1972) Malabsorption in *Plasmodium falciparum* malaria. *American Journal of Tropical Medicine and Hygiene,* 21, 1-5.

Kerlin, P., Ratnaike, R. N., Butler, R. et al (1978) Prevalence of giardiasis. *American Journal of Digestive Diseases,* 23, 940.

Klipstein, F. A., Samloff, I. M., Smarth, G. et al (1968) Malabsorption and malnutrition in rural Haiti. *American Journal of Clinical Nutrition,* 21, 1042.

Lasser, K. H., Lewin, K. J. & Tyning, F. W. (1979) Cryptosporidial enteritis in a patient with congenital hypogammaglobulinemia. *Human Pathology,* 10, 234-240.

Levine, N. D. (1973) *Protozoan Parasites of Domestic Animals and in Man* 2nd Edition. p. 118. Minneapolis: Burgess.

Levinson, J. D. & Nastro, L. J. (1978) Giardiasis with total villous atrophy. *Gastroenterology,* 74, 271.

Lindenbaum, J. (1969) Intestinal capillariasis. *Annals of Internal Medicine,* 70, 1277.

Mahalanabis, D., Jalan, K. N., Maitra, T. K. et al (1976) Vitamin A absorption in ascaris. *American Journal of Clinical Nutrition,* 29, 1372-1375.

Mahmoud, A. A. F. & Warren, K. S. (1975) Algorithms in the diagnosis and management of exotic disease. II. Giardiasis. *Journal of Infectious Diseases,* 131, 162.

Mayoral, L. G., Tripathy, K., Garcia, F. T. et al (1966) Intestinal malabsorption and parasitic disease. The role of protein malnutrition. *Gastroenterology,* 50, 856.

Mears, T. & Zinneman, H. H. (1969) *Giardia lamblia* as parasite in humans. *Minneapolis Medicine,* 52, 1107.

Meisel, J. L., Perea, D. R., Meligro, C. et al (1976) Overwhelming watery diarrhea associated with cryptosporidium in an immunosuppressed patient. *Gastroenterology,* 70, 1156.

Mettrick, D. F. & Podesta, R. B. (1974) Ecological and physiological aspects of helminth-host interactions in the mammalian gastrointestinal canal. *Advances in Parasitology,* 12, 183.

Meuten, D. J., van Kruiningen, H. J. & Lein, D. H. (1974) Cryptosporidiosis in a calf. *Journal of American Veterinary Medical Association,* 165, 915-917.

Migasena, P. & Maegraith, B. G. (1969) Intestinal absorption in malaria. *Annals of Tropical Medicine and Parasitology,* 63, 439.

Moore, G. T., Cross, W. M., McGuire, D. et al (1969) Epidemic giardiasis at a ski resort. *New England Journal of Medicine,* 281, 402.

Morecki, R. & Parker, J. G. (1967) Ultrastructural studies of the human: *Giardia lamblia* and subjacent mucosa in a subject with steatorrhea. *Gastroenterology,* 52, 151.

Nath, K., Sur, B. K., Samuel, K. C. et al (1971) Malabsorption in ankylostomiasis. *Indian Journal of Medical Research,* 59, 1090.

Nime, A., Burck, D., Page, D. et al (1976) Acute enterocolitis in a human being infected with the protozoan *Cryptosporidium. Gastroenterology,* 70, 592.

Nyberg, W. (1960) The influence of *Diphyllobothrium latum* on the vitamin B_{12} intrinsic factor complex. II. In vitro studies. *Acta Medica Scandinavica,* 167, 189.

Ochs, H. D., Ament, M. E. & Davis, S. D. (1972) Giardiasis with malabsorption in X-linked agammaglobulinemia. *New England Journal of Medicine,* 287, 341.

Olsson, R. A. & Johnston, E. H. (1969) Histopathologic changes and small-bowel absorption in falciparum malaria. *American Journal of Tropical Medicine and Hygiene,* 18, 355.

Petersen, H. (1972) Giardiasis. *Scandinavian Journal of Gastroenterology,* 7 (Supplement 14), 1.

Pitchumoni, C. S. & Folch, M. H. (1969) Hookworm disease, malabsorption, malnutrition. *American Journal of Clinical Nutrition,* 22, 813.

Pohlenz, J., Bemrick, W. J., Moon, H. W. et al (1978) Bovine cryptosporidiosis: a transmission and scanning electron microscopic study of some stages in the life cycle of the host-parasite relationship. *Veterinary Pathology,* **15,** 417-427.

Poley, J. R. & Rosenfield, S. (1981) Giardiasis and malabsorption: presence of an organic mucosal barrier. A scanning (SEM) and transmission (TEM) electron microscopic study of small bowel mucosa. *Gastroenterology,* **80,** 1254A.

Rogers, A. I. (1979) Giardia and steatorrhea. *Gastroenterology,* **76,** 224.

Saha, T. K. & Ghosh, T. K. (1977) Invasion of small intestinal mucosa by *Giardia lamblia* in man. *Gastroenterology,* **72,** 402.

Saraya, A. K., Tandon, B. N. & Ramachandran, K. (1971) Study of Vitamin B_{12} and folic acid deficiency in hookworm disease. *American Journal of Clinical Nutrition,* **24,** 3.

Scowden, E. B., Schaffner, W. & Stone, W. J. (1978) Overwhelming strongyloidiasis. *Medicine* (Baltimore), **57,** 527.

Shaw, P. T., Brodsky, R. E., Lyman, D. O. et al (1977) A community outbreak of giardiasis with evidence of transmission by a municipal water supply. *Annals of Internal Medicine,* **87,** 426.

Sheehy, T. W., Meroney, W. A., Cos, R. S. et al (1962) Hookworm disease in malabsorption. *Gastroenterology,* **42,** 148.

Siukumar, B. & Reddy, V. (1975) Absorption of vitamin A in children with ascaris. *American Journal of Tropical Medicine and Hygiene,* **78,** 114.

Sloper, K. S., Dourmashkin, R. R. Bird, R. B. et al (1982) Chronic malabsorption due to cryptosporidiosis in a child with immunoglobulin deficiency. *Gut,* **23,** 80-82.

Smitskamp, I. T. & Oey-muller, E. (1966) Geographical distribution and clinical significance of human coccidiosis. *Tropical and Geographical Medicine,* **18,** 133.

Stemmerman, G. N., Hayashi, T., Glober, G. A. et al (1980) Cryptosporidiosis. Report of a fatal case complicated by disseminated toxoplasmosis. *American Journal of Medicine,* **69,** 637-642.

Strickland, G. T. & Kostinas, J. E. (1970) Folic acid deficiency complicating malaria. *American Journal of Tropical Medicine and Hygiene,* **19,** 910.

Tandon, B. N., Kohli, R. K., Saraya, A. K. et al (1969) Role of parasites in the pathogenesis of intestinal malabsorption in hookworm disease. *Gut,* **10,** 293.

Tandon, B. N., Tandon, R. K., Satpathy, B. K. et al (1977) A study of bacterial flora and bile salt deconjugation in upper jejunum. *Gut,* **18,** 176.

The Medical Letter (1982) Drugs for parasitic infections. **24,** 5-12.

Toh, C. C. S. & Chow, K. W. (1969) Malabsorption syndrome in a patient infected with *Strongyloides stercoralis. Annals of Tropical Medicine and Parasitology,* **63,** 493.

Tomkins, A. M., Wright, S. G., Draser, B. S. et al (1978) Bacterial colonization of jejunal mucosa in giardiasis. *Transactions of Royal Society of Tropical Medicine and Hygiene,* **72,** 33-36.

Toskes, P. P. & Doren, J. J. (1973) Vitamin B_{12} absorption and malabsorption. *Gastroenterology,* **65,** 662.

Trier, J. S., Moxey, P. C. & Schimmel, E. M. (1974) Chronic intestinal coccidiosis in man. Intestinal morphology and response to treatment. *Gastroenterology,* **66,** 923.

Tripathy, K., Gonzalez, F., Lotero, H. et al (1971) Effects of ascaris infection on human nutrition. *American Journal of Tropical Medicine and Hygiene,* **20,** 212.

Tripathy, K., Duque, E., Bolanos, O. et al (1972) Malabsorption syndrome in ascaris. *American Journal of Clinical Nutrition,* **25,** 1276.

Tzipori, S., Angus, K. W., Campbell, I. et al (1980a) *Cryptosporidium:* evidence for a single-species genus. *Infection and Immunity,* **30,** 884-886.

Tzipora, S., Angus, K. W., Gray, E. W. et al (1980b) Vomiting and diarrhea associated with *Cryptosporidium* infection. *New England Journal of Medicine,* **303,** 818.

Tzipori, S., Angus, K. W., Campbell, I. et al (1982) Experimental infection of lambs with *Cryptosporidium* isolated from a human patient with diarrhea. *Gut,* **23,** 71-74.

Vehelyli, P. (1939) Celiac disease imitated by giardiasis. *American Journal of Diseases of Children,* **57,** 894.

Vetterling, J. M., Takevchi, A. & Madden, P. A. (1971) Ultrastructure of *Cryptosporidium wrairi* from the guinea pig. *Journal of Protozoology,* **18,** 248-260.

Warren, K. S. (1974) Helminthic disease endemic in the United States. *American Journal of Tropical Medicine and Hygiene,* **23,** 723-730.

Warren, K. S. & Mahmoud, A. A. F. (1977) Algorithms in the diagnosis and management of exotic diseases. XXII. Ascaris and toxocariasis. *Journal of Infectious Diseases,* **135,** 868-872.

Watten, R. H., Beckner, W. M., Cross, J. H. et al (1972) Clinical studies of *Capillariasis philippinensis. Transactions of the Royal Society of Tropical Medicine and Hygiene,* **66,** 828.

Weinstein, L., Edelstein, S. M., Madara, et al (1981) Intestinal cryptosporidiosis complicated by disseminated cytomegalovirus infection. *Gastroenterology,* **81,** 584-591.

Weisberger, W. R., Hutcheon, D. F., Yardley, J. H. et al (1979) Cryptosporidiosis in an immunosuppressed renal transplant recipient with IgA deficiency. *American Journal of Clinical Pathology,* **72,** 473-478.

Whalen, G. E., Strickland, G. T., Cross, J. H. et al (1969) Intestinal capillariasis. *Lancet,* **i,** 13.

Wolfe, M. S. (1975) Giardiasis. *Journal of the American Medical Association,* **233,** 1262.

Yardley, J. B. & Bayless, T. M. (1967) Giardiasis. *Gastroenterology,* **52,** 301.

Yardley, J. H., Takano, J. & Hendrix, T. R. (1965) Epithelial and other mucosal lesions of the jejunum in giardiasis. Jejunal biopsy studies. *Bulletin of the Johns Hopkins Hospital,* **115,** 389.

Zaman, V. (1968) Observation on human isospora. *Transactions of the Royal Society of Tropical Medicine and Hygiene,* **62,** 556.

12

Inflammatory and Malignant Diseases of the Small Bowel Causing Malabsorption

JOHN P. CELLO

This chapter will focus on those inflammatory and malignant conditions involving the small bowel wherein malabsorption is a major clinical manifestation of the disorders. Some common clinical conditions associated with nutrient maldigestion and malabsorption will be covered elsewhere in this volume and will not be considered here.

LYMPHOMA AND MALABSORPTION

Weight loss, steatorrhoea and severe nutrient malabsorption are commonly encountered in patients with abdominal lymphoma. These clinical manifestations of lymphoma may represent either late consequences of disseminated lymphoma or the presenting clinical symptoms of primary lesions originating in the small bowel or mesenteric nodes. In western society (referring herein, for epidemiological purposes, to North America and Europe) primary small intestinal lymphoma appears to develop largely as a late consequence of adult non-tropical sprue (coeliac disease) or the 'idiopathic' steatorrhoea syndrome. In Israel, Iran and South Africa, intestinal lymphoma develops in underprivileged young patients. This latter lymphoma has been termed 'Mediterranean' lymphoma.

Western Small Bowel Lymphoma and Malabsorption

Small bowel is second only to the stomach as the major site of primary intestinal lymphoma. Histologically, small intestinal lymphoma is usually diffuse histiocytic lymphoma originating within the small bowel wall with only limited regional lymph node involvement.

Pathogenesis

Primary small bowel lymphoma in western society appears to develop predominantly as a consequence of long-standing well-documented coeliac disease or idiopathic steatorrhoea (Holmes et al, 1976; Selby and Gallagher,

0300-5089/83/1202-511 $05.00©1983 W. B. Saunders Company Ltd

1979). In the majority of instances, the diagnosis of adult coeliac disease has been well established for many years' duration and the patients have been previously in good health with stable nutrition on a gluten-free diet. On occasion, the nature of a long-standing diarrhoeal illness has not been well defined and there has been variable responsiveness over a long period of time to gluten withdrawal. Over a nine-year period in one study, approximately 10 per cent of patients with adult coeliac disease developed gastrointestinal tract malignancy, with oesophageal cancer and primary small bowel lymphoma most commonly documented (Selby and Gallagher, 1979). Where tested, these patients have HLA phenotypes similar to those noted in patients with coeliac disease who do not develop lymphoma (Freeman et al, 1977). The development of malignancy appears to be a direct consequence of long-standing coeliac disease. There is no evidence that strict gluten withdrawal lessens the likelihood of developing intestinal malignancies in coeliac disease (Selby and Gallagher, 1979).

Pathology

On gross examination of the specimen, the small intestine is thickened diffusely with scattered areas of mucosal ulceration. The most prominent areas of involvement are in the jejunum, although duodenal and ileal involvement have been seen. Adjacent mesenteric nodes are also commonly involved. However, large bulky retroperitoneal lymphadenopathy together with liver and spleen involvement are uncommon. Microscopically, the most common histological type appears to be a reticulum cell sarcoma or a diffuse histiocytic lymphoma (Holmes et al, 1976; Freeman et al, 1977; Selby and Gallagher, 1979). The lymphoma involvement of small bowel may take the form of large focal tumour masses or, more commonly, diffuse small bowel thickening with microscopic foci of malignancy. The ulcerated mucosa, particularly in the jejunum, has an underlying heavy infiltrate consisting of a mixture of lymphocytes, histiocytes, polymorphonuclear leucocytes, eosinophils and plasma cells (Isaacson and Wright, 1978a). Malignant cells may be difficult to find on a single pathological section. The surface epithelium may be normal or there may be a loss of nuclear polarity (Figure 1). On occasion, this diffusely-infiltrative histiocytic tumour can be best described as 'histiocytic medullary reticulosis' rather than a malignant histiocytic lymphoma. In this former process there is, in addition to the small bowel diseases, a diffuse infiltration of sinuses, sinusoids and medullary cords of lymph nodes, liver, spleen and bone marrow without giving rise to any cohesive solid tumour except in the very late stage of the disease (Isaacson and Wright, 1978b).

Clinical features and diagnosis

The majority of patients with intestinal lymphoma associated with adult coeliac disease or 'idiopathic steatorrhoea' have been observed for many years, often 20 to 30 years, most of them in good control. They insidiously and relentlessly develop progressive weight loss and steatorrhoea in spite of maintenance of a gluten-free diet (Holmes et al, 1976; Selby and Gallagher, 1979). The coeliac disease may be occult in some patients developing

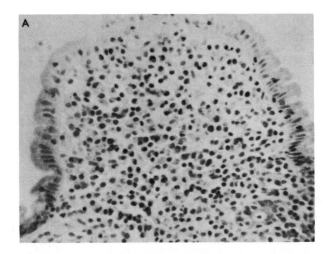

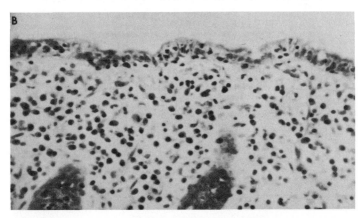

Figure 1. Histopathology of small bowel in primary intestinal lymphoma (A) and coeliac sprue (B). In lymphoma, the epithelium retains a normal columnar shape with villi widened by infiltrate but present. In sprue, the mucosa is flat without villi. The overlying epithelium is stunted. From Gray et al (1982), with kind permission of the authors and the editor of *Gastroenterology*.

lymphoma, with small bowel biopsy in areas away from the tumour demonstrating classic changes of adult coeliac disease. Weight loss, diarrhoea, steatorrhoea, vague abdominal discomfort with some additional systemic features such as fever and malaise may be noted in many patients. Postprandial abdominal distension, nausea and vomiting may suggest partial small bowel obstruction. Occasionally, a large abdominal mass may be noted on initial presentation (Gray et al, 1982). Clinically significant gastrointestinal tract bleeding is uncommon. However, occult blood in the stools with associated iron-deficiency anaemia may be seen. Prior to the insidious development of these symptoms, most patients have had excellent control of their coeliac disease for many years. The majority of these patients are middle-aged adults. In some patients, the clinical manifestations of diffuse intestinal lymphoma may mimic a relapse of coeliac sprue brought about by gluten exposure. Gastrointestinal tract radiography may suggest lymphoma (Figure 2). Diagnosis by peroral small bowel capsule biopsy may be extremely difficult in some patients, given the patchy nature of the malignancy and the variability of finding malignant cells in a dense infiltrate. Multiple biopsies distal to the ligament of Treitz must be made, preferably using the hydraulic multipurpose biopsy equipment. Even with such techniques, open surgical full thickness biopsies of small bowel together with lymph node biopsies may be necessary to establish the diagnosis.

Therapy and prognosis

In patients with well-documented coeliac sprue, the lymphoma-like symptoms do not respond to strict gluten withdrawal. In some lymphoma

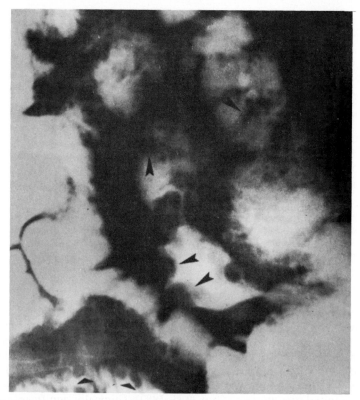

Figure 2. Barium radiography of small bowel in a patient with lymphoma. Multiple nodules (arrows) indent the column of barium. From Gray et al (1982), with kind permission of the authors and the editor of *Gastroenterology*.

patients with previously undocumented coeliac disease, however, there may be an apparent response to gluten restriction early in the course of the disease. In patients with diffuse primary intestinal lymphoma, the diagnosis may be made at surgery but extensive surgical resection should not be undertaken. Whole abdominal radiation (3500-4000 rads) with kidney shielding and shielding of the liver after an initial dose of 2500 rads is recommended (Gray et al, 1982). The radiation therapy alone may be curative in 75 per cent of patients with disease limited to the small intestine or adjacent mesenteric nodes (stage IE). With involvement of regional nodes (stage IIE), a combination radiation therapy and chemotherapy programme should be undertaken. For patients with extensive disease (stage IIIE or stage IV), chemotherapy alone should be employed. The chemotherapy for these diffuse intestinal lymphomas has had only limited experience. The combination of cyclophosphamide, adriamycin, vincristine and prednisone has been studied in a small series from Stanford University (Gray et al, 1982). The vincristine must be used with caution, since an acute intestinal paralytic ileus has been associated with its usage.

'Mediterranean' Lymphoma

Diffuse small intestinal lymphoma, reported in patients from Capetown, South Africa, Israel and Iran, has been termed Mediterranean lymphoma (Novis et al, 1971; Ramot, 1971; Kahn, Selzer and Kaschula, 1972; Rappaport et al, 1972; Eiderman, 1974; Nasr et al, 1976; Gray et al, 1982). This entity appears quite distinct in epidemiology and clinical presentation from the diffuse intestinal lymphoma encountered in 'western' society discussed above. Mediterranean lymphoma affects predominantly teenagers and young adults with a male-to-female ratio of 1.2:1 as opposed to the 3:1 ratio as noted in western lymphoma (Rappaport et al, 1972). Moreover, Mediterranean lymphoma involves predominantly the duodenum and proximal jejunum, with decreasing involvement of the distal small bowel, while western lymphoma is largely a mid-jejunal to distal small bowel malignancy.

Pathogenesis

The clustering of diffuse intestinal lymphoma in young individuals in certain societies of the world suggests a pathogenesis related to environmental and/or genetic factors. Mediterranean lymphoma is a disease of underprivileged communities, occasionally within well-developed nations. However, it is infrequently encountered in developing countries in Latin America where tropic sprue is endemic. The underprivileged societies with the high incidence of this unique diffuse proximal intestinal lymphoma are characterized by poor nutrition, housing, hygiene and medical care (Ramot, 1971). For example, in southern Iran, it is concentrated around the Fars province and is noted in Moslems from low-income rural communities (Nasr et al, 1976). In Israel, Mediterranean lymphoma has been reported largely in the poorer Sephardic Jews of Asian and North African background. More affluent Jews of North European origin are not afflicted in

Israeli society (Ramot, 1971). In the South African reports, however, the majority of patients with intestinal lymphoma are of mixed racial (so-called 'Cape coloured') background. It has, however, been reported among white and black South Africans (Novis et al, 1971; Kahn, Selzer and Kaschula, 1972). The clustering of these cases in certain areas of the world and amongst certain ethnic groups suggest that diffuse primary intestinal lymphoma may represent the outcome of long-standing chronic antigenic stimulation from an intestinal microbial organism. These lymphoma patients also could be at risk for malignancy because of a nutritionally-related immune deficiency state (Novis et al, 1972).

Pathology

On pathological examination of the bowel in these young patients with Mediterranean lymphoma, the small intestine is diffusely infiltrated with a 'cobblestoned' mucosal surface (Rappaport et al, 1972). The mucosal surface has foci of extensive deep small bowel ulceration. Usually, the entire length of the small bowel is involved with somewhat less involvement encountered distally in ileum. The normal circular mucosal folds are obliterated in patients with lymphoma and replaced by multiple submucosal nodules. Occasionally, large single or multiple nodules may be noted. Adjacent mesenteric nodes may likewise be involved. On microscopic examination, the most characteristic histological feature is the diffuse infiltration of lamina propria throughout the proximal small bowel, infiltrates composed of mature, well-differentiated non-neoplastic plasma cells (Rappaport et al, 1972). The mucosa is flattened. Villi are present but markedly widened due to the infiltration by plasma cells. In some instances, the mucosal epithelial cells retain their normal columnar pattern as opposed to the stunted, bizarre epithelial cells often encountered in coeliac sprue (Gray et al, 1982). In some patients, the malignancy is found diffusely throughout the small bowel with malignant histiocytes encountered down through the muscularis propria extending into the serosa (Figure 3). In other patients, the malignancy is encountered only in a focal distribution, forming large tumour masses or confined exclusively to adjacent mesenteric nodes. The most common histological type of lymphoma in these patients is termed reticulum cell sarcoma, although Hodgkin's lymphoma and undifferentiated lymphomas have been reported to occur (Rappaport et al, 1972).

Clinical features and diagnosis

The most common presenting complaint in patients with Mediterranean lymphoma is diffuse, poorly-localized abdominal pain (Kahn, Selzer and Kaschula, 1972). Insidiously progressive weight loss and diarrhoea are also very common. Moreover, patients note anorexia, nausea and vomiting. Patients may develop and present with acute intestinal obstruction or small bowel perforation. On physical examination, these young patients with Mediterranean lymphoma will often be noted to have a poorly-localized abdominal mass and signs of significant weight loss. Hepatomegaly, splenomegaly and clubbing of the fingers are occasionally encountered, together with peripheral oedema due to severe protein-losing enteropathy (Nasr et

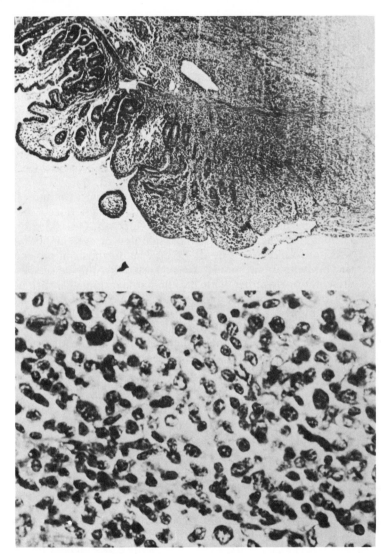

Figure 3. Reticulum cell sarcoma of the small bowel in a patient from Iran with intestinal lymphoma. The mucosa is infiltrated with tumour cells and ulcerated. Normal villus and crypt architecture are destroyed. From Nasr et al (1976), with kind permission of the authors and the editor of *Digestive Diseases*.

al, 1976). Peripheral lymphadenopathy is, however, rare. Modest steatorrhoea in the order of 10 g per 24 hours is commonly noted. Abnormal D-xylose and Schilling tests are observed in one-third to one-half of the patients, together with low serum albumin and carotene levels (Novis et al, 1971; Nasr et al, 1976). In the few patients carefully studied, a paraprotein has been shown in serum, jejunal secretions and plasma cells in the lamina propria. In a quarter or more of these patients, this paraprotein has been classified as an alpha-heavy chain related to immunoglobulin A. The paraprotein is devoid of kappa or lambda light chains (Rappaport et al, 1972; Gray et al, 1982). This heavy chain fragment may represent a congenital or acquired defect in IgA production with associated plasma cell proliferation. The immune deficiency might then predispose to the lymphoma (Rappaport et al, 1972). Alternatively, chronic antigenic stimulation, possibly from a ubiquitous intestinal microbe, could result in the appearance of an abnormal clone of plasma cells. Larger numbers of patients with lymphoma need to be studied. Moreover, immunological studies of individuals from the same environment need to be done before the significance of the paraprotein can be determined.

On barium upper gastrointestinal radiography, the most common finding is a 'non-specific, diffuse malabsorption pattern' with flocculation and puddling of the barium with flattening of the mucosa. Occasionally, focal changes such as thickened mucosal folds, nodules, or even circumferential mass lesions are found (Novis et al, 1971). The diagnosis in patients with Mediterranean lymphoma should be suggested by the above-described clinical presentation together with barium radiography. Confirmation is often made by an exploratory laparotomy. In most instances, the small bowel capsule biopsy specimens demonstrate only partial or total villous atrophy, diffuse plasma cell infiltration, without malignant cells. In a few patients, however, the lymphoma tissue itself may be encountered on the small bowel biopsy (Novis et al, 1971; Eidelman, 1974). In a few patients, malignancy can be demonstrated only in adjacent mesenteric nodes. Extensive involvement of organs outside the small bowel is uncommon in these patients with Mediterranean lymphoma.

Therapy and prognosis

The majority of the patients reported with Mediterranean lymphoma are nutritionally compromised at the time of diagnosis. However, the prognosis of this diffuse primary intestinal lymphoma type is reasonably good. Many patients will have some symptoms for months or years prior to definitive diagnosis. Extensive bowel resection is generally not necessary or indicated. The primary form of therapy is radiation therapy with usual doses of 3500 to 4000 rads (Gray et al, 1982). The kidneys must be shielded throughout radiation therapy while the liver may be shielded after the first 2500 rads. There is limited experience with chemotherapy but use of cyclophosphamide, vincristine, adriamycin and prednisone has been recommended by some researchers (Gray et al, 1982).

EOSINOPHILIC GASTROENTERITIS

Since eosinophilic gastroenteritis was first described by Kaijser in 1937, little more than 100 case reports have appeared describing patients with peripheral eosinophilia, eosinophilic infiltration of a portion of the gastrointestinal tract, and abnormalities of gastrointestinal function. In most patients described, the antrum, pylorus and proximal small bowel were involved with eosinophilic gastroenteritis. Oesophagus, colon, peritoneum and gall-bladder involvement has been described.

Pathogenesis

Since its initial description, eosinophilic gastroenteritis has been assumed to be an allergic or immunological disease. The extensive infiltration of the bowel with eosinophils, together with decreases in elevated peripheral eosinophil counts and exacerbation of gastrointestinal symptoms upon specific food challenge has suggested in many patients a unique allergic reaction (Caldwell, Tennenbaum and Bronstein, 1975). A number of mechanisms have been postulated to explain the development of the eosinophilic infiltration of the bowel wall and the onset of gastrointestinal symptoms with food allergies (Cello, 1979). One mechanism that has been proposed is shown in Figure 4. The specific antigens in certain foods may react within the gut wall with specific IgE antibodies bound to mast cell Fc receptors. Degranulation of the mast cells results in a release of histamine and eosinophilic chemotactic factor of anaphylaxis (ECF-A). These agents are capable of drawing the eosinophils to the site of injury. The local injury to the gut may, therefore, be due to the toxic substance released from the mast cells rather than to damage by infiltrating eosinophils. Tissue eosinophils may actually inactivate these toxic mediators and restore homeostasis.

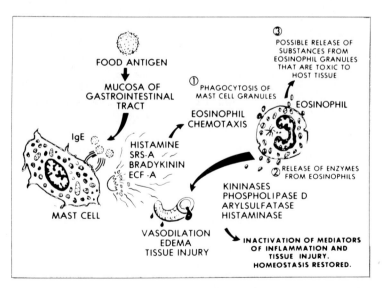

Figure 4. Hypothetical scheme of the pathophysiology of eosinophilic gastroenteritis. The eosinophils play a homeostatic role by neutralizing toxins released by the mast cells. From Cello (1979), with kind permission of the editor of *American Journal of Medicine.*

Pathology and diagnosis

Diagnosis in patients with predominantly mucosal eosinophilic gastroenteritis is often suggested by radiography but confirmed by mucosal biopsy
specimens obtained at endoscopy or peroral suction biopsy (Figures 5 and
6). The involvement with eosinophilic gastroenteritis may be patchy, and
multiple mucosal biopsies, perhaps six to eight, should be undertaken
before excluding the diagnosis of eosinophilic gastroenteritis (Perera,
Weinstein and Rubin, 1975). For patients with involvement of the
muscularis propria, such as those with extensive involvement with the
pylorus, and for patients with eosinophilic involvement of the serosa
(producing eosinophilic ascites) the diagnosis will probably require
operative transmural biopsy.

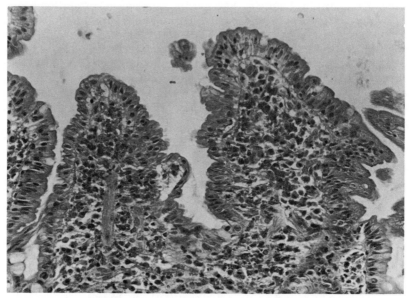

Figure 5. Jejunal biopsy in eosinophilic gastroenteritis. The epithelium is normal. A dense
infiltrate of eosinophils is noted within the lamina propria. From Cello (1979), with kind
permission of the editor of *American Journal of Medicine.*

Clinical presentation

The proximal small bowel and the stomach are the most commonly involved
regions, with rare involvement of oesophagus and colon (Klein et al, 1970;
Leinbach and Rubin, 1970; Dobbins, Sheahan and Behar, 1977; Levinson,
Ramanathan and Nozick, 1977). In addition to eosinophilic infiltration of
the bowel, peripheral eosinophilia must be present to make the diagnosis of
eosinophilic gastroenteritis. Patients develop nausea, vomiting,
periumbilical abdominal pain, and loose water stools. On occasion, weight
loss with profound cachexia occurs in some patients with widespread

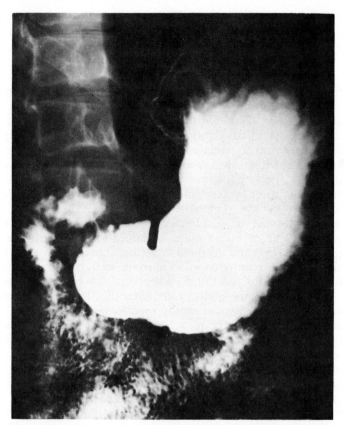

Figure 6. Barium radiograph of stomach and duodenum in eosinophilic gastroenteritis. The pylorus is thickened and narrowed while the duodenal folds are diffusely nodular in appearance. From Cello (1979), with kind permission of the editor of *American Journal of Medicine*.

diffuse mucosal and submucosal eosinophilic gastroenteritis. Charcot-Leyden crystals, presumably from mucosal eosinophils, may be noted on microscopic examination of the stools. The peripheral eosinophilia is occasionally up to 55 per cent of the total white cells on peripheral blood smear. The erythrocyte sedimentation rate is normal, however. Malabsorption of moderate severity commonly complicates the course in patients who have extensive proximal small bowel mucosal involvement with eosinophilic gastroenteritis. Abnormal D-xylose absorption tests, hypoalbuminaemia and significant steatorrhoea are not infrequent in patients with small bowel mucosal involvement.

The diffuse mucosal nature of the disease is suggested by barium radiography with nodular polypoid intraluminal masses, diffuse thickening of the valvulae conniventes, luminal narrowing and segmental bowel distension. Gastric involvement is suggested by cobblestoning of the mucosa in the antrum or by large polypoid filling masses. Biopsy is important to exclude gastric cancer, Crohn's disease or lymphoma mimicking eosinophilic gastroenteritis.

Therapy and prognosis

Although usually unrewarding on a long-term basis, a trial of elimination diets should be undertaken, especially in patients with an atopic history (Leinbach and Rubin, 1970). Substances known or suspected by the patient to exacerbate the symptoms should be rigidly excluded. Skin testing for an immediate hypersensitivity reaction to food substances is unreliable. In the absence of a known or suspected food allergy, a trial of sequentially eliminating milk, eggs, pork, beef and gluten flour products should be considered. On occasion, exacerbations of the disease occur even while on a strict dietary programme (Leinbach and Rubin, 1970). Clinical deterioration should suggest an inadvertent break in abstinence, changing sensitivity of the gut, or even a more fundamental absence of relationship between food ingestion and the disease. Steroids have been used in patients with eosinophilic gastroenteritis who fail to respond to an elimination diet. There are, however, no controlled clinical trials of patients treated with steroids for severe eosinophilic gastroenteritis. The doses commonly employed range from 20 to 40 mg of prednisone given daily in divided doses. In some instances, the responses are prompt and a short course lasting from seven to ten days may produce dramatic clinical remission. The limited experience with cromolyn sodium has been unfavourable (Elkon, Sher and Sejtel, 1977).

The long-term outlook is generally favourable for patients with eosinophilic gastroenteritis, with a course characterized by waxing and waning symptoms, sometimes unaffected by a variety of therapeutic manoeuvres (Gregg and Luna, 1973). Mortality related to the disease is rare. However, profound weight loss may occur in some patients. Many of the deaths reported with alleged eosinophilic gastroenteritis may actually have been due to polyarteritis nodosa, visceral lymphoma, gastric cancer or the 'hyper-eosinophilic' syndrome which can mimic eosinophilic gastroenteritis. Patients with eosinophilic gastroenteritis appear to have no increased risk of gastrointestinal malignancy.

SYSTEMIC MASTOCYTOSIS

Mastocytosis, characterized by increased proliferation of tissue mast cells, most commonly involves the skin where isolated nodules, diffuse macules or diffusely thickened skin with telangiectasias are noted (Dantzig, 1975) (Figure 7). Less than 10 per cent of patients with cutaneous mastocytosis have systemic mastocytosis in which other organs such as liver, spleen, gastrointestinal tract and bone marrow are infiltrated with mast cells.

Pathogenesis

Several theories have been proposed to explain the development of malabsorption and steatorrhoea in patients with systemic mastocytosis. Some,

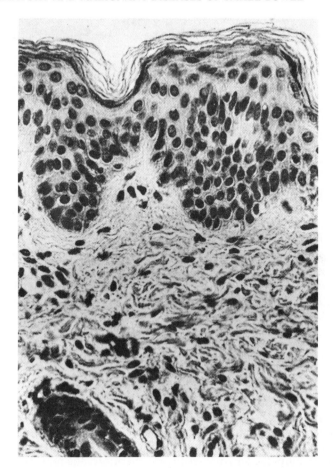

Figure 7. Skin biopsy in a patient with mastocytosis showing increased numbers of mast cells in the dermis. From Dantzig (1975), with kind permission of the author and the editor of *Archives of Internal Medicine.*

but not all, patients with systemic mastocytosis have gastric acid hypersecretion, and excess acid might inactivate pancreatic lipase, precipitate bile salt or cause jejunal mucosal injury (Bredfeldt et al, 1980). However, there is no good correlation between gastric acid secretion and faecal fat in patients with mastocytosis. Moreover, there is no evidence of significant pancreatic exocrine dysfunction or decreased intraluminal enzyme concentration in patients with systemic mastocytosis, although pancreatic fibrosis has been reported. A systemic effect of histamine on the bowel has not been documented. Some patients with steatorrhoea have no significant elevation of serum or urinary histamine levels. The most likely explanation for the proximal small bowel malabsorption and steatorrhoea in patients with systemic mastocytosis appears to be some direct injury of the small bowel

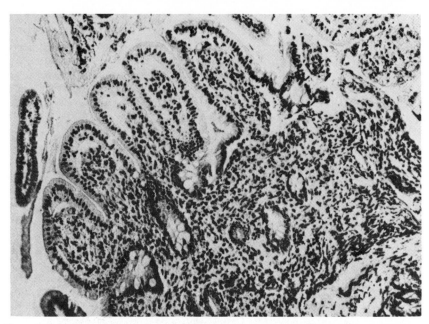

Figure 8. Small bowel biopsy in a patient with systemic mastocytosis. The villi are oedematous and atrophic, with dense infiltration of the lamina propria (consisting of lymphocytes, plasma cells and eosinophils). From Dantzig (1975), with kind permission of the author and the editor of *Archives of Internal Medicine*.

mucosa by chemical mediators released from adjacent tissue mast cells in the lamina propria (Bredfeldt et al, 1980). This mechanism postulated for mastocytosis and steatorrhoea is quite similar to that proposed for the tissue injury in eosinophilic gastroenteritis. Furthermore, the mast cell damage to the jejunal mucosa is probably responsible for the partial villous atrophy on small bowel histology found in patients with systemic mastocytosis.

Pathology

Peroral capsule biopsy of the jejunum in patients with systemic masto-cytosis demonstrates a lamina propria heavily infiltrated with mature mast cells, lymphocytes, plasma cells and eosinophils (Figure 8). The small bowel villi are oedematous and atrophic. The mast cell infiltration may be patchy with large concentrations of cells producing small nodules in the mucosa. The mast cell infiltration decreases in prominence in the distal small bowel. Mast cell infiltration of the lamina propria and muscularis mucosa of the rectum has likewise been documented.

Clinical features and diagnosis

Patients with systemic mastocytosis commonly present with urticaria, facial flushing, nausea, vomiting, cramping abdominal pains, and diarrhoea. The cutaneous manifestations of the disease described above are often quite prominent, with Darier's sign seen in many. Profound hypocalcaemia and hypomagnesaemia have been reported, with patients manifesting Chvostek and Trousseau's signs. The diarrhoea in systemic mastocytosis is often episodic, with five to ten loose watery stools per day. Modest weight loss is also noted in patients with systemic mastocytosis and malabsorption. Routine clinical laboratory tests demonstrate depressed serum calcium, magnesium, potassium, carotene, iron and albumin. The plasma pro-thrombin time is occasionally elevated as well. D-Xylose absorption tests are often abnormal, together with abnormal glucose tolerance and lactose tolerance tests. Steatorrhoea may be severe, with up to 30 g in 24 hours (Dantzig, 1975; Bredfeldt et al, 1980). Upper gastrointestinal series in patients with systemic mastocytosis may evidence a tubular appearance to the small bowel with scattered nodules throughout the proximal gut.

The diagnosis of steatorrhoea and malabsorption should be suspected in patients with systemic mastocytosis and significant gastrointestinal complaints, including diarrhoea and weight loss.

Therapy and prognosis

Histamine-1 antagonists, steroids and cromolyn sodium have not been effective in the treatment of systemic mastocytosis. Cimetidine in doses of 300 mg every four to six hours has, however, been associated with complete suppression of the gastrointestinal tract symptoms (Bradfeldt et al, 1980). The decrease in the abdominal complaints with cimetidine may not be associated with significant improvement in objective tests of absorptive function. The diarrhoea and increased stool weights do, however, normalize on cimetidine therapy in patients with systemic mastocytosis.

MALABSORPTION IN PATIENTS WITH CROHN'S DISEASE

Pathogenesis

Nutritional disturbances commonly complicate the management of patients with Crohn's disease (Dyer and Dawson, 1973). Multiple factors, including malabsorption, have been implicated in the development of malnutrition in these patients: (a) anorexia with decreased food intake; (b) active inflammation with altered metabolic balance; (c) malabsorption of nutrients; and (d) gastrointestinal fluid and protein loss. Decreased food intake should be anticipated in patients with intermittent cramping postprandial abdominal pain due to the active inflammatory process of Crohn's disease. Weight loss from decreased food intake can be attributed either to anorexia or to actual fear of aggravating the cramping abdominal pain by eating. The active inflammatory process of Crohn's disease, transmural in character, ranging in location from oesophagus to anorectal junction is associated with a toxic depression of metabolic activity together with an enhanced need for nutrients. The active inflammatory process will therefore be associated with a net nutritional deficit in so many patients.

Malabsorption in patients with Crohn's disease is most commonly due to the loss of functioning small bowel. This loss of bowel may be a result of the inflammation destroying normal mucosa, or resection or bypass of small bowel. In addition, the stagnant loop syndrome with bacterial overgrowth brought about by the strictures, fistulas, or surgically created blind loop may occur. Minor factors contributing to the malabsorption and maldigestion in Crohn's disease are rapid intestinal transit and impaired small bowel function proximal to the obstructing lesion. Gastrointestinal loss of blood, protein, water and electrolytes is also commonly encountered in patients with Crohn's disease (Dawson, 1972; Warshaw, Waldmann and Laster, 1972). This loss correlates only roughly with the length of intestine involved. Indeed, a short segment of intestine involved by Crohn's disease can be associated with substantial gastrointestinal loss, particularly of protein (Warshaw, Waldmann and Laster, 1972). Profound hypoprotein-aemia, anaemia and electrolyte depletion may be noted in these patients with Crohn's disease.

Pathology

Crohn's disease of the small bowel is largely, but not exclusively, limited to the distal ileum. In nearly half the patients with ileal Crohn's disease, the small bowel inflammatory process extends into the right colon with focal areas of involvement of the ascending and transverse colon (Dawson, 1972). The small bowel is grossly thickened with superficial discrete ulcerations and confluent linear ulcerations (Cook and Dixon, 1973). Deep transverse and longitudinal fissures create a cobblestoning of the mucosa on gross inspection. 'Skip areas' with neither macroscopic nor microscopic involvement are characteristic in patients with Crohn's disease. Both small bowel lumen and ileocaecal valve are narrowed by inflammation and fibrosis with extensive fistulas often encountered between adjacent loops of large and small bowel. On microscopic examination, there is extensive transmural inflammation with submucosal thickening and marked increase in submucosal mononuclear cells (Cook and Dixon, 1973). Transmural fibrosis ensues, leading to a further narrowing of the lumen. Non-caseating granulomas in the submucosa are often found, particularly on examining large specimens of tissue obtained at surgery. The finding of granulomas is not, however, essential to making the diagnosis of Crohn's disease.

Clinical features and diagnosis

Patients with small bowel Crohn's disease characteristically present with recurrent episodes of cramping right lower quadrant abdominal pain (Dawson, 1972). Intermittent partial small bowel obstruction may be encountered in those patients presenting with abdominal distension, nausea, vomiting and the inability to pass stool or flatus. Malnutrition with variable degrees of weight loss may be noted in up to 20 per cent of patients with ileal Crohn's disease. Enterocutaneous fistulas, perianal fistulas and rectal bleeding may be encountered in 10 per cent of patients with ileal Crohn's disease. In children wtih ileal Crohn's disease, growth retardation may be the sole manifestation of the small bowel inflammatory process.

With involvement of the colon in addition to the small bowel in Crohn's disease, a larger number of patients will manifest rectal bleeding and perianal fissures and fistulas. In those patients with radiographic evidence of extensive ileocaecal disease, some consideration should be given to other diseases which may mimic Crohn's disease. In patients from endemic areas of tuberculosis, this disease entity must be considered in the differential diagnosis. Small bowel malignancies, particularly lymphomas and carcinoid tumours, may likewise mimic extensive Crohn's disease of the small bowel.

Small intestinal absorptive tests in patients with Crohn's disease demonstrate profound changes in vitamin B_{12} and fat absorption. In 65 patients with documented Crohn's disease in one study, an inverse correlation was demonstrated between B_{12} absorption and the length of small bowel diseased or resected (Gerson, Cohen and Janowitz, 1973) (Figures 9 and 10). All patients with more than 100 cm of ileum involved had abnormal results on a standard Schilling test. In a second study of 70 patients with Crohn's disease, only 20 per cent of patients with less than 30 cm of ileal disease had an abnormal Schilling test (Filipsson, Hulten and Lindstedt, 1978). Forty-eight per cent of patients had abnormal B_{12} absorption with

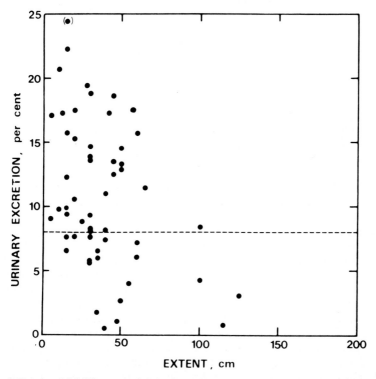

Figure 9. Results of Schilling tests related to the extent of ideal Crohn's disease (n = 55). From Filipsson, Hulten and Lindstedt (1978), with kind permission of the authors and the editor of *Scandinavian Journal of Gastroenterology.*

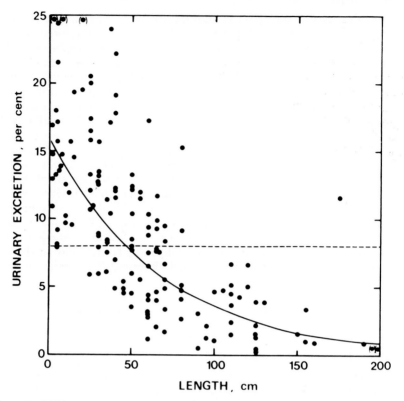

Figure 10. Schilling test results compared to the length of ileum *resected* for Crohn's disease (n = 145). From Filipsson, Hulten and Lindstedt (1978), with kind permission of the authors and the editor of *Scandinavian Journal of Gastroenterology.*

intestinal involvement ranging from 30 to 60 cm, while 60 per cent of patients had abnormal Schilling tests with more than 60 cm of ileal involvement.

There is considerable variability in the correlation between faecal fat and the length of ileal disease and/or resection (Figures 11 and 12). Of patients with 60 cm or less of ileal involvement, only a quarter had substantial steatorrhoea, while over 90 per cent of patients with 60 to 100 cm or more of ileal involvement had steatorrhoea (Filipsson, Hulten and Lindstedt, 1978). The correlation between faecal fat and ileal dysfunction has been more clearly demonstrated in the postoperative state where, in over 130 observations, all patients with more than 90 cm of ileal resection had steatorrhoea (Filipsson, Halten and Lindstedt, 1978). Postoperatively, faecal fat and Schilling test results tended to improve with time, but not significantly. Absorption of D-xylose in patients with Crohn's disease appears to be unchanged. No good correlation exists between the length of Crohn's disease and/or resection and D-xylose absorption. Thus jejunal

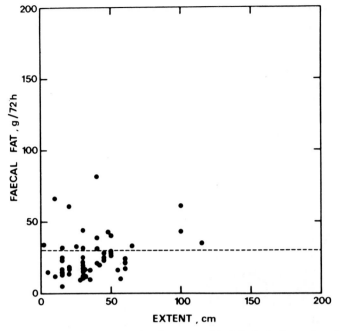

Figure 11. Faecal fat excretion compared to the extent of ileal Crohn's disease (n = 52). From Filipsson, Hulten and Lindstedt (1978), with kind permission of the authors and the editor of *Scandinavian Journal of Gastroenterology*.

function appears to be normal in most patients with Crohn's disease, while a correlation does exist between the length of ileal resection and/or disease and impaired absorption of vitamin B_{12} and ingested fat.

Pathogenesis of steatorrhoea and diarrhoea in ileal resection

Severe small bowel Crohn's disease may be associated with substantial diarrhoea or steatorrhoea as stated above. Generally these patients fall into two groups which actually represent a continuum from predominantly 'fatty acid diarrhoea' to 'bile acid diarrhoea'. Commonly, patients with 90 cm or more of ileal disease and/or resection develop profound steatorrhoea — in excess of 20 g of faecal fat per day. These patients generally have no increased bile acids in the aqueous phase of the stool (Poley and Hoffman, 1976). Moreover, those patients with ileal resection and fatty acid malabsorption respond to decreased dietary fat. The mechanism of fatty acid malabsorption and steatorrhoea in those patients with extensive ileal resection has been investigated (Poley and Hoffman, 1976). These patients have a dramatic *decrease* in the jejunum of both total bile acid and aqueous phase bile acid concentrations. Much of the jejunal bile acids are also not in solution in these patients and can be ultracentrifuged out. The administration of cholestyramine to those patients with fatty acid malabsorption appears to further decrease the jejunal total bile acid and aqueous phase bile

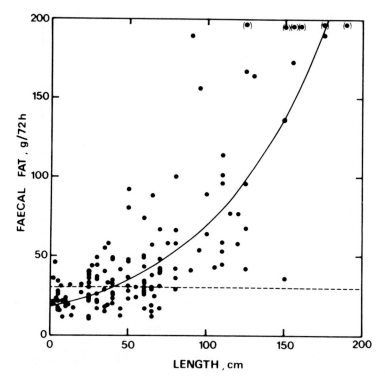

Figure 12. Good correlation exists between faecal fat excretion and the extent of ileum *resected* (n = 137). From Filipsson, Hulten and Lindstedt (1978), with kind permission of the authors and the editor of *Scandinavian Journal of Gastroenterology*.

acid concentrations, while administration of bile acids results in worsening diarrhoea due to the cathartic effect of malabsorbed bile acids. Future studies with individual bile salts, such as chenodeoxycholylglycine, may suggest, however, that specific bile acid replacement could provide benefit to these patients with extensive ileal resection.

Patients with less than 100 cm of ileal resection or ileal Crohn's disease often develop profound diarrhoea in addition to mild steatorrhoea (less than 20 g of faecal fat per day). Stool samples in these patients have substantially *elevated* aqueous phase bile acid concentrations. Moreover, jejunal aspirates in these patients demonstrate essentially normal bile acid concentrations, in both total concentration and aqueous phase concentration (Poley and Hoffman, 1976). These patients do respond clinically to cholestyramine with a clinical improvement and a demonstrable decrease in jejunal total bile acid concentration. The final meal of the day in patients with less than 100 cm of ileal resection probably has the lowest available bile acids in the jejunum for digestion. These patients with 'bile acid diarrhoea' often have mild steatorrhoea in addition to bile acid diarrhoea. Some of the steatorrhoea is undoubtedly due to the decreased intraluminal concentration of bile acids falling below the critical micellar concentration during digestion of the third and often largest meal of the day. However, other factors may be implicated. Rapid gastric emptying in these patients may contribute to decreased fatty acid absorption by overwhelming the precarious fatty acid solubilization in those patients with ileal resection. It has been postulated that the slightly decreased micellar solubilization of dietary lipid and the decreased fat absorption by the enterocytes leads to decreased release of the hormone enterogastrone. The decreased levels of enterogastrone might be associated with the accelerated gastric emptying which may further overwhelm the fatty acid absorptive mechanism. These two features may be contributing to the steatorrhoea encountered in patients with smaller ileal resections. Patients with bile acid diarrhoea who have less than 100 cm of ileal resection/disease do respond to cholestyramine. Dietary changes are also needed. The largest amounts of dietary fat and the larger doses of cholestyramine should be given during the morning meal. Successive meals during the day in patients with subtotal ileal resection should be tailored so as to decrease the amount of ingested dietary fat.

Therapy and prognosis

As stated above in the section dealing with the pathogenesis of steatorrhoea and diarrhoea in patients with ileal Crohn's disease, patients with 90 cm or more of ileal disease and/or resection are incapable of handling substantial dietary fats. Other nutritional supplements should be encouraged, particularly higher carbohydrate and protein intake in these patients. There is *no* rationale for orally-administered bile salts in these patients since the lack of functioning ileal receptors will inevitably lead to bile acid malabsorption and worsening of the diarrhoeal state. Patients with extensive ileal involvement are likewise incapable of absorbing normal vitamin B_{12}. Total body stores of B_{12} are sufficient for several years; however, these patients should be treated with 1000 μg of aqueous B_{12} intramuscularly every month. Patients with ileal resection or ileal Crohn's disease of 30 to 60 cm tends to have mild steatorrhoea but substantial bile acid diarrhoea. Judicious administration of cholestyramine will result in some clinical improvement. As stated above, larger amounts of dietary fat should be administered earlier in the day, together with cholestyramine. Later in the day these patients should be encouraged to limit the intake of dietary fat.

REFERENCES

Bredfeldt, J. E., O'Laughlin, J. C., Durham, J. B. & Blessing, L. D. (1980) Malabsorption and gastric hyperacidity in systemic mastocytosis. *American Journal of Gastroenterology,* **74,** 133-137.

Caldwell, J. H., Tennenbaum, J. I. & Bronstein, H. A. (1975) Serum IgE in eosinophilic gastroenteritis. *New England Journal of Medicine,* **26,** 1388-1390.

Cello, J. P. (1979) Eosinophilic gastroenteritis — a complex disease entity. *American Journal of Medicine,* **67,** 1097-1·104.

Cook, M. G. & Dixon, M. F. (1973) An analysis of the reliability of detection and diagnostic value of various pathological features in Crohn's disease and ulcerative colitis. *Gut,* **14,** 255-262.

Dantzig, P. I. (1975) Tetany, malabsorption, and mastocytosis. *Archives of Internal Medicine,* **135,** 1514-1518.

Dawson, A. M. (1972) Nutritional disturbances in Crohn's disease. *British Journal of Surgery,* **59,** 817-819.

Dobbins, J. W., Sheahan, D. G. & Behar, J. (1977) Eosinophilic gastroenteritis with esophageal involvement. *Gastroenterology,* **72,** 1312-1316.

Dyer, N. H. & Dawson, A. M. (1973) Malnutrition and malabsorption in Crohn's disease with reference to the effect of surgery. *British Journal of Surgery,* **60,** 134-140.

Eidelman, S. (1974) Abdominal lymphoma with malabsorption. *Journal of the American Medical Association,* **229,** 1103-1104.

Elkon, K. B., Sher, R. & Seftel, H. C. (1977) Immunological studies of eosinophilic gastroenteritis and treatment with disodium cromoglycate and beclomethasone dipropionate. *South Africa Medical Journal,* **52,** 838.

Farmer, R. G., Hawk, W. A. & Turnbull, R. B. Jr (1975) Clinical patterns in Crohn's disease: a statistical study of 615 cases. *Gastroenterology,* **68,** 627-635.

Filipsson, S., Hulten, L. & Lindstedt, G. (1978) Malabsorption of fat and vitamin B$_{12}$ before and after intestinal resection for Crohn's disease. *Scandinavian Journal of Gastroenterology,* **13,** 529-536.

Freeman, H. J., Weinstein, W. M., Shnitka, T. K. et al (1977) Primary abdominal lymphoma. *American Journal of Medicine,* **63,** 585-594.

Gerson, C. D., Cohen, N. & Janowitz, H. D. (1973) Small intestinal absorptive function in regional enteritis. *Gastroenterology,* **64,** 907-912.

Gray, G., Rosenberg, S., Cooper, A. et al (1982) Lymphomas involving the gastrointestinal tract. *Gastroenterology,* **82,** 143-152.

Gregg, J. A. & Luna, L. (1973) Eosinophilic gastroenteritis — report of a case with protein-losing enteropathy. *American Journal of Gastroenterology,* **59,** 41-47.

Holmes, G. K. T., Stokes, P. L., Sorahan, T. M. et al (1976) Coeliac disease, gluten-free diet, and malignancy. *Gut,* **17,** 612-619.

Isaacson, P. & Wright, D. H. (1978a) Intestinal lymphoma associated with malabsorption. *Lancet,* **i,** 67-70.

Isaacson, P. & Wright, D. H. (1978b) Malignant histiocytosis of the intestine. *Human Pathology,* **9,** 661-677.

Kahn, L. B., Selzer, G. & Kaschula, R. O. C. (1972) Primary gastrointestinal lymphoma. *Digestive Diseases,* **17,** 219-232.

Klein, N. C., Hargrove, R. L., Sleisenger, M. H. & Jeffries, G. H. (1970) Eosinophilic gastroenteritis. *Medicine,* **49,** 299-319.

Leinbach, G. E. & Rubin, C. E. (1970) Eosinophilic gastroenteritis: a simple reaction to food allergens? *Gastroenterology,* **59,** 874-888.

Levinson, J. D., Ramanathan, V. R. & Nozick, J. H. (1977) Eosinophilic gastroenteritis with ascites and colon involvement. *American Journal Gastroenterology,* **68,** 603-607.

Nasr, K., Haghighi, P., Kiumars, B. et al (1976) Primary upper small intestinal lymphoma. *Digestive Diseases,* **21,** 313-323.

Novis, B. H., Bank, S., Marks, I. N. et al (1971) Abdominal lymphoma presenting with malabsorption. *Quarterly Journal of Medicine, New Series,* **XL,** 521-540.

Perera, D. R., Weinstein, W. M. & Rubin, C. E. (1975) Small intestinal biopsy. *Human Pathology,* **6,** 157-217.

Poley, J. R. & Hoffman, A. F. (1976) Role of fat maldigestion in pathogenesis of steatorrhea in ileal resection. *Gastroenterology,* **71,** 38-44.

Ramot, B. (1971) Malabsorption due to lymphomatous disease. *Annual Review of Medicine,* **22,** 19-24.

Rappaport, H., Ramot, B., Hulu, N. & Park, J. K. (1972) The pathology of so-called Mediterranean abdominal lymphoma with malabsorption. *Cancer,* **29,** 1502-1511.

Selby, W. S. & Gallagher, N. D. (1979) Malignancy in a 19-year experience of adult celiac disease. *Digestive Diseases and Sciences,* **24,** 684-688.

Warshaw, A. L., Waldmann, T. A. & Laster, L. (1972) Protein-losing enteropathy and malabsorption in regional enteritis. *Annals of Surgery,* **178,** 578-580.

13

A Diagnostic Approach to Malabsorption Syndromes: A Pathophysiological Approach

MICHAEL E. RYAN
WARD A. OLSEN

Our approach in discussing the diagnosis of malabsorption will be to consider the problem within a framework of the mechanisms of fat absorption. This seems like a reasonable approach because fat malabsorption is not only common in patients with the diseases we are considering but is often responsible for the predominent manifestations. Although this approach is convenient and hopefully satisfies the authors' desires for clarity and simplicity, it should be pointed out that fat malabsorption is not a universal feature of these diseases; thus, coeliac sprue or Whipple's disease may result in an isolated deficiency of a mineral such as iron or a vitamin even when fat absorption is normal. The manifestations of fat malabsorption may also be relatively minimal when compared to other symptoms: for example, the patient with cholestasis is more apt to be concerned with his jaundice and pruritus than with an increase in number of bowel movements. Finally, we should point out that carbohydrate malabsorption most commonly occurs as an isolated defect and not as manifestation of pancreatic or generalized intestinal disease and needs therefore to be discussed separately.

NORMAL DIGESTION AND ABSORPTION

Normal fat assimilation

Usually malabsorption syndromes are characterized by steatorrhoea with an abnormality in either digestion or absorption of lipid. Thus, some knowledge of the mechanisms by which fat is absorbed is crucial in the rational evaluation and diagnosis of patients with malabsorption. Dietary fats are mainly in the form of triglycerides, water-insoluble compounds made up of three molecules of fatty acids esterified to a glycerol backbone. The first step in triglyceride breakdown probably occurs with the release of lingual lipase from glands at the base of the tongue, i.e., von Ebner's glands

(Hamosh and Burns, 1977). The quantitative role of this enzyme in fat digestion is not known; however, it has a relatively low pH optimum, suggesting that it may be responsible for intragastric hydrolysis of triglycerides (Hamosh et al, 1975). The major contribution of the stomach to lipid digestion, however, is the controlled and relatively slow delivery of the meal to the duodenum — of considerable importance because the capacity of the small bowel to digest and absorb the meal may be overwhelmed if it is delivered too rapidly. When the chyme does reach the duodenum, bile and pancreatic juice are added to the luminal contents through both hormonal (cholecystokinin and secretin) and nervous mechanisms.

The alkaline bile and pancreatic juice neutralize the hydrochloric acid secreted by the stomach and provide an optimal environment for the activity of pancreatic enzymes. Pancreatic lipase is responsible for hydrolysis of triglyceride at the 1- and 3-positions, resulting in the formation of two molecules of fatty acids and 2-monoglyceride. An additional pancreatic factor is also required for adequate triglyceride hydrolysis: a protein called colipase which stabilizes lipase at the water-triglyceride interface (preventing displacement by bile salts) and reduces the pH optimum of lipase to a more physiological level (Borgstrom, Erlanson-Albertsson and Wieloch, 1979). Although the products of lipolysis (fatty acids and monoglycerides) are more polar than the parent triglyceride they are still relatively insoluble in water and therefore require the presence of bile salts for solubilization and dispersal in the aqueous environment of the small intestine. Bile salts possess both hydrophilic and hydrophobic portions, i.e., they are amphipaths; when present at or above a critical concentration, not surprisingly called the critical micelle concentration, they exist as small water-soluble aggregates known as micelles which are able to solubilize fatty acids and monoglycerides much as laundry soaps dissolve grease. The mixed micelles are then responsible for the delivery of these lipolytic products to the intestinal surface, maintaining maximal concentrations in the adjacent aqueous phase from which passive diffusion into the intestinal absorptive cells occurs. The bile salt micelle is not absorbed as such during this process, apparently, but returns to the lumen to continue its work. Substantial intestinal absorption of bile salts does go on (by passive diffusion throughout the small intestine and by active transport in the distal ileum), with reabsorbed bile salts returning to the liver in an enterohepatic circulation. This is an important conservation mechanism since the liver's capacity to synthesize bile salts is limited.

Within the enterocyte, triglyceride is reformed from fatty acids and 2-monoglycerides, covered with a coat of cholesterol, phospholipid, and protein, and released into the lamina propria by reverse pinocytosis as chylomicrons. The chylomicrons are taken up by the lymphatics of the villi and from there reach the general circulation.

Normal protein assimilation

Although protein malabsorption is common in a variety of diseases, signs of severe protein malnutrition are relatively uncommon. Therefore digestion and absorption of protein will be reviewed only briefly. After ingestion of a meal, pepsinogen is released from the chief cells of the stomach and converted to its active form, pepsin, which begins the breakdown of protein; peptic digestion is not important for overall protein digestion but may be important in the release of certain micronutrients like vitamin B_{12} from food. The more significant part of protein digestion begins in the duodenum with the action of a number of proteolytic enzymes (trypsin, chymotrypsin, exopeptidase, carboxypeptidase and elastase) of pancreatic origin. These proteases result in the hydrolysis of protein to a mixture of small peptides and amino acids. Amino acids, as well as di- and tripeptides, to a large extent, can be absorbed intact into the enterocyte. Other peptides require hydrolysis at the surface of the enterocyte by membrane-bound peptidases. Free amino acids (and some small peptides) exit into the portal circulation.

Normal carbohydrate assimilation

Dietary carbohydrates are primarily starch (a mixture of the polysaccharides amylose and amylopectin), sucrose (table sugar), and lactose (the sugar in milk). Amylose is a straight chain glucose polymer with bonds between the first carbon atom of one glucose molecule and the fourth carbon of the next. Amylopectin is a branching glucose polymer with alpha-1,4 linear chains which are joined at periodic branch points via 1,6 bonds. Although digestion of starch begins with release of salivary amylase, the bulk of digestion occurs because of the action of the amylase in pancreatic juice. Amylase readily catalyses the breakdown of the interior 1,4 bonds of both amylose and amylopectin but is not very effective against the external bonds or those adjacent to the branch points, and is ineffective against the 1,6 bonds themselves. Amylase is also not effective at hydrolysis of beta linkages and therefore cellulose, another glucose polymer, is not digested. Thus intraluminal starch digestion results in the formation of a disaccharide (maltose), a trisaccharide (maltotriose), and a series of branched oligosaccharides called the alpha-limit dextrins. These carbohydrates, together with the dietary disaccharides sucrose and lactose, must be further hydrolysed before intestinal absorption occurs.

Further hydrolysis occurs at the surface membrane of the enterocyte in reactions catalysed by enzymes called disaccharidases. Maltose and maltotriose are hydrolysed to glucose by several maltases, the alpha-limit dextrins to glucose by a single alpha-dextrinase, sucrose to glucose and fructose by sucrase, and lactose to glucose and galactose by lactase. The monosaccharide products then are rapidly transported into the enterocytes and subsequently into the portal circulation — glucose and galactose by the same active transport mechanism and fructose by a passive mechanism which has great capacity.

Absorption of vitamins

Vitamins A, D, E and K are quite insoluble in aqueous solutions and consequently are very dependent upon micellar solubilization for adequate absorption. Thus conditions which impair the formation of bile salt micelles frequently decrease absorption of fat-soluble vitamins. Although water-soluble vitamins are not dependent upon micellar solubilization for optimal absorption, they frequently require specialized digestive and transport mechanisms which are often altered in intestinal diseases. Folic acid and cobalamin (vitamin B_{12}) are two important examples. Folic acid exists in food as free folate (pteroylmonoglutamate) conjugated to many glutamate molecules. Dietary folate, pteroyl*poly*glutamate, must be first hydrolysed to free folate before intestinal absorption can occur; this reaction occurs at the surface of enterocytes because of the presence of another brush border enzyme called folic acid conjugase (Rosenberg, 1981). Free folate is then absorbed by both diffusion and a carrier-mediated transport mechanism. One might predict, then, that folate deficiency is a frequent problem in patients with intestinal disease.

Cobalamin malabsorption is also common in intestinal disease. The vitamin is present in animal protein sources from which it is liberated by the action of gastric pepsin. Subsequent events are really quite remarkable and have become understood only in the last few years (Allen et al, 1978a,b). Within the stomach, the free vitamin binds to a ubiquitous binding protein called R protein which possesses an even greater affinity for cobalamin than does the intrinsic factor secreted by gastric parietal cells. Unlike B_{12} bound to intrinsic factor, neither free B_{12} nor B_{12} bound to R protein is absorbable, so that the R protein must be removed and intrinsic factor allowed to attach. This event occurs in the proximal small intestine, apparently the result of pancreatic proteases which alter the R protein in a way which decreases its affinity for cobalamin; this allows intrinsic factor to successfully compete for the vitamin. Subsequently the intrinsic factor-B_{12} complex attaches to specific receptors on the surface of enterocytes in the ileum and B_{12} is absorbed.

DISORDERS OF DIGESTION AND ABSORPTION

Disorders of fat assimilation

The breakdown of dietary triglycerides to fatty acids and β-monoglycerides with subsequent absorption is complex, and disorders at any stage may lead to steatorrhoea. Table 1 lists each stage and classifies the major causes of steatorrhoea according to physiological defect. Alterations in lipolysis are common and may occur because of disorders in delivery of substrate (the triglyceride meal), the secretion of enzyme (lipase), or the environment in which the reaction takes place. Rapid gastric emptying because of a partial gastrectomy or antrectomy for peptic ulcer disease causes precipitous delivery of a large amount of triglyceride to the small intestine which may result in inadequate mixing of the triglyceride substrate with the enzyme and impair lipolysis. The substrate may be delivered adequately but won't be hydrolysed if the enzyme is not delivered; for example, if cholecystokinin release is impaired because of diffuse proximal small intestinal disease such as coeliac sprue, or because of significant bypass of the duodenum with partial gastrectomy and a Bilroth 2 or Polya anastomosis or with a gastroenterostomy, lipase delivery may not be optimal. Lipase delivery is even more defective with severe pancreatic acinar destruction from chronic pancreatitis or pancreatic duct obstruction from pancreatic cancer and results in marked steatorrhoea. Even if substrate and enzyme reach the duodenum at sufficient rates, the environment must be appropriate for optimal lipolysis. Thus a low pH within the duodenal lumen, the result of the excessive secretion of gastric acid in patients with gastrinoma, will result in steatorrhoea because lipase is not effective in an acid environment. A deficiency of colipase might also prevent adequate lipolysis, and recently two patients have been described who appeared to have steatorrhoea because of isolated colipase deficiency (Hildebrand et al, 1982).

Table 1. *Typical disorders of fat absorption*

I.   *Defects in lipolysis*
   A. Altered delivery of triglyceride substrate: partial gastrectomy
   B. Decreased secretion of lipase:
      1. Diminished release of cholecystokinin: diffuse proximal intestinal disease or bypass
      2. Pancreatic acinar disease from chronic pancreatitis
      3. Pancreatic duct obstruction from carcinoma
   C. Altered environment limiting lipolysis
      1. Low pH from excessive gastric acid secretion with gastrinoma
      2. Colipase deficiency

II. *Defects in incorporation of lipolytic products into bile salt micelles*
   A. Hepatic/biliary disease with diminished secretion of bile salts
      1. Intrahepatic cholestasis: cirrhosis, hepatitis
      1. Bile duct obstruction: neoplasma or gallstone
   B. Ileal resection/disease with significant defect in the enterohepatic circulation
   C. Intraluminal defects with alteration of bile salts
      1. Certain drugs, especially cholestyramine
      2. Intestinal bacterial overgrowth

III. *Defects in intestinal absorption*
   A. Impaired uptake by enterocytes: intestinal mucosal disease, resection, or bypass
   B. Altered chylomicron formation: abetalipoproteinaemia
   C. Decreased transport through the lamina propria: Whipple's disease
   D. Diminished uptake by lymphatic system: intestinal lymphangiectasia or lymphoma

Altered incorporation of fatty acids and monoglyceride into micelles may slow the rate of lipolysis and also diminish dispersal through the aqueous environment of the intestinal lumen. The resultant fat malabsorption is relatively modest compared to the severe steatorrhoea seen with either impaired lipolysis or extensive intestinal mucosal disease; this is probably because fatty acid and monoglyceride possess some water-solubility and can be slowly absorbed over an intact small bowel. On the other hand, significant problems with absorption of fat-soluble vitamins are common when micellar solubilization is impaired because these micronutrients are insoluble in the absence of micelles. Bile salt concentrations may be insufficient for adequate micelle formation because of intrahepatic cholestasis (for example, cirrhosis, viral hepatitis, cholestatic hepatitis from drugs like chlorpromazine, and alcoholic hepatitis) or extrahepatic bile duct obstruction from an obstructing neoplasm or gallstone. The delivery system may be patent but bile salt secretion will be low if there is impairment in ileal reabsorption of bile salts to the point where increased hepatic synthesis of bile salts cannot compensate for the losses. Thus surgical resection or bypass of the ileum and extensive ileal mucosal disease are common causes of fat malabsorption. Even if bile salts are secreted normally they may not be effective because of binding to a drug like cholestyramine or because of bacterial metabolism in patients with intestinal bacterial overgrowth. Certain bacterial species which may colonize the intestine under circumstances of chronic stasis (for example, strictures, pseudo-obstruction) or seeding (multiple small bowel diverticula, enterocolonic fistula) are capable of removing the glycine and taurine from bile salts. This renders them less capable of solubilizing lipolytic products and more readily absorbable by passive diffusion from the proximal intestine (undesirable because intraluminal concentrations may prematurely fall below the critical micelle concentration).

Sufficient numbers of intact enterocytes are necessary for optimal absorption of the products of lipolysis. Intestinal mucosal diseases, such as coeliac and tropical sprue, invasive giardiasis, and large intestinal resections, are examples of conditions where steatorrhoea may occur because of decreases in mucosal uptake. No clear example of steatorrhoea from alterations in triglyceride resynthesis exists, but impaired chylomicron formation has been recognized in the rare disorder called abetalipoprotein-aemia. Decreased transport of the chylomicrons through the laminia propria appears, in part, responsible for the fat malabsorption often seen in Whipple's disease where large macrophages may hinder the movement of chylomicrons. (Diminished numbers and function of absorptive cells also contribute in this disease.) Finally, the chylomicrons must be taken up by the lymphatic system, a process that is impaired in conditions where there is lymphatic obstruction like intestinal lymphangiectasia or lymphoma.

Disorders of carbohydrate assimilation

Decreased absorption of carbohydrates may lead to their accumulation within the intestinal lumen and delivery to the colon where bacterial fermentation to monosaccharides, short-chain fatty acids, molecular hydrogen, and carbon dioxide occurs at variable rates. Although the short-chain fatty acids are absorbed fairly rapidly from the colon, the carbo-hydrates themselves are not and may lead to diarrhoea because of osmotic retention of water within the colonic lumen. Thus the clinical manifestations of carbohydrate malabsorption are watery diarrhoea, abdominal cramps and bloating, and often excessive flatus after ingestion of the appropriate carbohydrate(s).

Disorders of intraluminal carbohydrate digestion are exceedingly rare in adults because of the great excess of secreted amylase; they are seen only with total pancreatic duct obstruction and probably never with pancreatic acinar disease, even when extensive. On the other hand, transient amylase deficiency is physiological in the newborn state and, of course, is the reason starch is not fed to neonates. A doubtful example of impaired starch hydrolysis is the effect of an amylase inhibitor derived from kidney beans which has recently enjoyed heavy sales in the United States as an aid to weight reduction. There are no acceptable published data to support or refute the drug's presumed ability to inhibit starch digestion in man, but the apparent lack of symptoms of carbohydrate malabsorption with its use suggest that it is not effective.

Although abnormalities of intraluminal starch digestion are rare, abnormalities of surface digestion of oligosaccharides are very common. So-called lactase deficiency is the normal state for most adults in the world. Because milk and its products are common foods in man, lactase deficiency is a relatively common cause of diarrhoea. Sucrase and alpha-dextrinase activities reside on the same brush border protein which is sometimes missing in the uncommon genetic disease, sucrase-alpha-dextrinase (iso-maltase) deficiency. This disease results in symptoms with sucrose ingestion, but interestingly there is less trouble with starch, presumably because the higher molecular weight alpha-dextrins exert less osmotic force. Since several brush border proteins can hydrolyse maltose, isolated maltase deficiency has not been described. It is important to point out that a variety of intestinal diseases, including coeliac sprue, bacterial overgrowth, inflammatory bowel disease, viral gastroenteritis, and cancer chemotherapy (Hyams, Krause and Gleason, 1981; Hyams et al, 1982) may cause isolated lactase deficiency or even a generalized disaccharidase deficiency. Finally both acquired (intestinal disease) and congenital abnormalities of the glucose/galactose transport system have been described with intolerance to all carbohydrates save fructose.

DIAGNOSTIC TESTS IN MALABSORPTION

Assessment of Fat Absorption

Qualitative faecal fat

Microscopic examination of a random stool sample may provide a clue to the presence of steatorrhoea. A sample of stool (5 mm diameter) is placed on a glass slide to which several drops of glacial acetic acid and Sudan III or IV stain are added. This is mixed, gently heated to boiling (but not to dryness) and examined while still warm for fat (orange globules). The examiner determines the number of droplets per high-power field as well as the size (compared to a red blood cell). Normal values are up to 100 particles/high-power field, each from 1-4 μm in diameter. Drummey, Benson and Jones (1961) found a reasonable correlation between microscopic fat analysis and quantitative assay of a 72-hour collection, with some variability when there was only mild steatorrhoea (6-11 g of fat/day). A potential problem with the test exists in patients with ileal dysfunction who may progressively deplete their bile salt pool during the day because of gallbladder contraction with meals; an isolated stool sample might not be representative of the 24-hour period. Examination of a sample from a

24-hour collection has therefore been advocated (Simko, 1981), but in our opinion, this would diminish whatever attractiveness the test has. A much more serious problem is that the test is generally performed by the least experienced person, i.e., student, intern, or novice laboratory technician, so that the results are often not reliable. Although the test is quick, inexpensive, and easy to perform, we do not feel that diagnostic or therapeutic decisions should be based on it unless done by someone with experience.

Quantitative faecal fat

The gold standard continues to be the 72-hour faecal fat determination (van de Kamer, Huinink and Weyers, 1949) with a fat intake of 70-110 g a day. Although this test is unaesthetic and requires more dedication on the part of patient, nursing staff, and laboratory personnel than most tests, it is frequently the most valuable study obtained in suspected malabsorption. We have not used a disposable collection unit which fits onto the toilet seat to collect stool and separate urine as described by Krejs and Fordtran (1978), but their photograph suggests that it would work well, and together with a large covered paint-can which can be refrigerated might be a convenient method of collecting 72-hour stool samples on outpatients. The degree of steatorrhoea is often a clue to the diagnosis. Thus severe steatorrhoea, 40 g or more of faecal fat per day, suggests defective lipolysis, often from chronic pancreatitis or carcinoma of the pancreas, or massive small bowel resection; moderate steatorrhoea (25-35 g per day) is more common with intestinal mucosal diseases like coeliac sprue, and mild steatorrhoea (less than 25 g per day) is commonly seen with defects in micelle formation. The 72-hour stool weight which is obtained during this study may also be very helpful even if steatorrhoea is not found; a normal stool weight (less than 200 g a day) in a patient complaining of diarrhoea might suggest irritable colon, while passage of 2000 g or more of watery stool would suggest the possibility of pancreatic cholera or laxative abuse.

$^{14}CO_2$ breath tests

Because of the difficulties in obtaining 72-hour stool collections for faecal fat, investigators have sought easier methods to determine the presence or absence of fat malabsorption. In 1962, Schwabe et al measured $^{14}CO_2$ in expired air after the oral administration of triglyceride containing ^{14}C-fatty acid to determine the degree to which fat was absorbed. The idea was that the oxidation of ^{14}C-fatty acid (and production of $^{14}CO_2$) might be proportional to the rate of absorption of fatty acid. Subsequently, efforts have been made to use the test to distinguish between disorders of fat digestion and fat absorption by comparing results using labelled free fatty acid with those with labelled triglyceride (Burrows et al, 1974; Adlung and Grazikowske, 1979; Pedersen et al, 1979). The use of a stable isotope like ^{13}C allows this test to be performed in children and women of childbearing age where the use of radioactivity is undesirable (Watkins et al, 1977; Schoeller et al, 1981), although the additional necessity of mass spectrometry makes it unlikely that this modification will be generally used for some time to come.

The $^{14}CO_2$ breath test would seem to be a relatively easy approach to establishing fat malabsorption. However, the six-hour duration of the study together with the necessity for isotope administration and measurement are certainly obvious disadvantages. More importantly, the test may have some built-in limitations. The oxidation of fatty acids is obviously dependent upon factors other than the rate of fatty acid absorption, and it seems likely that disorders like diabetes mellitus, thyroid disease, liver disease, or fever might result in an unreliable test (Newcomer et al, 1979). It is also likely that a variety of disorders of fat metabolism like hyperlipaemia or obesity, where the specific radioactivity (radioactive/total) of absorbed ^{14}C-fatty acid might be abnormal because of differences in the quantity of endogenous fatty acids, would also affect the test. Finally, the test should be inaccurate in patients with abnormal retention of carbon dioxide. Because of these limitations and conflicting results in the literature, we believe that it is not yet ready for general use.

Tests of Intestinal Mucosa Integrity

Jejunal mucosa: D-xylose absorption test

D-Xylose is a 5-carbon sugar which, unlike glucose, is incompletely absorbed from the jejunum, is not metabolized by mammalian cells, and is quantitatively excreted in the urine (Fordtran, Soergel and Ingelfinger, 1962). Xylose absorption has had considerable use as a test of the functional integrity of the intestinal mucosa with measurements of urinary excretion or blood levels after oral administration. Our personal experience has been with the test based upon urinary excretion and is similar to the results of Sladen and Kumar (1973), that is, the test is not very sensitive. The results using blood levels seem better, however, especially in children (Rolles et al, 1973; Buts et al, 1978) although there is no universal agreement (Lamabadusuriya, Packer and Harries, 1975; Christie, 1978; Hill et al, 1981). Administration of 5 g rather than the usual 25 g may eliminate the occasional nausea and vomiting seen which of course invalidate the test. This dose with a one-hour blood level may result in higher sensitivity and specificity (Haeney et al, 1978). It must be pointed out that low values for xylose absorption are frequent in intestinal bacterial overgrowth syndromes because of bacterial metabolism of the sugar (Goldstein et al, 1970; Krawitt and Beeken, 1975) and that there are other causes of apparent low xylose absorption in the absence of mucosal disease; these include slow gastric emptying, ascites, advanced age (Kendall, 1970; Webster and Leeming, 1975), and abnormal renal function (Kendall and Nutter, 1970), although the measurement of blood levels ought to eliminate the problems in the last two situations.

We think that the xylose test, although it may miss mild mucosal disease, is not an unreasonable test to perform, especially if a one-hour blood level is measured after a 5 g dose. At least in the adult patient we believe that it should never be accepted as strong evidence against intestinal mucosal disease; we believe that only a small bowel biopsy provides that evidence.

Jejunal mucosa: small bowel biopsy

The small bowel biopsy is the only way to exclude intestinal mucosal disease with reasonable assurance (though it may miss patchy lesions of the mucosa). For this reason, and because intestinal diseases like coeliac sprue and Whipple's disease can be effectively treated, we believe that all patients with unexplained malabsorption should be biopsied, even if xylose absorption is normal. We also believe that patients with unexplained nutritional deficiencies, even without steatorrhoea, should be biopsied because many will turn out to have treatable intestinal mucosal disease. Biopsies have usually been obtained in the past with the use of a swallowed capsule or a fluoroscopically directed biopsy tube, but some have switched to the use of endoscopic biopsies as a more convenient and fast alternative, although the specimens are somewhat more difficult to orient properly.

Ileal mucosa

The functional integrity of the ileum can also be evaluated because the distal ileum is the only segment of intestine capable of active bile salt transport and vitamin B_{12} absorption. Absorption tests for both substances have been devised and used not only to assess the function of the distal ileum, but as tests for intestinal bacterial overgrowth as well. We will defer discussion of the bile breath test until the section on bacterial overgrowth syndromes and review here only the vitamin B_{12} absorption test. Originally described by Schilling (1953), the test ordinarily involves the oral administration of radiolabelled cobalamin and the measurement of radioactivity of a 24-hour urine collection as an index of absorption (normally greater than 7 per cent of the administered dose). A large amount of 'cold' vitamin is injected intramuscularly so that the absorbed radioactive B_{12} is excreted rather than used by the body. Normal B_{12} absorption implies secretion of intrinsic factor, removal of R protein by pancreatic proteases, an intact distal ileum, and the absence of sufficient intraluminal bacteria (or parasites) to successfully compete for the vitamin. An abnormal test should be repeated successively with each of the missing ingredients in an effort to determine the nature of the absorptive defect. Thus correction with intrinsic factor implies pernicious anaemia, with pancreatic enzymes pancreatic insufficiency, and after antibiotics (tetracycline has usually been used) intestinal bacterial overgrowth syndrome. Failure to correct suggests ileal dysfunction. Interestingly, cobalamin malabsorption correctable with oral bicarbonate has been described in the Zollinger-Ellison syndrome (Shimoda, Saunders and Rubin, 1968), but we do not know how commonly that occurs. These concepts are summarized in Table 2. Although some have questioned the reliability and reproducibility of the test (Adams and Cartwright, 1963), it has been valuable in our experience. The test obviously depends upon normal renal function and is relatively contraindicated in children and in women of childbearing age (especially if pregnant). A recent modification of the vitamin B_{12} absorption test has been described which studies simultaneous absorption of intrinsic factor-bound B_{12} and R protein-bound B_{12} by a double label technique (Brugge et al, 1980). This test can apparently distinguish between ileal dysfunction/bacterial overgrowth and pancreatic insufficiency (the B_{12} bound to R protein will be poorly absorbed compared to that bound to intrinsic factor in pancreatic insufficiency.

Table 2. *Schilling test*

Disease resulting in abnormal test	Test corrected by administration of
Pernicious anaemia	Intrinsic factor
Bacterial overgrowth	Antibiotics
Pancreatic insufficiency	Pancreatic enzymes
Gastrinoma	Bicarbonate
Ileal dysfunction or resection	Nothing

Pancreatic Insufficiency

Severe steatorrhoea occurring in the setting of chronic alcoholic pancreatitis with obvious pancreatic calcifications (seen in some 30 per cent according to Reber, 1978) is usually not an especially difficult diagnostic challenge. On the other hand, mild degrees of pancreatic insufficiency are difficult to detect because steatorrhoea and creatorrhoea do not occur until output of lipase and trypsin have diminished to 10 per cent of normal (DiMagno, Go and Summerskill, 1973). A number of tests have been devised for use in the recognition of these patients.

Tests involving collection of duodenal fluid for pancreatic enzymes

These tests involve duodenal intubation and collection of fluid after the administration of a stimulus to pancreatic secretion. Usually trypsin or amylase activity, but sometimes total protein or bicarbonate, is measured in a series of aspirates obtained over a period of several hours. The best of these tests is probably the measurement of pancreatic enzymes after the Lundh test meal which contains 6 per cent fat, 5 per cent protein and 15 per cent carbohydrate (Lundh, 1962; Thaysen et al, 1964). The test does appear to work (Cook et al, 1967; Mottaleb et al, 1973; Zeitlin and Sircus, 1974; Lake-Bakaar et al, 1979), with the claim of 90 per cent sensitivity in a review by James (1973).

The other approach has been to stimulate pancreatic secretion by injection of secretin-cholecystokinin. Since bicarbonate measurements have been thought more useful than enzyme concentrations in this approach (Rolny and Jagenburg, 1978), one must simultaneously aspirate and discard gastric juice which might otherwise contaminate the duodenal fluid. Reasonable correlations have been reported between secretin-cholecystokinin tests and Lundh meal tests (Lurie et al, 1973; Gyr et al, 1975; Braganza and Rao, 1978). Since these tests require relatively prolonged intubation and a considerable amount of technical support they have never become very popular, at least in the United States, and we do not use them.

B-T-PABA test

In 1972 Imondi, Stradley and Wolgemuth described the use of a synthetic peptide, *N*-benzoyl-L-tyrosyl-*p*-aminobenzoic acid (B-T-PABA), to evaluate pancreatic function in animals. After reaching the duodenum the peptide is normally cleaved by chymotrypsin to form *p*-aminobenzoic acid (PABA) which is absorbed, conjugated by the liver, and excreted in the urine where it can be measured (see Figure 1). B-T-PABA is apparently free of acute toxicity (Lang et al, 1980) and the test has been shown to compare favourably to the Lundh test meal or the secretin-cholecystokinin test in the detection of moderate to severe pancreatic insufficiency (Arvanitakis and Greenberger, 1976; Gyr et al, 1976; Imamura et al, 1978; Nousia-Arvanitakis et al, 1978; Sacher, Kobsa and Shmerling, 1978; Harada et al, 1979; Hoek et al, 1981; Kimura, Wakasugi and Ibayashi, 1981; Lang et al, 1981). Because the test as originally described depends upon intestinal absorption and hepatic conjugation, small bowel disease and severe liver disease may give false positive results. For this reason Mitchell et al (1979 and 1981) have described the use of the B-T-PABA test combined with study of absorption of free PABA to detect those patients with impaired absorption or conjugation of PABA. The two tests were done either on two successive days or on the same day using radiolabelled PABA. The test does require normal renal function, but looks very promising. At present, however, it is not approved for use in the United States.

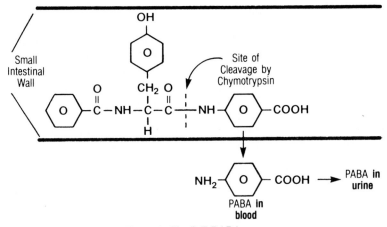

Figure 1. The B-T-PABA test.

General comment

As indicated earlier, the majority of patients with malabsorption from pancreatic insufficiency can be recognized fairly easily. In a patient with massive steatorrhoea (more than 40 g of faecal fat a day), a history suggestive of recurrent pancreatitis, especially if pancreatic calcifications are found by ordinary x-rays or by CT scan, would certainly suggest pancreatic insufficiency. A normal xylose test and small intestinal barium x-ray study might be reassuring enough so that further evaluation would not have to be carried out. A clinical response to pancreatic enzymes, especially if diminished faecal fat can be documented, is also often helpful. Only a small number of patients turn out to have unsuspected pancreatic insufficiency as a cause for malabsorption and it is in the recognition of these patients that the more specific tests of pancreatic function are most useful.

Bacterial Overgrowth Syndrome

Small intestinal culture

Although small intestinal culture remains the definitive test for bacterial overgrowth syndromes (patients with the syndrome have bacterial concentrations of 10^6/ml, often 10^8/ml), it is unusual in our experience for this test to be done except by groups with a research interest in the syndrome. This is because the test requires not only intubation of the jejunum, but fairly rigorous attention to the bacteriology, especially if anaerobes are to be measured. Fortunately there are some reasonably easy alternatives, including a test that has already been discussed (the Schilling test) before and after antibiotics.

^{14}C-Glycocholate breath test

In 1971, bile breath tests for the detection of intestinal bacterial overgrowth and also ileal dysfunction were described (Fromm and Hofmann, 1971; Sherr et al, 1971) and have since been used extensively. The test involves the oral administration of glycocholate in which the glycine moiety is labelled with ^{14}C. As shown in Figure 2, if the amide bond is cleaved by bacterial enzymes, labelled glycine is released which can then be metabolized to ^{14}CO$_2$ by either bacterial or human cells; ^{14}CO$_2$ is then collected in expired air by techniques similar to those used with the ^{14}C-fat absorption test. The source of the enzymes to deconjugate glycocholate can be either bacteria within the lumen of the small intestine (bacterial overgrowth syndrome) or the normal

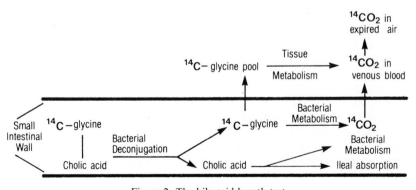

Figure 2. The bile acid breath test.

flora of the colon (when ileal absorption of bile salts is defective). The test, however, has not proved to be especially useful in the detection of ileal dysfunction (Lauterburg, Newcomer and Hofmann, 1978), but has been helpful in the diagnosis of intestinal bacterial overgrowth (Parkin et al, 1972; James, Agnew and Bouchier, 1973; Farivar et al, 1979). Our experience with the test at our institution indicates that the test is very specific but not very sensitive, so that a normal test does not disprove the diagnosis.

^{14}C-D-Xylose breath test

King et al (1979) have devised a breath test for the detection of intestinal bacterial overgrowth based upon the observation that intestinal bacteria metabolize xylose. They report that the test is more sensitive and specific than the bile breath test (King et al, 1980); with further experience, this test may become a practical approach to diagnosis of bacterial overgrowth syndromes.

Carbohydrate Intolerance

The usual manifestation of carbohydrate malabsorption is watery diarrhoea, the result of the intraluminal load of unabsorbed carbohydrate and derivative short-chain fatty acids and consequent osmotic retention of water. Two screening tests for carbohydrate malabsorption based upon the pathophysiology of the diarrhoea have been suggested (Krejs and Fordtran, 1978) and have been useful in our hands. A stool water pH of less than 6 obtained with ordinary pH paper, together with the finding of a large 'osmotic gap', is very suggestive. An 'osmotic gap' is indirect evidence of the presence of carbohydrate and short-chain fatty acids and is found by measuring the osmolality of stool water (with particulate matter removed by filtration or centrifugation) and subtracting the osmolality contributed by sodium, potassium, and their anions. In practice, the osmolality contributed by these electrolytes can be conveniently estimated by simply doubling (to account for the anions) the sum of sodium and potassium concentrations of stool water. It must be pointed out that these screening studies probably have no value in the absence of watery diarrhoea and in examination of stool that is not fresh or refrigerated (because of continuing carbohydrate fermentation in vitro (Shiau et al, 1982).

A more specific diagnosis can be made by means of a tolerance test using the suspected disaccharide; the classical test is the lactose tolerance test where 50 g of lactose are given orally and blood glucose measured at intervals. Lactase deficiency is suggested by a failure to increase blood glucose concentrations by 20 mg per cent over fasting levels and by precipitation of the patient's symptoms. Delayed gastric emptying or decreased glucose absorption may cause false positive results so that an abnormal study should be repeated with a glucose/galactose mixture. The same approach can be used for suspected sucrase-isomaltase deficiency.

A more sensitive and specific test for carbohydrate malabsorption is the measurement of breath hydrogen concentrations after administration of the suspected sugar (Levitt and Donaldson, 1970; Bond and Levitt, 1977). Although a few individuals appear to lack the colonic organisms responsible for hydrogen production, the test has been remarkably successful. The recent availability of relatively cheap and simple gas chromatographs dedicated to breath hydrogen measurements makes this approach very attractive. The ultimate diagnostic test is to measure the levels of disaccharidases in an intestinal mucosal biopsy. It is unlikely, however, that this approach is necessary in ordinary clinical practice.

DIAGNOSTIC WORKUP OF MALABSORPTION

Patients with malabsorption may present with one of a multitude of manifestations which do not immediately suggest intestinal disease; these range from unexplained weight loss (not as common as one would suppose unless anorexia is also present) or deficiency of a specific vitamin or mineral. Bowel symptoms are usually present, however, even if they consist only of passage of unusually large, bulky or sticky stools. Ordinarily the cornerstone of a diagnostic workup is to determine if steatorrhoea is present; if it is not the physician must consider other causes for the symptoms, including carbohydrate malabsorption (especially if watery diarrhoea is present). If steatorrhoea is found, the cause may be fairly obvious because of a history of previous surgery or pancreatic disease or because cholestasis is very apparent. An extensive diagnostic evaluation may not be warranted in that case. Assuming that the diagnosis is not obvious, one should begin with a few simple studies: a plain abdominal x-ray looking for pancreatic calcifications; a barium meal x-ray with small bowel examination to look for specific anatomical lesions like diverticula, fistulas, and surgical alterations as well as the dilatation and mucosal changes suggestive of intestinal mucosal diseases; and a xylose absorption test or the B-T-PABA test. Either form of the B_{12} absorption test with the appropriate attempts to correct B_{12} malabsorption could probably be added to that list because of its general utility. Further studies would depend on the results obtained. We emphasize that it is important to make the correct diagnosis because most of these diseases can be satisfactorily treated.

REFERENCES

Adams, J. F. & Cartwright, J. (1963) The reliability and reproducibility of the Schilling test in primary malabsorptive disease and after partial gastrectomy. *Gut,* **4,** 32-36.
Adlung, J. & Grazikowske, H. (1979) Diagnosis of fat absorption with ^{14}C-tripalmitate/ ^{3}H-palmitic acid. *Scandinavian Journal of Gastroenterology,* **14,** 587-592.
Allen, R. H., Seetharam, B., Podell, E. & Alpers, D. H. (1978a) Effects of proteolytic enzymes on the binding of cobalamin to R protein and intrinsic factor. In vitro evidence that a failure to partially degrade R protein is responsible for cobalamin malabsorption in pancreatic insufficiency. *Journal of Clinical Investigation,* **61,** 47-54.
Allen, R. H., Seetharam, B., Allen, N. C. et al (1978b) Correction of cobalamin malabsorption in pancreatic insufficiency with a cobalamin analogue that binds with high affinity to R protein but not to intrinsic factor. In vivo evidence that a failure to partially degrade R protein is responsible for cobalamin malabsorption in pancreatic insufficiency. *Journal of Clinical Investigation,* **62,** 1628-1634.

Arvanitakis, C. & Greenberger, N. J. (1976) Diagnosis of pancreatic disease by a synthetic peptide. A new test of exocrine pancreatic function. *Lancet,* **i,** 663-666.

Bond, J. H. & Levitt, M. D. (1977) Use of breath hydrogen (H_2) in the study of carbohydrate absorption. *American Journal of Digestive Diseases,* **22,** 379-382.

Borgstrom, B., Erlanson-Albertsson, C. & Wieloch, T. (1979) Pancreatic colipase: chemistry and physiology. *Journal of Lipid Research,* **20,** 805-816.

Braganza, J. M. & Rao, J. J. (1978) Disproportionate reduction in tryptic response to endogenous compared with exogenous stimulation in chronic pancreatitis. *British Medical Journal,* **ii,** 392-394.

Brugge, W. R., Goff, J. S., Allen, N. C. et al (1980) Development of a dual label Schilling test for pancreatic exocrine function based on the differential absorption of cobalamin bound to intrinsic factor and R protein. *Gastroenterology,* **78,** 937-949.

Burrows, P. J., Fleming, J. S., Garnett, E. S. et al (1974) Clinical evaluation of the ^{14}C fat absorption test. *Gut,* **15,** 147-150.

Buts, J. P., Morin, C. L., Roy, C. C. et al (1978) One-hour blood xylose test: a reliable index of small bowel function. *Journal of Pediatrics,* **92,** 729-733.

Christie, D. L. (1978) Use of the one-hour blood xylose test as an indicator of small bowel mucosal disease. *Journal of Pediatrics,* **92,** 725-728.

Cook, H. B., Lennard-Jones, J. E., Sherif, S. M. & Wiggins, H. S. (1967) Measurement of tryptic activity in intestinal juice as a diagnostic test of pancreatic disease. *Gut,* **8,** 408-414.

DiMagno, E. P., Go, V. L. W. & Summerskill, W. H. J. (1973) Relations between pancreatic enzyme outputs and malabsorption in severe pancreatic insufficiency. *New England Journal of Medicine,* **288,** 813-815.

Drummey, G. D., Benson, J. A. & Jones, C. M. (1961) Microscopical examination of the stool for steatorrhea. *New England Journal of Medicine,* **264,** 85-87.

Farivar, S., Fromm, H., Schindler, D. & Schmidt, F. W. (1979) Sensitivity of bile acid breath test in the diagnosis of bacterial overgrowth in the small intestine with and without the stagnant (blind) loop syndrome. *Digestive Diseases and Sciences,* **24,** 33-40.

Fordtran, J. S., Soergel, K. H. & Ingelfinger, F. J. (1962) Intestinal absorption of D-xylose in man. *New England Journal of Medicine,* **267,** 274-279.

Fromm, H. & Hofmann, A. F. (1971) Breath test for altered bile-acid metabolism. *Lancet,* **ii,** 621-625.

Goldstein, F., Karacadag, S., Wirts, C. W. & Kowlessar, O. D. (1970) Intraluminal small-intestinal utilization of D-xylose by bacteria. A limitation of the D-xylose absorption test. *Gastroenterology,* **59,** 380-386.

Gyr, K., Agrawal, N. M., Felsenfeld, O. & Font, R. G. (1975) Comparative study of secretin and Lundh tests. *American Journal of Digestive Diseases,* **20,** 506-512.

Gyr, K., Stadler, G. A., Schiffmann, I. et al (1976) Oral administration of a chymotrypsin-labile peptide — a new test of exocrine pancreatic function in man (PFT). *Gut,* **17,** 27-32.

Haeney, M. R., Culank, L. S., Montgomery, R. D. & Sammons, H. G. (1978) Evaluation of xylose absorption as measured in blood and urine: a one-hour blood xylose screening test in malabsorption. *Gastroenterology,* **75,** 393-400.

Hamosh, M. & Burns, W. A. (1977) Lipolytic activity of human lingual glands (Ebner). *Laboratory Investigation,* **37,** 603-608.

Hamosh, M., Klaeveman, H. L., Wolf, R. O. & Scow, R. O. (1975) Pharyngeal lipase and digestion of dietary triglyceride in man. *Journal of Clinical Investigation,* **55,** 908-913.

Harada, H., Mishima, K., Shundo, T. et al (1979) Exocrine pancreatic function test by a synthetic peptide. *American Journal of Gastroenterology,* **71,** 45-52.

Hildebrand, H., Borgstrom, B., Bekassy, A. et al (1982) Isolated co-lipase deficiency in two brothers. *Gut,* **23,** 243-246.

Hill, R., Cutz, E., Cherian, G. et al (1981) An evaluation of D-xylose absorption measurements in children suspected of having small intestinal disease. *Journal of Pediatrics,* **99,** 245-247.

Hoek, F. J., Sanders, G. T. B., Teunen, A. & Tijtgat, G. N. (1981) In vitro and in vivo analysis of the PABA test compared with the Lundh test — influence of intraluminal pH. *Gut,* **22,** 8-14.

Hyams, J. S., Krause, P. J. & Gleason, P. A. (1981) Lactose intolerance following rotavirus infection in young children. *Journal of Pediatrics,* **99,** 916-918.

Hyams, J. S., Batrus, C. L., Grand, R. J. & Sallan, S. E. (1982) Cancer chemotherapy-induced lactose malabsorption in children. *Cancer,* **49,** 646-650.

Imamura, K., Nakamura, T., Miyazawa, T. et al (1978) Oral administration of chymotrypsin labile peptide for a new test of exocrine pancreatic function (PFT) in comparison with pancreozymin-secretin test. *American Journal of Gastroenterology,* **69,** 572-578.

Imondi, A. R., Stradley, R. P. & Wolgemuth, R. (1972) Synthetic peptides in the diagnosis of exocrine pancreatic insufficiency in animals. *Gut,* **13,** 726-731.

James, O. (1973) The Lundh test. *Gut,* **14,** 582-591.

James, O., Agnew, J. E. & Bouchier, I. A. D. (1973) Assessment of the ^{14}C-glycocholic acid breath test. *British Journal of Medicine,* **3,** 191-195.

Kendall, M. J. (1970) The influence of age on the xylose absorption test. *Gut,* **11,** 498-501.

Kendall, M. J. & Nutter, S. (1970) The influence of sex, body weight and renal function on the xylose test. *Gut,* **11,** 1020-1023.

Kimura, T., Wakasugi, H. & Ibayashi, H. (1981) Clinical study of exocrine pancreatic function test by oral administration of N-benzoyl-L-tyrosyl-p-aminobenzoic acid. *Digestion,* **21,** 133-139.

King, C. E., Toskes, P. P., Spivey, J. C. et al (1979) Detection of small intestine bacterial overgrowth by means of a ^{14}C-D-xylose breath test. *Gastroenterology,* **77,** 75-82.

King, C. E., Toskes, P. P., Guilarte, T. R. et al (1980) Comparison of the one-gram D-[^{14}C]xylose breath test to the [^{14}C] bile acid breath test in patients with small-intestine bacterial overgrowth. *Digestive Diseases and Sciences,* **25,** 53-58.

Krawitt, E. L. & Beeken, W. L. (1975) Limitations of the usefulness of the D-xylose absorption test. *American Journal of Clinical Pathology,* **63,** 261-263.

Krejs, G. J. & Fordtran, J. S. (1978) Physiology and pathophysiology of ion and water movement in the human intestine. In *Gastrointestinal Disease* (Ed.) Sleisenger, M. H. & Fordtran, J. S. pp. 297-335. Philadelphia: W. B. Saunders.

Lake-Bakaar, G., McKavanagh, S., Redshaw, M. et al (1979) Serum immunoreactive trypsin concentration after a Lundh meal. Its value in the diagnosis of pancreatic disease. *Journal of Clinical Pathology,* **32,** 1003-1008.

Lamabadusuriya, S. P., Packer, S. & Harries, J. T. (1975) Limitations of xylose tolerance test as a screening procedure in childhood celiac disease. *Archives of Disease in Childhood,* **50,** 34-39.

Lang, C., Gyr, K., Kraehenmann, J. A. & Arenz, F. (1980) The oral pancreatic function test with N-benzoyl-L-tyrosyl-p-aminobenzoic acid: acute toxicity and effects of renal function on this test. *Journal of Clinical Chemistry and Clinical Biochemistry,* **18,** 551-555.

Lang, C., Gyr, K., Stadler, G. A. & Gillessen, D. (1981) Assessment of exocrine pancreatic function by oral administration of N-benzoyl-L-tyrosyl-p-aminobenzoic acid (Bentiromide): 5 years' clinical experience. *British Journal of Surgery,* **68,** 771-775.

Lauterburg, B. H., Newcomer, A. D. & Hofmann, A. F. (1978) Clinical value of the bile acid breath test. Evaluation of the Mayo Clinic experience. *Mayo Clinic Proceedings,* **53,** 227-233.

Levitt, M. D. & Donaldson, R. M. Jr (1970) Use of respiratory hydrogen [H$_2$] excretion to detect cabohydrate malabsorption. *Journal of Laboratory and Clinical Medicine,* **75,** 937-945.

Lundh, G. (1962) Pancreatic exocrine function in neoplastic and inflammatory disease; a simple and reliable new test. *Gastroenterology,* **42,** 275-280.

Lurie, B., Brom, B., Bank, S. et al (1973) Comparative response of exocrine pancreatic secretion following a test meal and secretin-pancreozymin stimulation. *Scandinavian Journal of Gastroenterology,* **8,** 27-32.

Mitchell, C. J., Humphrey, C. S., Bullen, A. W. et al (1979) Improved diagnostic accuracy of a modified oral pancreatic function test. *Scandinavian Journal of Gastroenterology,* **14,** 737-741.

Mitchell, C. J., Field, H. P., Simpson, F. G. et al (1981) Preliminary evaluation of a single-day tubeless test of pancreatic function. *British Medical Journal,* **ii,** 1751-1753.

Mottaleb, A., Kapp, F., Noguera, E. C. A. et al (1973) The Lundh test in the diagnosis of pancreatic disease: a review of five years' experience. *Gut,* **14,** 835-841.

Newcomer, A. D., Hofmann, A. F., DiMagno, E. P. et al (1979) Triolein breath test. A sensitive and specific test for fat malabsorption. *Gastroenterology,* **76,** 6-13.

Nousia-Arvanitakis, S., Arvanitakis, C., Desai, N. & Greenberger, N. (1978) Diagnosis of exocrine pancreatic insufficiency in cystic fibrosis by the synthetic peptide N-benzoyl-L-tyrosyl-p-aminobenzoic acid. *Journal of Pediatrics,* **92,** 734-737.

Parkin, D. M., Cussons, D. J., Rooney, P. et al (1972) Evaluation of the 'breath test' in the detection of bacterial colonization of the upper gastrointestinal tract. *Lancet,* **ii,** 777-780.

Pedersen, N. T., Marquersen, J., Skjoldborg, H. & Jensen, E. (1979) Serum radioactivity of ^{14}C-triolein and ^{3}H-oleic acid ingested in a test meal. A rapid test of pancreatic exocrine insufficiency. *Scandinavian Journal of Gastroenterology,* **14,** 529-534.

Reber, H. A. (1978) Chronic pancreatitis. In *Gastrointestinal Disease* (2nd edition) (Ed.) Sleisenger, M. H. & Fordtran, J. S. pp. 1439-1456. Philadelphia: W. B. Saunders.

Rolles, C. J., Nutter, S., Kendall, M. J. & Anderson, C. M. (1973) One-hour blood-xylose screening-test for coeliac disease in infants and young children. *Lancet,* **ii,** 1043-1045.

Rolny, P. & Jagenburg, R. (1978) The secretin-CCK test and a modified Lundh test. A comparative study. *Scandinavian Journal of Gastroenterology,* **13,** 927-931.

Rosenberg, I. H. (1981) Intestinal absorption of folate. In *Physiology of the Gastrointestinal Tract* (Ed.) Johnson, L. R., Christensen, J., Grossman, M. I. et al. pp. 1221-1230. New York: Raven Press.

Sacher, M., Kobsa, A. & Shmerling, D. H. (1978) PABA screening test for exocrine pancreatic function in infants and children. *Archives of Diseases in Childhood,* **53,** 639-641.

Schilling, R. F. (1953) Intrinsic factor studies. II. The effect of gastric juice on the urinary excretion of radioactivity after the oral administration of radioactive vitamin B_{12}. *Journal of Laboratory and Clinical Medicine,* **42,** 860-866.

Schoeller, D. A., Klein, P. D., MacLean, W. C. Jr & Watkins, J. B. (1981) Faecal ^{13}C analysis for the detection and quantitation of intestinal malabsorption. Limits of detection and application to disorders of intestinal cholylglycine metabolism. *Journal of Laboratory and Clinical Medicine,* **97,** 439-448.

Schwabe, A. D., Cozzetto, F. J., Bennett, L. R. & Mellinkoff, S. M. (1962) Estimation of fat absorption by monitoring of expired radioactive carbon dioxide after feeding a radioactive fat. *Gastroenterology,* **42,** 285-291.

Sherr, H. P., Sasaki, Y., Newman, A. et al (1971) Detection of bacterial deconjugation of bile salts by a convenient breath-analysis technic. *New England Journal of Medicine,* **285,** 656-661.

Shiau, Y. F., Feldman, G. M., Resnick, M. A. & Coff, P. M. (1982) Pitfalls of stool osmolality and electrolyte measurements. *Gastroenterology,* **82,** 1178 (Abstract).

Shimoda, S. S., Saunders, D. R. & Rubin, C. E. (1968) The Zollinger-Ellison syndrome with steatorrhoea. II. The mechanisms of fat and vitamin B_{12} malabsorption. *Gastroenterology,* **55,** 705-723.

Simko, V. (1981) Faecal fat microscopy. Acceptable predictive value in screening for steatorrhoea. *American Journal of Gastroenterology,* **75,** 204-208.

Sladen, G. E. & Kumar, P. J. (1973) Is the xylose test still a worthwhile investigation? *British Medical Journal,* **iii,** 223-226.

Thaysen, E. H., Mullertz, S., Worning, H. & Bang, H. O. (1964) Amylase concentration of duodenal aspirates after stimulation of the pancreas by a standard meal. Clinical evaluation in gastrointestinal disorders. *Gastroenterology,* **46,** 23-31.

Van de Kamer, J. H., Huinink, H. T. B. & Weyers, H. A. (1949) Rapid method for the determination of fat in feces. *Journal of Biological Chemistry,* **177,** 347-355.

Watkins, J. B., Schoeller, D. A., Klein, P. D. et al (1977) ^{13}C-Trioctanoin: a non-radioactive breath test to detect fat malabsorption. *Journal of Laboratory and Clincial Medicine,* **90,** 422-430.

Webster, S. G. P. & Leeming, J. T. (1975) Assessment of small bowel function in the elderly using a modified xylose tolerance test. *Gut,* **16,** 109-113.

Zeitlin, I. J. & Sircus, W. (1974) Factors influencing duodenal trypsin levels following a standard test meal as a test of pancreatic function. *Gut,* **15,** 173-179.

14

Nutrition and Absorption in Diseases of the Pancreas

JAMES H. GRENDELL

The pancreas is the master exocrine digestive gland of the alimentary tract, secreting approximately two litres of protein- and bicarbonate-rich fluid into the duodenum each day. Approximately 90 per cent of the protein content of pancreatic juice consists of digestive enzymes (Scheele, Bartelt and Bieger, 1981) which are responsible for much of the intraluminal digestion of complex nutrients in the small intestine. The most important of these in man are *amylase*, which splits starches into maltose, maltotriose and limit dextrins; *lipase*, which splits triglycerides into fatty acids and mono-glycerides; and the proteolytic enzymes (*trypsin, chymotrypsin, elastase,* and the *carboxypeptidases*) which cleave proteins and polypeptides into oligopeptides and free amino acids. The bicarbonate secreted in pancreatic juice neutralizes hydrochloric acid delivered to the small intestine from the stomach, raising the pH to levels at which the pancreatic digestive enzymes are catalytically active (pH > 3.5-4.0). In addition, neutralization of stomach acid by pancreatic bicarbonate probably has a protective effect on small intestinal mucosa.

NUTRITIONAL FACTORS AS AETIOLOGICAL AGENTS IN DISEASES OF THE PANCREAS

Pancreatitis

Ethanol. The most important nutritional factor in the aetiology of pancreatic disease is excessive consumption of ethanol which is associated with the great majority of cases of chronic pancreatitis and pancreatic insufficiency in the industrialized world and, together with gall stone disease, is responsible for most cases of acutely symptomatic pancreatitis in these same geographic areas. The question of how ethanol causes pancreatic disease in man has not been fully answered. However, chronic excessive ethanol use results in abnormalities in both pancreatic juice (Sahel and Sarles, 1979; Renner et al, 1980; DeCaro et al, 1981) and pancreatic duct anatomy (Nagata et al, 1981). Several theories have been proposed to explain the role of ethanol in the development of pancreatitis (Sarles, 1971; Allan and White, 1974; Wakabayashi and Takeda, 1976).

Clinics in Gastroenterology — Vol. 12, No. 2, May 1983
0300-5089/83/1202-551 $05.00©1983 W. B. Saunders Company Ltd

Malnutrition. An increased incidence of pancreatic exocrine insufficiency (tropical chronic pancreatitis) has been reported in both children and adults in areas where protein-calorie malnutrition is endemic (Barbezat and Hansen, 1968; Tandon et al, 1970). Histological studies demonstrate that the pancreatic acinar cells first show a decrease in the numbers of zymogen granules and mitochondria and in the amount of endoplasmic reticulum. Eventually the cells undergo atrophy and replacement by fibrous tissue (Blackburn and Vinijchaikul, 1969). The pancreactic dysfunction in this setting is associated with hypoproteinaemia and appears to be due to an inadequate supply of amino acids for pancreatic enzyme synthesis. In most patients pancreatic enzyme secretion returns to normal after nutritional repletion (Barbezat and Hansen, 1968; Tandon et al, 1970).

Pancreatic cancer

Various studies have shown a positive correlation between the incidence of pancreatic cancer and meat consumption (Ishii et al, 1973), per capita consumption of fat, sugar, animal proteins, eggs, and milk (Lea, 1967), and coffee drinking (MacMahon et al, 1981). Studies of the relationship between ethanol consumption and cancer of the pancreas have yielded conflicting results (Burch and Ansari, 1968; Monson and Lyon, 1975; MacMahon et al, 1981). The data favouring a significant aetiological role for any of these potential risk factors are neither unequivocal nor convincing.

MALABSORPTION IN DISEASES OF THE PANCREAS

Pathophysiology

Malabsorption in the setting of pancreatic disease is due to inadequate intraluminal digestion in the small intestine which results from an insufficient quantity of pancreatic digestive enzymes. In clinical practice this is most frequently the result of a failure of the pancreas to secrete a normal amount of all of its digestive enzymes (Table 1). There are rare reports in the paediatric age group of patients with congenital isolated enzyme deficiencies or the failure to activate in the small intestine proteolytic enzymes — which are secreted by the pancreas in inactive (zymogen) forms — due to a congenital absence of the small intestine mucosal enzyme enterokinase (Table 1). These unusual congenital abnormalities in pancreatic digestive function have been reviewed recently (Stafford and Grand, 1982) and will not be considered further here.

Significant impairment in the pancreatic secretion of digestive enzymes may exist in the absence of clinical malabsorption. Studies by DiMagno, Go and Summerskill (1973) have demonstrated that approximately 90 per cent of the secretory capacity of the pancreas must be lost before significant steatorrhoea or azotorrhoea is observed (Figure 1). Thus the pancreas possesses a remarkable reserve capacity for enzyme secretion. However, once secretory capacity falls below 5 per cent of normal, a rapid increase in the amount of steatorrhoea is found (Figure 2) (Regan et al, 1977).

Table 1. *Causes of exocrine pancreatic insufficiency*

Reduction in all digestive enzymes
    Chronic pancreatitis
    Cystic fibrosis
    Neoplasms obstructing pancreatic duct
    Major pancreatic resection
    Protein-calorie malnutrition
    Schwachman's syndrome

Isolated enzyme deficiency
    Lipase
    Trypsin
    Amylase

Failure of enzyme activation in the small intestine
    Enterokinase deficiency

Dietary fat and protein may be absorbed to a greater degree than would seem possible based upon the amount of pancreatic enzymes available for digestion. Thus in a group of patients studied by DiMagno et al (1977), 20 to 40 per cent of dietary fat and protein was absorbed despite mean outputs of lipase and trypsin which were 0.2 per cent of normal. Experiments in animals (Imondi, Stradley and Wolgemuth, 1972) in which all pancreatic juice was diverted from the intestinal tract have yielded similar results. This residual digestive capability in the absence of pancreatic digestive enzymes has been attributed to alternative sources of small amounts of digestive enzymes (e.g., salivary amylase, pharyngeal and gastric lipase, gastric pepsin, peptidases located in the brush border of the small intestine).

Vitamin, iron, or calcium deficiencies are rarely observed in pancreatic exocrine insufficiency, unlike the case in some of the disorders of the small bowel associated with malabsortpion, such as coeliac sprue (Evans and Wollaeger, 1966). This is probably the result of the persistence of intact small bowel absorptive capacity and the preservation of the enterohepatic circulation of bile salts in pancreatic insufficiency. One exception to this general rule is that at least 50 per cent of patients with severe pancreatic insufficiency malabsorb cobalamin (vitamin B_{12}), although overt cobalamin deficiency rarely develops. Impaired cobalamin absorption is due to an alteration in the function of a non-specific binding protein (R protein) which is present in saliva, gastric juice, and bile. R protein competes with intrinsic factor for the binding of cobalamin in the stomach. At the normal acid pH of the stomach and proximal duodenum, R protein binding to cobalamin is altered by pancreatic proteases. This results in the release of cobalamin which then binds to intrinsic factor which resists proteolytic digestion. In pancreatic insufficiency, some of the cobalamin remains attached to R protein, and this complex does not bind to the ileal receptor specific for the cobalamin-intrinsic factor complex.

Assessment of the patient with malabsorption due to pancreatic exocrine insufficiency

Patients with significant malabsorption due to pancreatic insufficiency will usually present to the physician complaining of diarrhoea (or steatorrhoea)

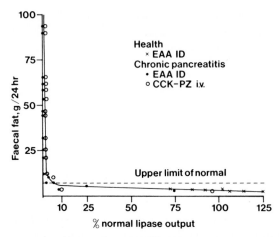

Figure 1. The relationship between 24-hour faecal fat excretion and pancreatic lipase output in healthy individuals following intraduodenal perfusion with essential amino acids (× EAA ID) and in patients with chronic pancreatitis following intraduodenal perfusion with essential amino acids (● EAA ID) or intravenous injection of cholecystokin-pancreozymin (○ CCK-PZ i.v.). Note that faecal fat excretion remains normal (below broken line) until lipase output falls to less than 10 per cent of normal. From DiMagno, Go and Summerskill (1973) *New England Journal of Medicine,* **288,** 813, reprinted with permission.

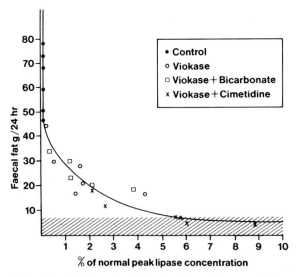

Figure 2. The relationship of 24-hour faecal fat excretion and pancreatic lipase concentration in patients with pancreatic insufficiency. The shaded area represents the normal range of faecal fat excretion. Symbols represent various treatment regimens as denoted in the inset. Note that for peak lipase concentrations less than 5 per cent of normal, faecal fat excretion increased markedly for even small decrements in lipase concentration. From Regan et al (1977) *New England Journal of Medicine,* **297,** 857, reprinted with permission.

and weight loss. When the patient attempts to compensate for malabsorption by overeating, the increased fat intake may result in increased fat absorption, but at the expense of more abdominal cramping associated with more voluminous diarrhoea. In contrast, an increase in protein intake will lead to considerable additional nitrogen absorption with no increase in symptoms (Wollaeger et al, 1948). Symptomatic carbohydrate malabsorption with flatulence and watery diarrhoea is rare with pancreatic insufficiency for two reasons: (1) salivary amylase secretion remains unimpaired; and (2) pancreatic amylase secretion has to be reduced by more than 97 per cent before the rate of intraluminal starch digestion is slowed (Fogel and Gray, 1973).

The diagnosis of significant malabsorption in a patient with suspected pancreatic insufficiency is made on the basis of direct measurement of increased faecal fat excretion on a fat balance study. Because of the great reserve capacity of the pancreas, the finding of reduced pancreatic enzyme output alone does not constitute evidence of insufficiency. The quantification of fat loss in the stool not only establishes the presence of steatorrhoea but also provides a baseline with which to assess the response to therapy. A three-day stool collection is usually obtained with the patient consuming 70 to 100 g of fats per day. The normal faecal fat excretion is less than 5 to 7 g per day (depending on the daily fat intake) and is exceeded in pancreatic insufficiency usually by a large margin. Indeed, some of the highest values for faecal fat excretion are found in patients with pancreatic insufficiency. Azotorrhoea (>2.5 g faecal nitrogen per day on a daily diet of about 120 g protein) (Wollaeger, Comfort and Osterberg, 1947) usually accompanies steatorrhoea. However, the stool nitrogen determination is cumbersome and adds little information useful to the clinician.

Fat or nitrogen balance studies do not distinguish between malabsorption due to impaired intraluminal digestion resulting from pancreatic disease and impaired absorption due to diseases of the small intestine (Comfort et al, 1953). Pancreatic disease is suggested by a compatible history (e.g., of chronic pancreatitis, cystic fibrosis, or previous pancreatic resection); the finding of calcification in the region of the pancreas on abdominal x-ray, abdominal sonography, or computed tomography; abnormal pancreatic duct architecture on endoscopic retrograde pancreatography; and abnormalities in a variety of tests of pancreatic exocrine function (Arvanitakis and Cooke, 1978; Goff, 1981). Patients with steatorrhoea and weight loss who do not have evidence of significant pancreatic disease, and patients diagnosed as having pancreatic insufficiency who do not respond to appropriate medical management, should be evaluated thoroughly for possible primary disease of the small intestine.

Pancreatic enzyme replacement therapy

Because the basis of malabsorption due to pancreatic enzyme insufficiency is evident — inadequate delivery of pancreatic digestive enzymes to the small intestine — replacement of the deficient enzymes is the logical mainstay of therapy. However, success with enzyme supplementation is not always easily achieved and requires some understanding of the factors that determine the enzyme activities which will occur in the lumen of the small intestine following ingestion of the supplement (DiMagno, 1979, 1982). Four important points must be considered:

1. The commercially available enzyme preparations are rather low in potency. Thus, if *none* of the contained lipase were inactivated, six to eight tablets or capsules of such commonly used preparations as pancreatin (Viokase) or pancreatolipase (Cotazym) with meals would be necessary to abolish steatorrhoea. This amount roughly equals 5 to 10 per cent of the total amount of lipase secreted after maximal stimulation of the pancreas. Administration of smaller amounts of enzyme will reduce faecal fat excretion but will not return it to normal levels (DiMagno, Go and Summerskill, 1973; Graham, 1977).
2. Once ingested, lipase is rapidly inactivated at a pH below 4.0, whereas trypsin inactivation proceeds more slowly and is mediated by pepsin at a pH less than 3.5 (Heizler, Cleveland and Iber, 1965).
3. The duodenal pH in patients with chronic pancreatitis is lower than in controls late in the postprandial period (DiMagno et al, 1977) and is frequently less than 5.0 — a pH at which bile acids precipitate. This reduced availability of conjugated bile acids for fat solubilization and micelle formation is an additional cause of impaired fat absorption (Regan et al, 1979; Zenler-Munro et al, 1981).
4. Because enzyme supplementation is expensive and must be taken with every meal and snack to be maximally effective, compliance is often poor, especially in alcoholics.

Clinical studies have shown that eight pancreatin tablets taken with a meal result in the delivery to the duodenum of only 8 per cent of the lipase activity contained in the tablets, amounting to less than 1 per cent of the normal output of meal-stimulated lipase (Figure 3). The corresponding values for trypsin are 22 per cent and 1.4 per cent respectively. However, even these small increments in duodenal digestive enzyme content are sufficient to reduce stool fat by about 50 per cent and stool nitrogen output by about 75 per cent (DiMagno et al, 1977). In addition, other studies have demonstrated that the efficiency of enzyme supplementation therapy decreases in parallel with the mean postprandial pH in stomach and duodenum.

These observations have led to recent efforts to improve the efficacy of therapy in patients who do not have an adequate response to enzyme supplementation by avoiding the inactivation of the oral enzyme preparations by the acid pH in the stomach and proximal small intestine. Two different approaches have been tried: (1) the use of antacids or cimetidine to raise the gastric and intestinal pH; or (2) the administration of pancreatic enzymes in microencapsulated enteric-pH-coated preparations.

The use of antacids has yielded mixed results. Whereas coadministration of enzyme tablets with either sodium bicarbonate or aluminium hydroxide resulted in a greater reduction of steatorrhoea than did enzyme tablets alone, the use of calcium carbonate or magnesium-aluminium hydroxide actually tended to worsen steatorrhoea (Graham, 1982; Regan et al, 1977).

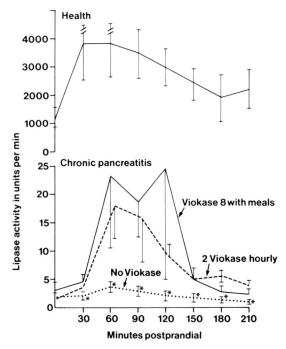

Figure 3. The delivery of lipase activity to the ligament of Trietz following a meal in healthy individuals (upper panel, solid line), patients with pancreatic insufficiency not receiving enzyme supplementation (dotted line), and patients with pancreatic insufficiency receiving enzyme supplementation with Viokase (pancreatin) either given with meals (lower panel, solid line) or hourly (broken line). Note that while Viokase administration results in a marked increase in lipase delivery to the small intestine compared to that observed for the untreated patients, the absolute amount is less than 1 per cent of that seen in healthy individuals. The hourly administration of Viokase was no more effective in increasing lipase delivery than was giving the supplement with meals. From DiMagno et al (1977) *New England Journal of Medicine,* **296,** 1319, reprinted with permission.

Sodium hydroxide was effective only if given prior to or at the beginning of the meal rather than following the meal (Regan et al, 1979). The worsening of steatorrhoea with the use of calcium carbonate may be due to the formation of calcium soaps (Drenick, 1961) or the intraluminal precipitation of glycine conjugates of bile salts (Hofmann and Small, 1967). The adverse effects of magnesium-aluminium hydroxide are due to the presence of magnesium hydroxide (DiMagno et al, 1977). The mechanism is unknown.

The use of cimetidine (300 mg 30 min before meals) as an adjunct to pancreatic enzyme supplementation has also produced mixed results. Modest-to-major reductions in steatorrhoea have been reported in some studies (Regan et al, 1977; Cox et al, 1979; Boyle et al, 1980; Durie et al, 1980; Gow et al, 1981), while no effect was observed in another (Graham, 1982). It appears that the use of cimetidine is more likely to be beneficial in patients with hyperchlorhydria than in patients with relatively low rates of gastric acid secretion and when given in conjunction with large amounts of pancreatic enzymes (approximately 30 000 i.u. of lipase per meal) (DiMagno, 1982). In addition to reducing inactivation of pancreatic enzymes by maintaining gastric and duodenal pH greater than 4.0, cimetidine may also be effective in reducing steatorrhoea by decreasing the total volume of fluid in the duodenum (by reducing gastric secretion), thus resulting in less dilution of ingested pancreatic enzymes (Regan et al, 1977).

In a different approach to the prevention of pH-dependent inactivation of enzyme, a lipase-enriched pancreatic extract is enclosed by a pH-dependent polymer to yield granules 1.5-2.5 mm in diameter (Pancrease). When swallowed in capsule form, the granules are released in the stomach; but their protective coating dissolves only when the pH is 6.0 or higher. Thus the enzymes are designed to go into solution only in the duodenum or upper jejunum. Unlike some previous enteric-coated 'delayed-release' preparations, Pancrease is effective in reducing steatorrhoea due to pancreatic insufficiency (Graham, 1979; Valerio, 1981). However, it has not been shown to be more effective than comparable doses of potent conventional enzyme preparations (Regan et al, 1977; Graham, 1979; Dutta, Rubin and Harvey, 1983) which are generally significantly cheaper. The failure of this type of enteric-coated preparation to be more effective than conventional forms may be due to incomplete release of enzyme in the duodenum in patients with chronic pancreatitis who may have an intra-luminal pH for extended periods of time which is less than the value of 6.0 required for dissolution of the enzyme-containing granules, or to delayed emptying of the granules from the stomach (Dutta, Rubin and Harvey, 1983). It has been suggested that patients with relative hyperchlorhydria (as is often present in children with cystic fibrosis) may benefit from this enteric-coated preparation (DiMagno, 1981).

Despite the potential complexity of enzyme replacement therapy in chronic pancreatitis, most patients will respond to treatment with conventional preparations (e.g., Viokase, six tablets; Cotazym, five capsules; or Ilozyme, three tablets per meal) with stabilization or gain of weight and a reduction in diarrhoea, abdominal cramps, and bloating. Administration of pancreatic enzyme supplements at regular intervals (e.g., every two hours) instead of with meals does not appear to be a therapeutically more effective dosage schedule (Figure 3) (DiMagno et al, 1977) and is less convenient for the patient. The efficacy of therapy can be assessed objectively by comparing the 24-hour stool fat excretion on enzyme supplementation to that measured prior to enzyme therapy. If this regimen is unsuccessful, then the dose of the original preparation should be increased. If the exocrine insufficiency remains substantially unimproved, then use of the enteric-coated preparation (Pancrease, two to three capsules per meal) or addition of cimetidine (300 mg taken 30 min before meals) should then be tried. Continued failure should lead one to consider other potential causes of malabsorption (e.g., parasitic disease, coeliac sprue) which might be present instead of, or in addition to, pancreatic insufficiency.

Pancreatic extracts contain 8 to 10 per cent by weight of nucleic acids. When given in therapeutic doses, this increased dietary purine content results in an additional uric acid load of up to 500 mg per day. This explains why considerable hyperuricosuria and occasional hyperuricaemia has been reported in children with cystic fibrosis receiving large amounts of supplemental pancreatic enzymes (Stapleton et al, 1976). Renal urate stone formation, however, has not been noted. This issue has yet to be investigated in adult patients with pancreactic insufficiency.

Medium-chain triglycerides

In patients with weight loss refractory to diet and enzyme supplementation, the addition of medium-chain triglycerides (MCT) to the diet is theoretically an attractive step. MCT is derived from coconut oil and consists of approximately 75 per cent trioctanoate (C_8) and 24 per cent tridecanoate (C_{10}). MCT differs from the typical dietary long-chain triglycerides (LCT) in the following ways (Greenberger and Skillman, 1969):

1. MCT is partly water-soluble.
2. Hydrolysis by gastric and pancreatic lipase proceeds much faster for MCT than for LCT.
3. Some MCT is absorbed intact.
4. Absorbed medium-chain fatty acids enter the portal vein rather than the intestinal lymph.
5. More MCT than LCT is metabolized to CO_2 and ketone bodies.

MCT may be used to replace part of the dietary LCT and to increase total fat intake as high as tolerated. However, about 25 per cent of patients develop nausea and increased diarrhoea when consuming 40 g or more of MCT per day. The coefficient of fat absorption invariably rises when MCT is added to the diet, but weight gain is achieved with regularity only in children with cystic fibrosis, and rarely in adults with advanced chronic pancreatitis (Greenberger and Skillman, 1969). MCT is available in a formula diet (Portagen), but many patients prefer to use pure MCT oil in food preparations (Schizas et al, 1967).

Hyperoxaluria

An additional risk of untreated steatorrhoea is increased renal oxalate excretion. When the concentration of long-chain fatty acids in the colon is high, intraluminal calcium is bound by the formation of insoluble calcium soaps. As a result, less calcium is available for the precipitation of unabsorbed dietary oxalate as calcium oxalate. The oxalate remains in solution and passively diffuses across the colonic mucosa, ultimately being excreted in the urine. The net result is that patients with steatorrhoea of any cause exhibit hyperoxaluria (greater than 40-50 g per day of urinary oxalate) provided their colon is intact. The hyperoxaluria can be corrected by four different approaches: a low dietary oxalate intake; a diet low in long-chain triglycerides; pancreatic enzyme supplementation; and an increased intake of either calcium (2-3 g per day) or aluminium in the form of antacids (3.5 g of aluminium per day). With severe steatorrhoea (greater than 30 g faecal fat per day) any two of these four modalities should be employed (Earnest et al, 1974; Stauffer, 1977). The risk of renal oxalate stone formation in patients with pancreatic insufficiency is not known but is probably quite low. The detection and specific treatment of hyper-oxaluria may, therefore, be reserved for those few patients who develop nephrolithiasis.

Nutritional support

Although many patients with pancreatic insufficiency are able to maintain weight and strength due to good appetite, high caloric intake, pancreatic enzyme supplementation, and the use of medium-chain triglycerides, some require more extensive measures to achieve or maintain an acceptable nutritional state. For those who have become severely debilitated or whose nutrition may be jeopardized by an acute complication of their underlying disease (e.g., exacerbation of chronic pancreatitis, development of pancreatic ascites) enteral feeding or total parentaral nutrition may be necessary for extended periods of time. Similarly enteral or parenteral nutritional support may be advisable to prepare a patient for surgery or to maintain the patient following an operation.

Surgery to improve pancreatic exocrine function in chronic pancreatitis

It has been proposed that, in chronic pancreatitis, operations designed to facilitate drainage of pancreatic juice into the small intestine might result in improved exocrine function. Whether any significant long-term improve-ment in digestive function actually accrues from such operations remains in dispute (Priestley et al, 1965; Arnesjo et al, 1975; Warshaw, Popp and Schapiro, 1980). Therefore, exocrine insufficiency must not be the sole indication for surgery in chronic pancreatitis.

REFERENCES

Allan, J. & White, T. T. (1974) Alternate mechanism for the formation of protein plugs in chronic calcifying pancreatitis. *Digestion,* **11,** 428-431.
Arnesjo, B., Ishe, I., Kugelberg, C. & Tyler, U. (1975) Pancreatico-jejunostomy in chronic pancreatitis. An appraisal of 29 cases. *Acta Chirurgica Scandinavica,* **141,** 139-148.
Arvanitakis, C. & Cook, A. R. (1978) Diagnostic tests of exocrine pancreatic function and disease. *Gastroenterology,* **74,** 932-948.
Barbezat, G. O. & Hansen, J. D. L. (1968) The exocrine pancreas and protein-calorie malnutrition. *Pediatrics,* **42,** 77-92.
Blackburn, W. R. & Vïnijchaikul, K. (1969) The pancreas in kwashiorkor. An electron microscope study. *Laboratory Investigation,* **20,** 305-318.
Boyle, B. J., Long, W. B., Balisteri, W. F. et al (1980) Effect of cimetidine and pancreatic enzymes on serum and fecal bile acids and fat absorption in cystic fibrosis. *Gastro-enterology,* **78,** 950-953.
Brugge, W. R., Goff, J. S., Allen, N. C. et al (1980) Development of a dual label Schilling test for pancreatic exocrine function based on the differential absorption of cobalamin bound to intrinsic factor and R protein. *Gastroenterology,* **78,** 937-949.
Burch, G. E. & Ansari, A. (1968) Chronic alcoholism and carcinoma of the pancreas — a correlative hypothesis. *Archives of Internal Medicine,* **122,** 273-275.
Comfort, M. W., Wollaeger, E. E., Taylor, A. B. & Power, M. H. (1953) Non-tropical sprue: observations on absorption and metabolism. *Gastroenterology,* **23,** 155-178.

Cox, K. L., Isenberg, J. W., Asher, A. B. & Dooley, R. R. (1979) The effect of cimetidine on maldigestion in cystic fibrosis. *Journal of Pediatrics,* **94,** 488-492.

DeCaro, A., Guy, O., Adrich, Z. & Sarles, H. (1981) Pancreatic lithogenesis. *Gastroenterology,* **80,** 1133 (Abstract).

DiMagno, E. P. (1979) Medical treatment of pancreatic insufficiency. *Mayo Clinic Proceedings,* **54,** 435-442.

DiMagno, E. P. (1982) Controversies in the treatment of exocrine pancreatic insufficiency. *Digestive Diseases and Sciences,* **27,** 481-484.

DiMagno, E. P., Go, V. L. W. & Summerskill, W. H. J. (1973) Relations between pancreatic enzyme outputs and malabsorption in severe pancreatic insufficiency. *New England Journal of Medicine,* **288,** 813-815.

DiMagno, E. P., Malagelada, J. R., Go, V. L. W. & Moertel, C. G. (1977) Fate of orally ingested enzymes in pancreatic insufficiency. Comparison of two dosage schedules. *New England Journal of Medicine,* **296,** 1318-1322.

Drenick, E. J. (1961) The influence of the ingestion of calcium and other soap-forming substances on fecal fat. *Gastroenterology,* **41,** 242-244.

Durie, P., Bell, L., Linton, W. et al (1980) Effect of cimetidine and sodium bicarbonate on pancreatic replacement therapy in cystic fibrosis. *Gut,* **21,** 778-786.

Dutta, S. K., Rubin, J. & Harvey, J. (1983) Comparative evaluation of the therapeutic efficacy of a pH sensitive enteric coated pancreatic enzyme preparation with conventional pancreatic enzyme therapy in the treatment of exocrine pancreatic insufficiency. *Gastroenterology,* **84,** 476-482.

Earnest, D. L., Johnson, G., Williams, H. E. & Admirand, W. H. (1974) Hyperoxaluria in patients with ileal resection: an abnormality in dietary calcium in regulating intestinal oxalate absorption. *Gastroenterology,* **66,** 1114-1122.

Evans, W. B. & Wollaeger, E. E. (1966) Incidence and severity of nutritional deficiency states in chronic pancreative insufficiency: comparison with nontropical sprue. *American Journal of Digestive Diseases,* **11,** 594-606.

Fogel, M. R. & Gray, G. M. (1973) Starch hydrolysis in man: an intraluminal process not requiring membrane digestion. *Journal of Applied Physiology,* **35,** 263-267.

Goff, J. S. (1981) Pancreatic exocrine function testing. *Western Journal of Medicine,* **135,** 368-374.

Gow, R., Francis, P., Bradbear, R. & Shepherd, R. (1981) Comparative study of varying regimens to improve steatorrhoea and creatorrhoea in cystic fibrosis: effectiveness of an enteric-coated preparation with and without antacids and cimetidine. *Lancet,* **ii,** 1071-1074.

Graham, D. Y. (1977) Enzyme replacement therapy of exocrine pancreatic insufficiency in man. Relation between in vitro enzyme activities and in vivo potency in commercial pancreatic extracts. *New England Journal of Medicine,* **296,** 1314-1317.

Graham, D. Y. (1979) An enteric-coated pancreatic enzyme preparation that works. *Digestive Diseases and Sciences,* **24,** 906-909.

Graham, D. Y. (1982) Pancreatic enzyme replacement. The effect of antacid or cimetidine. *Digestive Diseases and Sciences,* **27,** 485-490.

Greenberger, N. J. & Skillman, T. G. (1969) Medium-chain triglycerides. Physiologic considerations and clinical implications. *New England Journal of Medicine,* **280,** 1045-1058.

Heizler, W. D., Cleveland, C. R. & Iber, F. L. (1965) Gastric inactivation of pancreatic supplements. *Bulletin of the Johns Hopkins Hospital,* **116,** 261-270.

Hofmann, A. F. & Small, D. M. (1967) Detergent properties of bile salts: correlation with physiological function. *Annual Review of Medicine,* **18,** 333-376.

Imondi, A. R., Stradley, P. & Wolgemuth, R. (1972) Enzyme replacement in the pancreatic duct ligated swine. *Proceedings of the Society for Experimental Biology and Medicine,* **141,** 367-372.

Ishii, K., Nakamura, K., Takeuchi, T. & Hirayama, T. (1973) Chronic calcifying pancreatitis and pancreatic carcinoma in Japan. *Digestion,* **9,** 429-473.

Lea, A. J. (1967) Neoplasms and environmental factors. *Annals of the Royal College of Surgeons of England,* **41,** 432-437.

MacMahon, B., Yen, S., Trichopoulos, D. et al (1981) Coffee and cancer of the pancreas. *New England Journal of Medicine,* **304,** 630-633.

Monson, R. R. & Lyon, J. L. (1975) Proportional mortality among alcoholics. *Cancer,* **36,** 1077-1079.

Nagata, A., Homma, T., Tamai, K. et al (1981) A study of chronic pancreatitis by serial endoscopic pancreatography. *Gastroenterology,* **81,** 884-891.

Priestley, J. T., Remine, W. H., Barber, K. W. Jr & Gambill, E. E. (1965) Chronic relapsing pancreatitis: treatment by surgical drainage of the pancreas. *Annals of Surgery,* **161,** 838-844.

Regan, P. T., Malagelada, J. R., DiMagno, E. P. et al (1977) Comparative effects of antacids, cimetidine and enteric coating on the therapeutic response to oral enzymes in severe pancreatic insufficiency. *New England Journal of Medicine,* **297,** 854-858.

Regan, P. T., Malagelada, J. R., DiMagno, E. P. & Go, V. L. W. (1979) Reduced intraluminal bile acid concentrations and fat maldigestion in pancreatic insufficiency: correction by treatment. *Gastroenterology,* **77,** 285-291.

Renner, I. G., Rinderknecht, H., Valenzuela, J. E. & Douglas, A. P. (1980) Studies of pure pancreatic secretions in chronic alcoholic subjects without pancreatic insufficiency. *Scandinavian Journal of Gastroenterology,* **15,** 281-287.

Sahel, J. & Sarles, H. (1979) Modifications of pure human pancreatic juice induced by chronic alcohol consumption. *Digestive Diseases and Sciences,* **24,** 897-905.

Sarles, H. (1971) Alcoholism and pancreatitis. *Scandinavian Journal of Gastroenterology,* **6,** 193-198.

Scheele, G., Bartelt, D. & Bieger, W. (1981) Characterization of human exocrine pancreatic proteins by two-dimensional isoelectric focusing/sodium dodecyl sulfate gel electrophoresis. *Gastroenterology,* **80,** 461-473.

Schizas, A. A., Cremen, J. A., Larson, E. & O'Brien, R. (1967) Medium-chain triglycerides — use in food preparation. *Journal of the American Dietetic Association,* **51,** 228-272.

Stafford, R. J. & Grand, R. J. (1982) Hereditary disease of the exocrine pancreas. *Clinics in Gastroenterology,* **11,** 141-170.

Stapleton, F. B., Kennedy, J., Nousia-Arvanitakis, S. & Linshaw, M. A. (1976) Hyperuricosuria due to high-dose pancreatic extract therapy in cystic fibrosis. *New England Journal of Medicine,* **295,** 246-248.

Stauffer, J. Q. (1977) Hyperoxaluria and intestinal disease. The role of steatorrhea and dietary calcium in regulating intestinal oxalate absorption. *American Journal of Digestive Diseases,* **22,** 921-928.

Tandon, B. N., Banks, P. A., George, P. K. et al (1970) Recovery of exocrine pancreatic function in adult protein-calorie malnutrition. *Gastroenterology,* **58,** 358-362.

Valerio, D., Whyte, E. H. A., Schlamm, H. T. et al (1981) Clinical effectiveness of a pancreatic enzyme supplement. *Journal of Parenteral and Enteral Nutrition,* **5,** 110-114.

Wakabayashi, A. & Takeda, Y. (1976) The behavior of mucopolysaccharide in the pancreatic juice in chronic pancreatitis. *American Journal of Digestive Diseases,* **21,** 607-612.

Warshaw, A. L., Popp, J. W. Jr & Schapiro, R. H. (1980) Long-term patency, pancreatic function, and pain relief after lateral pancreatico-jejunostomy for chronic pancreatitis. *Gastroenterology,* **79,** 289-293.

Wollaeger, E. E., Comfort, M. W. & Osterberg, A. E. (1947) Total solids, fat and nitrogen in the feces. *Gastroenterology,* **74,** 932-948.

Wollaeger, E. E., Comfort, M. W., Claggett, O. T. & Osterberg, A. E. (1948) Efficiency of the gastrointestinal tract after resection of the head of the pancreas. *Journal of the American Medical Association,* **137,** 838-847.

Zentler-Munro, P. L., Fine, D. R., Gannon, M. & Northfield, T. C. (1981) Effect of cimetidine on intraduodenal bile acid precipitation, pancreatin inactivation, and lipid solubilization in pancreatic steatorrhea. *Gut,* **21,** A431 (Abstract).

15

Alcohol, Nutrition and Malabsorption

PETER H. R. GREEN

Chronic alcoholism is frequently associated with malnutrition and vitamin deficiencies. Malnutrition may be an important factor in the altered immune responses and increased incidence of infection seen in alcoholics (Smith and Palmer, 1976; Chandra, 1979). Although it is recognized that malnutrition may be due to poor dietary intake, less well recognized is the disturbed digestion and absorption that occurs in the alcoholic. Malabsorption in chronic alcoholics is due to several interacting factors, including folic acid deficiency, pancreatic insufficiency, liver disease, malnutrition and the direct effects of alcohol on absorption.

Malabsorption has been documented in approximately 50 per cent of recently hospitalized alcoholics, with and without cirrhosis (Fast et al, 1959; Small, Longarini and Zamcheck, 1959; Roggin et al, 1969; Mezey et al, 1970). In one study, 93 per cent of alcoholic patients had at least one abnormal parameter of absorption (Roggin et al, 1969). Studies performed on recently drinking malnourished alcoholics have demonstrated malabsorption of several substances (Table 1). D-Xylose malabsorption occurs in 16 to 76 per cent of those alcoholics studied (Small, Longarini and Zamcheck, 1959; Roggin et al, 1969; Mezey et al, 1970). Steatorrhoea has been documented in 35 to 60 per cent of alcoholics (Fast et al, 1959; Small, Longarini and Zamcheck, 1959; Rogin et al, 1969; Mezey et al, 1970). It is usually mild and subsides after hospitalization except when associated with severe hepatic or pancreatic disease (Mezey et al, 1970). Malabsorption of thiamine (Tomasulo, Kater and Iber, 1968; Thomson, Baker and Leevy, 1970), folic acid (Halsted et al, 1967, 1971), nitrogen (Roggin et al, 1969), vitamin A (Small, Longarini and Zamcheck, 1959) and vitamin B_{12} (Roggin et al, 1969) have also been demonstrated. Glucose, sodium and water transport can also be impaired (Halsted, Robles and Mezey, 1973; Krasner et al, 1974). These abnormalities reflect an impaired luminal phase of absorption and diffuse functional mucosal abnormalities.

Abnormalities usually return to normal after several weeks of hospitalization and alcohol withdrawal. During this period, nutritional status and hepatic and pancreatic function improve. Absorption may improve despite the continued ingestion of alcohol and alcohol ingestion for several weeks together with a nutritious diet (Halsted, Robles and Mezey, 1971, 1973; Lindenbaum and Lieber, 1975; Mezey, 1975) does not result in fat or xylose

Clinics in Gastroenterology — Vol. 12, No. 2, May 1983
0300-5089/83/1202-563 $05.00©1983 W. B. Saunders Company Ltd

Table 1. *Substances malabsorbed in chronic malnourished alcoholics*

D-Xylose
Folic acid
Vitamin A
Thiamine
Glucose
Sodium and water
Fat
Nitrogen
Vitamin B_{12}

malabsorption. In one study (Lindenbaum and Lieber, 1975) involving alcoholic volunteers the absorption of fat and xylose tended to increase when ethanol was given for several weeks along with a nutritious diet. The poor nutritional state, therefore, appears to be a major determinant of malabsorption in chronic alcoholics. Ethanol, however, has been demonstrated to alter the absorption of some nutrients in alcoholics without nutritional deficiency (Table 2). The malnourished alcoholic has several interacting factors which contribute to altered intestinal function and malabsorption (Table 3). These factors include direct effects of alcohol and indirect or related factors such as folate and protein deficiency. These indirect effects are of major clinical importance in the aetiology of malabsorption in alcoholics.

Table 2. *Effects of alcohol on absorption in the absence of nutritional deficiency experimental studies in man*

Absorption	Acute administration	Chronic administration
Decreased	D-xylose Thiamine L-Methionine Folic acid[b]	Folic acid[a] Vitamin B_{12} Sodium and water
Increased	Iron	D-xylose Fat

[a] Only two of seven subjects studied.
[b] Only one of five subjects studied.

MECHANISMS OF MALABSORPTION IN THE ALCOHOLIC
Direct Effects of Alcohol on the Intestine

Alcohol is rapidly absorbed from the stomach and upper small intestine. In order to study the concentrations of ethanol to which the intestinal mucosa is exposed, Halsted, Robles and Mezey (1973) administered alcohol orally and intravenously to alcoholic volunteers and measured the concentration of alcohol at various levels in the gastrointestinal tract. After the ingestion of alcohol (0.8 g/kg body weight), extremely high concentrations of alcohol are obtained in the stomach (7 to 8 g/100 ml) and upper small intestine (1 to

Table 3. *Factors contributing to malabsorption and diarrhoea in chronic alcoholics*

Mucosal factors	
Folate deficiency	— functional and morphological damage
Alcohol	— morphological damage (cellular and subcellular)
	— altered metabolism (Na-K ATPase)
	— malabsorption (vit. B_{12}, amino acids, thimaine)
	— inhibition Na/H_2 O transport
	— net secretion Na/H_2 O
	— disaccharidase deficiency
Protein malnutrition	— ? (not proven)
Luminal factors	
Pancreatic insufficiency	— direct effect alcohol
	— protein malnutrition
	— pancreatitis
Liver disease	— bile salt secretion
Altered intestinal mobility	

4 g/100 ml). High levels (> 400 mg/100 ml) are maintained in the upper intestine for more than one hour and result in blood levels of 100 to 150 mg/100 ml. Ethanol concentrations in the gastrointestinal tract rapidly decrease and reach levels similar to those in the vascular space by 120 minutes. After the intravenous administration of alcohol the concentrations of alcohol in the intestine and blood are similar. Ileal levels of alcohol tended to follow blood levels whether alcohol was given orally or intravenously.

As well as being absorbed, ethanol is metabolized by the intestine. Alcohol dehydrogenase (ADH), the major enzyme responsible for ethanol oxidation in the liver (Isselbacher and Greenberger, 1964), has been found in the stomach and small intestine (Mistilis and Garski, 1969; Carter and Isselbacher, 1971; Mezey, 1975). The role of intestinal ADH in ethanol metabolism is not known; however, the liver is considered to be the major site of ethanol oxidation in vivo (Mezey, 1975). Recently the mixed function microsomal oxidases, including the microsomal ethanol-oxidizing system described by Lieber and DiCarli in the liver (Lieber and DeCarli, 1970), have been found in the intestine and shown to be induced by ethanol (Seitz, Korsten and Lieber, 1978). These, however, are probably not major ethanol-oxidizing pathways in the intestine. The high concentrations of ethanol found in the intestinal lumen after the ingestion of alcoholic beverages are greater than those necessary to saturate known ethanol oxidizing systems. The effects of ethanol on the intestinal cell could, therefore, be due to either direct toxic effects of the high alcohol concentrations or metabolic imbalances produced by its oxidation.

Morphological effects of ethanol on the intestine

Abnormal intestinal function produced by ethanol may be related to structural and morphological changes seen within the intestinal mucosa as a result of ethanol. Ethanol, in concentrations similar to that obtained during drinking in human subjects, produced haemorrhagic erosions in the small intestinal villi of rats (Baraona, Pirola and Lieber, 1974). The lesions were most obvious proximally, were concentration-dependent, and were associated with decreased intestinal enzyme activity. Similar haemorrhagic erosions of villus tips have been seen in duodenal biopsy specimens from alcoholic volunteers after ingestion of a single dose (1 g/kg body weight) of ethanol (Gottfried, Korsten and Lieber, 1976). Long-term ingestion did not produce haemorrhagic lesions in rats but resulted in altered villous architecture, including fewer cells and villus shortening. This was associated with decreased disaccharidase activities (Baraona, Pirola and Lieber, 1974).

The long-term administration of ethanol in the absence of nutritional deficiencies produced ultrastructural changes in the small intestinal cells of both the rat and man (Rubin et al, 1972). Changes were seen in mitochondria, the endoplasmic reticulum and Golgi apparatus and are similar to those produced in the liver by ethanol. Morphological changes were not seen after chronic ethanol administration to monkeys (Halsted et al, 1979).

Enzyme defects induced by ethanol

On a subcellular level ethanol administration has been shown to alter several enzyme systems found in the intestinal mucosa. Ethanol administration to human volunteers for three to six days inhibited intestinal glycolytic and gluconeogenic enzyme activities. This effect was reversed by the administration of folic acid (Greene et al, 1974). In the rat, acute (single dose) and chronic (long-term) ethanol ingestion resulted in reduced intestinal lactase, sucrase and alkaline phosphatase activity associated with morphological changes in the intestine (Baraona, Pirola and Lieber, 1974). Reduced intestinal disaccharidase activity has also been found in intestinal biopsy specimens from chronic alcoholics (Perlow, Baraona and Lieber, 1977). Abstinence for two weeks resulted in a significant increase in the activity of both lactase and sucrase, and indicates reversibility of the lesion. Alcoholics appeared to exhibit a greater lactose intolerance and a higher incidence of adverse effects after the oral administration of lactose than controls. The reversible disaccharidase deficiency probably reflects cellular damage which may be a direct result of alcohol, or related to malnutrition or folate deficiency.

Ethanol, in concentrations found in the human gut, has been shown to reduce rat intestinal adenosine triphosphate (ATP) content (Carter and Isselbacher, 1973), and in some studies reduced the activity of sodium-potassium ATPase in jejunal basolateral membrane (Hoyumpa et al, 1977) and brush border membrane fractions (Mitjavila, Lacombe and Carrera, 1976). Reduction in sodium-potassium ATPase activity provides a probable mechanism for the reduction in absorption of actively transported substances.

Effect of alcohol on absorption in the absence of nutritional deficiency

A direct effect of alcohol has been demonstrated on the absorption of specific nutrients in experimental animals and in man in the absence of nutritional deficiency. Varying responses have been reported depending on the animal model used and on the dose and route of alcohol administration. The results of the studies in both experimental animals and man have been fully reviewed recently (Baraona and Lindenbaum, 1977; Wilson and Hoyumpa, 1979).

Ethanol interferes with the absorption of actively transported substances that require a carrier-mediated process. This may be due to a direct effect of alcohol on the physical properties of the cell membrane (membrane fluidity) or it may be due to damage to membrane-bound enzymes (e.g., sodium-potassium ATPase) (Wilson and Hoyumpa, 1979). Substances absorbed passively are either not affected or are enhanced by alcohol administration.

Animals studies. The acute administration of ethanol resulted in decreased absorption of actively transported amino acids, but not D-phenylalanine, which is passively absorbed (Chang, Lewis and Glazko, 1967; Israel, Salazar and Rosenmann, 1968). The absorption of ferrous iron (Tapper et al, 1968), calcium (Krawitt, 1974), thiamine (Hoyumpa et al, 1975) and glucose (Chang, Lewis and Glasko, 1967; Kuo and Shanbour, 1978) are reduced by the acute administration of ethanol, whereas fat (Baraona and Lieber, 1975) and manganese absorption (Schafer et al, 1974) are enhanced.

Chronic administration of ethanol in experimental animals reduced xylose absorption (Small et al, 1960), carbohydrate (Lindenbaum et al, 1972), vitamin B_{12} (Lindenbaum, Saha and Lieber, 1973), and calcium (Krawitt, 1975) absorption, but had no effect on fat (Baraona and Lieber, 1975) or iron absorptin (Tapper et al, 1968).

Human studies. Studies in man have been more limited. Most studies have been performed either on alcoholics after adequate nutritional repletion or on a few normal volunteers. The results of these studies are summarized in Table 2. The administration of ethanol as a single dose to healthy volunteers resulted in impaired absorption of the essential amino acid L-methionine (Israel et al, 1969), thiamine (Thomson, Baker and Leevy, 1970) and D-xylose (Mezey, 1975). In these studies, the doses of alcohol resulted in concentrations similar to those found in the upper intestine after the ingestion of moderate doses of alcohol. Folic acid absorption, however, was impaired in only one of five normal subjects after the administration of ethanol (Halsted, Griggs and Harris, 1967). Smaller single doses of alcohol had no effect on the absorption of calcium (Verdy and Caron, 1973) or ferrous iron (Charlton et al, 1964). Sodium and water transport were not affected (Mekhjian and May, 1977), whereas ferric iron absorption was enhanced by a single dose of ethanol (Charlton et al, 1964).

Long-term ethanol administration to normal volunteers resulted in a significant reduction in sodium and water transport in the perfused jejunum (Mekhjian and May, 1977). This effect was augmented by a folate-deficient diet and may be a contributing factor to the diarrhoea of the alcoholic. Long-term ethanol ingestion also interferes with vitamin B_{12} absorption (Lindenbaum and Lieber, 1969, 1975). This is not corrected by the administration of intrinsic factor or pancreatic supplements, suggesting interference with ileal function. Vitamin B_{12} deficiency is not, however, a clinical problem in alcoholics. Even though alcoholics may have an abnormal Schilling test, and serum levels of vitamin B_{12} are low in 10 per cent of them (Leevy et al, 1965), megaloblastic anaemia due to vitamin B_{12} deficiency has not been reported as a result of ethanol ingestion.

The long-term administration of alcohol to alcoholics in the presence of a nutritious diet does not significantly alter folate absorption, although reduced absorption was observed in two of the seven subjects studied by Halsted, Robles and Mezey (1971). However, the nutritional status of these two subjects was questioned (Halsted, Robles and Mezey, 1971).

Effect of ethanol on lipid metabolism

The mild steatorrhoea of the alcoholic appears to be related to impaired pancreatic function (Mezey et al, 1970, 1976) and not due to a mucosal lesion. Several animal studies have demonstrated enhanced intestinal lipid metabolism and lipid transport in mesenteric lymph due to ethanol.

Acute ethanol administration increases intestinal cholesterol and triglyceride synthesis (Carter and Drummey, 1971; Middleton et al, 1971) associated with increased activity of re-esterifying enzymes (Rogers and O'Brien, 1975). This is associated with increased intestinal very low density lipoprotein (VLDL) production (Mistilis and Ockner, 1972), mesenteric lymph flow (Baraona and Lieber, 1975), and lipid output by the intestine, especially when ethanol is present in the lumen (Carter, Drummey and Isselbacher, 1971; Middleton et al, 1971; Baraona and Lieber, 1975). In contrast, long-term ethanol administration failed to enhance lipid absorption and appeared to mildly inhibit it (Baraona and Lieber, 1975). Recent evidence has demonstrated that the intestine of both the rat (Glickman and Green, 1977; Tall et al, 1978) and man (Green et al, 1979, 1980) is an important source of plasma lipoprotein components, especially apoprotein A-I and A-IV and phospholipid for plasma high density lipoproteins (HDL). In view of the association of alcohol ingestion with elevation of plasma HDL levels (Yano, Rhoads and Kagan, 1977) further study is required to determine the effect of ethanol on intestinal lipoprotein and apoprotein formation.

Altered small intestinal motility

Alcohol administered to alcoholic and normal volunteers resulted in increased duodenal (Pirola and Davis, 1970), jejunal, and ileal motility (Robles et al, 1974). Ethanol, given either orally or intravenously, had similar effects. There was an increase in propulsive (type III) waves in the ileum, more marked than in the jejunum, and in inhibition of type I waves in the jejunum. Increased intestinal transit may contribute to diarrhoea and malabsorption in the alcoholic.

Indirect Effects of Alcohol on Intestinal Function

Folic acid deficiency

Folic acid deficiency is the most frequently seen nutritional defect in alcoholics (Leevy et al, 1965) and is considered to contribute to their high morbidity and mortality (Kaunitz and Lindenbaum, 1977). Uptake of dietary folate at low, physiological doses is probably by an active process, whereas at higher concentrations uptake is by passive diffusion (Halsted, Bhanthumnavin and Mezey, 1974). Folate deficiency in alcoholics is related to several interacting factors, for alcohol interferes with folate metabolism in several areas. Alcoholics ingest folate-deficient diets. Alcohol interferes, directly or indirectly, with absorption of folate and its transport to tissues, its storage and release by the liver (Eichner and Hillman, 1973; Hillman and Steinberg, 1982). A major effect of the acute ingestion of alcohol is the reversible sequestration of folate in the hepatocyte and a failure of release of folate into bile, thus disrupting the enterohepatic circulation of folate. This results in a rapid reversible fall in serum folate (Hillman and Steinberg, 1982). Thus the chronically folate-deficient alcoholic is subjected to an acute insult to folate metabolism each time alcohol is acutely ingested.

Severe folate deficiency may cause morphological changes in the intestine (Bianchi et al, 1970; Hermos et al, 1972). Changes include villus shortening, decreased mitoses in crypts, macrocytosis and enlargement of epithelial cell nuclei. Similar changes occur in vitamin B_{12} deficiency and are associated with defective absorption (Lindenbaum, Pezzimenti and Shea, 1974). Folate deficiency can alter intestinal function prior to the production of morphological changes. Studies in several subjects have also demonstrated a synergistic effect between alcohol and folic acid deficiency (Halsted, Robles and Mezey, 1971; Mekhjian and May, 1977). In one study, a folate-deficient diet augmented the abnormalities in sodium and water transport produced by ethanol, despite being normal in serum folate levels (Mekhjian and May, 1977), indicating that functional abnormalities occur early in folate deficiency.

Among the chronic alcoholics who have been studied there is a strong association between D-xylose, vitamin B_{12} and folic acid malabsorption and evidence of folate deficiency (Halsted, Robles and Mezey, 1973; Baraon and Lindenbaum, 1977). Jejunal perfusion studies performed in binge-drinking alcoholics demonstrated reduced absorption of tritiated folic acid. This occurred only in subjects who were folate-deficient (serum folate < 5 ng/ml) but not when folate levels were normal (Halsted, Robles and Mezey, 1973). In other studies, ethanol ingestion for two weeks in seven well-nourished volunteers did not reduce mean folate absorption (Halsted, Robles and Mezey, 1971). However, in two subjects induction of dietary folate deficiency, together with ethanol ingestion, resulted in decreased absorption of labelled folic acid, D-xylose, glucose, fluid and sodium (Halsted, Robles and Mezey, 1973), indicating the important role of folic acid deficiency in the aetiology of folate and other nutrient malabsorption. Folate deficiency together with the long-term alcohol ingestion can also cause a net secretion of fluid and sodium (Halsted, Robles and Mezey, 1973; Mekhjian and May, 1977). Dietary folate deficiency appears to be a major contributing factor to the diffuse mucosal abnormality seen in chronic alcoholics.

Protein malnutrition

Protein malnutrition is often present in chronic alcoholics. Dietary insufficiency and alcohol inhibition of intestinal amino acid transport may be contributing factors. The exact role of protein malnutrition as a contributing factor to the diffuse mucosal abnormality of alcoholics has not been established.

There is experimental evidence (Glickman and Kirsch, 1973), and evidence in protein-deficient children (James, 1968) and malnourished adults (Mayoral et al, 1967), that intestinal function is impaired by protein deficiency. Severe protein malnutrition can produce a flat mucosal biopsy specimen (Brunser et al, 1966). Biopsy findings of lipid-laden cells, similar to those in abetalipoproteinaemia, have been seen in human protein-calorie malnutrition (Theron, Wittmann and Prinslov, 1971). This suggests that apoprotein synthesis and lipid transport can be impaired by protein deficiency. It is well established experimentally that protein synthesis inhibitors interfere with intestinal lipid transport into lymph (Glickman and Kirsch, 1973).

Studies in protein-deficient children have shown malabsorption of xylose, glucose (James, 1968) and fat (Viteri, Flores and Alvarado, 1973). The severity of steatorrhoea in malnourished children is directly related to the degree of protein deficiency, and affects both triglycerides and fatty acids, indicating that deficient lipolysis is not the primary cause of fat malabsorption in protein-deficient states (Viteri, Flores and Alvardo, 1973). Protein deficiency also reduces pancreatic exocrine secretion in rats and man (Lemire and Iber, 1967; Tandon et al, 1970), and subclinical protein malnutrition has been incriminated as a cause of the reversible pancreatic insufficiency which was seen in a group of alcoholics studied by Mezey et al (1970). Protein deficiency may, therefore, contribute to malabsorption in the chronic alcoholic by altering both the luminal phase of absorption as well as affecting mucosal function. Its exact role, however, remains to be determined.

Pancreatic and hepatic dysfunction

Malabsorption in alcoholics may result from disturbance of the luminal phase of digestion secondary to pancreatic and hepatic dysfunction. Experimentally, ethanol reduces water, bicarbonate and protein secretion by the rabbit pancreas (Solomon et al, 1974). The presence of steatorrhoea in alcoholics correlates with a low pancreatic lipase output following cholecystokinin-pancreozymin (CCK-PZ) and secretin stimulation (Mezey and Potter, 1976). It is well known that acute and chronic pancreatitis occur in alcoholics. In addition, subclinical pancreatic dysfunction as assessed by an abnormal response to secretin stimulation was present in 44 per cent of a group of chronic alcoholics admitted because of their alcoholism (Mezey et al, 1970). In most subjects, the test returned to normal after institution of a normal diet with or without alcohol, suggesting nutritional factors may be an important cause of pancreatic dysfunction.

Ethanol alters bile secretion in the rat. There is depression of bile flow. However, long-term administration results in increased flow and secretion of bile salts, and an increase in the non-bile salt-dependent flow (Maddrey and Boyer, 1973). In addition, protein-deficient states result in decreased bile salt pool size (Schneider and Viteri, 1974). Cirrhosis is also associated with a decreased excretion of bile salts (Vlahcevic et al, 1972) and a subnormal concentration of intraduodenal bile salt (Badley et al, 1970), indicating that alcoholic subjects may have several reasons for an altered micellar phase of digestion contributing to malabsorption of fat.

SUMMARY

Malabsorption occurs frequently in chronic alcoholics. Alcoholics may malabsorb fat, nitrogen, sodium, water, thiamine, folic acid, vitamin B_{12} and D-xylose. Malabsorption is due to an abnormal luminal phase of digestion as well as a diffuse functional mucosal abnormality. Malabsorption may, therefore, contribute to clinically significant malnutrition, diarrhoea, folate-deficiency and to abnormalities in tests of xylose and vitamin B_{12} absorption. Factors producing malabsorption in alcoholics include dietary folic acid and protein deficiency, pancreatic insufficiency, abnormalities of biliary secretions and direct effects of alcohol on the gastrointestinal tract. Many of the absorptive abnormalities are reversed when alcoholics are given a nutritious diet, even with continued intake of alcohol. This highlights the causal role of nutritional deficiencies in the malabsorption of chronic alcoholics.

REFERENCES

Badley, B. W. D., Murphy, G. M., Bouchier, I. A. D. et al (1970) Diminished micellar phase lipid in patients with chronic nonalcoholic liver disease and steatorrhea. *Gastroenterology,* **58,** 781.

Baraona, E. & Lieber, C. S. (1975) Intestinal lymph formation and fat absorption: stimulation by acute ethanol administration and inhibition by chronic ethanol feeding. *Gastroenterology,* **68,** 495.

Baraona, E. & Lindenbaum, J. (1977) Metabolic effects of alcohol on the intestine. *Metabolic Aspects of Alcoholism* (Ed.) Lieber, C. S. p. 81. Baltimore, Maryland: University Park Press.

Baraona, E., Pirola, R. C. & Lieber, C. S. (1974) Small intestinal damage and changes in cell population produced by ethanol ingestion in the rat. *Gastroenterology,* **66,** 226.

Bianchi, A., Chipman, S. Q., Dreskin, A. et al (1970) Nutritional folic acid deficiency with megaloblastic changes in the small-bowel epithelium. *New England Journal of Medicine,* **282,** 859.

Brunser, O., Reid, A., Monckeberg, F. et al (1966) Jejunal biopsies in infant malnutrition with special reference to mitotic index. *Pediatrics,* **38,** 605.

Carter, E. A. & Isselbacher, K. J. (1971) The metabolism of ethanol to carbon dioxide by stomach and small intestinal slices. *Proceedings: Society of Experimental Biology and Medicine,* **138,** 817.

Carter, E. A. & Isselbacher, K. J. (1973) Effect of ethanol on intestinal adenosine triphosphate (ATP) content. *Proceedings: Society of Experimental Biology and Medicine,* **142,** 1171.

Carter, E. A. & Drummey, G. B. & Isselbacher, K. J. (1971) Ethanol stimulates triglyceride synthesis by the intestine. *Science,* **174,** 1241.

Chandra, R. K. (1979) Interactions of nutrition, infection and immune response. Immunocompetence in nutritional deficiency, methodological considerations and intervention strategies. *Acta Paediatrica Scandinavica,* **68,** 137.

Chang, T., Lewis, J. & Glazko, A. J. (1967) Effect of ethanol and other alcohols on the transport of amino acids and glucose by everted sacs of rat small intestine. *Biochimica et Biophysica Acta,* **135,** 1000.

Charlton, R. W., Jacobs, P., Seftel, H. et al (1964) Effect of alcohol on iron absorption. *British Medical Journal,* **ii,** 1427.

Eichner, E. D. & Hillman, R. S. (1973) Effect of alcohol on serum folate level. *Journal of Clinical Investigation,* **52**, 584.

Fast, B. B., Wolfe, S. J., Stormont, J. M. et al (1959) Fat absorption in alcoholics with cirrhosis. *Gastroenterology,* **37**, 321.

Glickman, R. M. & Green, P. H. R. (1977) The intestine as a source of apolipoprotein A-I. *Proceedings of the National Academy of Sciences, USA,* **74**, 2569.

Glickman, R. M. & Kirsch, K. (1973) Lymph chylomicron formation during protein synthesis inhibition. Studies of chylomicron apoproteins. *Journal of Clinical Investigation,* **52**, 2910.

Gottfried, E. B., Korsten, M. A. & Lieber, C. S. (1976) Gastritis and duodentitis induced by alcohol: an endoscopic and histologic assessment. *Gastroenterology,* **70**, 890.

Green, P. H. R., Glickman, R. M. & Riley, J. W. (1980) Human apolipoprotein A-IV. Intestinal origin and distribution in plasma. *Journal of Clinical Investigation,* **65**, 911.

Green, P. H. R., Glickman, R. M., Saudek, C. D. et al (1979) Human intestinal lipoproteins — studies in chyluric subjects. *Journal of Clinical Investigation,* **64**, 233.

Greene, H. L., Stifel, F. B., Herman, R. H. et al (1979) Ethanol-induced inhibition of human intestinal enzyme activities: reversal by folic acid. *Gastroenterology,* **67**, 434.

Halsted, C. H., Bhanthumnavin, K. & Mezey, E. (1974) Jejunal uptake of tritiated folic acid in the rat studied by in vivo perfusion. *Journal of Nutrition,* **104**, 1674.

Halsted, C. H., Griggs, R. G. & Harris, J. W. (1967) The effect of alcoholism on the absorption of folic acid (³H-PGA) evaluated by plasma levels and urine excretion. *Journal of Laboratory and Clinical Medicine,* **69**, 116.

Halsted, C. H., Robles, E. A. & Mezey, E. (1971) Decresed jejunal uptake of labelled folic acid (³H-PGA) in alcoholic patients. Roles of alcohol and nutrition. *New England Journal of Medicine,* **285**, 701.

Halsted, C. H., Robles, E. A. & Mezey, E. (1973) Intestinal malabsorption in folate-deficient alcoholics. *Gastroenterology,* **64**, 526.

Halsted, C. H., Robles, E. A. & Mezey, E. (1973) Distribution of ethanol in the human gastro-intestinal tract. *American Journal of Clinical Nutrition,* **26**, 831.

Halsted, C. M., Romero, J. J., Tamura, T., Ruebrer, B. & French, S. (1979) Folate metabolism in the alcoholic monkey. *Gastroenterology,* **76** (5), 1149.

Hermos, J. A., Adams, W. H., Lin, Y. K. et al (1972) Mucosa of the small intestine in folate deficient alcoholics. *Annals of Internal Medicine,* **76**, 957.

Hillman, R. S. & Steinberg, S. E. (1982) The effects of alcohol on folate metabolism. *Annual Review of Medicine,* **33**, 345.

Hoyumpa, A. M. Jr, Breen, K. J., Schenker, S. et al (1975) Thiamine transport across the rat intestine. II. Effect of ethanol. *Journal of Laboratory and Clinical Medicine,* **86**, 803.

Hoyumpa, A. M., Nichols, S. G., Wilson, F. A. et al (1977) Effect of ethanol on intestinal (Na,K) ATPase and intestinal thiamine transport in rats. *Journal of Laboratory and Clinical Medicine,* **90**, 1086.

Israel, Y., Salazar, I. & Rosenmann, E. (1968) Inhibitory effects of alcohol on intestinal amino acid transport in vivo and in vitro. *Journal of Nutrition,* **96**, 499.

Israel, Y., Valenzuela, J. E., Salazar, I. et al (1969) Alcohol and amino acid transport in the human small intestine. *Journal of Nutrition,* **98**, 222.

Isselbacher, K. J. & Greenberger, N. J. (1964) Metabolic effects of alcohol on the liver. *New England Journal of Medicine,* **270**, 351.

James, W. P. T. (1968) Intestinal absorption in protein calorie malnutrition. *Lancet,* **i**, 333.

Kaunitz, J. D. & Lindenbaum, J. (1977) The bioavailability of folic acid added to wine. *Annals of Internal Medicine,* **87**, 542.

Krasner, N., Cochran, K. M., Thompson, C. G. et al (1974) Effects of ethanol on small intestinal absorption. *Gut,* **15**, 831.

Krawitt, E. L. (1974) Effect of acute ethanol administration on duodenal calcium transport. *Proceedings of the Society of Experimental Biology and Medicine,* **146**, 406.

Krawitt, E. L. (1975) Effect of ethanol ingestion on duodenal calcium transport. *Journal of Laboratory and Clinical Medicine,* **85**, 665.

Kuo, Y-J. & Shanbour, L. L. (1978) Effects of ethanol on sodium, 3-*O*-methyl glucose and L-alanine transport in the jejunum. *American Journal of Digestive Diseases,* **23**, 51.

Leevy, C. M., Baker, H., TenHove, W. et al (1965) B-complex vitamins in liver disease of the alcoholic. *American Journal of Clinical Nutrition,* **16**, 339.

Lemire, S. & Iber, F. L. (1967) Pancreatic secretion in rats with protein malnutrition. *Johns Hopkins Medical Journal,* **120,** 21.

Lieber, C. S. & DeCarli, L. M. (1970) Hepatic microsomal ethanol-oxidizing system. In vitro characteristics and adaptive properties in vivo. *Journal of Biological Chemistry,* **245,** 2505.

Lindenbaum, J. & Lieber, C. (1969) Alcohol-induced malabsorption of vitamin B_{12} in man. *Nature,* **224,** 806.

Lindenbaum, J. & Lieber, C. S. (1975) Effects of chronic ethanol administration on intestinal absorption in man in the absence of nutritional deficiency. *Annals of the New York Academy of Sciences,* **252,** 228.

Lindenbaum, J., Pezzimenti, J. F. & Shea, N. (1974) Small-intestinal function in vitamin B_{12} deficiency. *Annals of Internal Medicine,* **80,** 326.

Lindenbaum, J., Saha, J. R. & Lieber, C. S. (1973) Mechanism of alcohol-induced malabsorption of vitamin B_{12}. *Gastroenterology,* **64,** 762.

Lindenbaum, J., Shea, N., Saha, J. R. et al (1972) Alcohol-induced impairment of carbohydrate absorption. *Clinical Research,* **20,** 459.

Maddrey, W. C. & Boyer, J. L. (1973) The acute and chronic effects of ethanol administration on bile secretion in the rat. *Journal of Laboratory and Clinical Medicine,* **82,** 215.

Mayoral, L. G., Tripathy, K., Garcia, F. T. et al (1967) Malabsorption in the tropics: a second look. *American Journal of Clinical Nutrition,* **20,** 866.

Mekhjian, H. S. & May, E. S. (1977) Acute and chronic effects of ethanol on fluid transport in the human small intestine. *Gastroenterology,* **72,** 1280.

Mezey, E. (1975) Intestinal function in chronic alcoholism. *Annals of the New York Academy of Sciences,* **252,** 215.

Mezey, E. (1979) Ethanol: metabolism and adverse effects. *Viewpoints on Digestive Diseases,* **II,** 2.

Mezey, E. & Potter, J. J. (1976) Changes in exocrine pancreatic function produced by altered dietary protein intake in drinking alcoholics. *Johns Hopkins Medical Journal,* **138,** 7.

Mezey, E., Jow, E., Slavin, R. E. et al (1970) Pancreatic function and intestinal absorption in chronic alcoholism. *Gastroenterology,* **59,** 657.

Middleton, W. R. J., Carter, E. A., Drummey, G. D. et al (1971) Effect of oral ethanol administration on intestinal cholesterogenesis in the rat. *Gastroenterology,* **60,** 880.

Mistilis, S. P. & Garski, A. (1969) Induction of alcohol dehydrogenase in liver and gastrointestinal tract. *Australasian Annals of Medicine,* **18,** 227.

Mistilis, S. P. & Ockner, R. K. (1972) Effects of ethanol on endogenous lipid and lipoprotein metabolism in the small intestine. *Journal of Laboratory and Clinical Medicine,* **80,** 34.

Mitjavila, S., Lacombe, C. & Carrera, G. (1976) Changes in activity of rat brush border enzymes incubated with a homologous series of aliphatic alcohols. *Biochemistry and Pharmacology,* **25,** 625.

Perlow, W., Baraona, E. & Lieber, C. S. (1977) Symptomatic intestinal disaccharidase deficiency in alcoholics. *Gastroenterology,* **71,** 680.

Pirola, R. C. & Davis, A. E. (1970) Effects of intravenous alcohol on motility of the duodenum and sphincter of Oddi. *Australasian Annals of Medicine,* **19,** 1.

Robles, E. A., Mezey, E., Halsted, C. H. et al (1974) Effect of ethanol on motility of the small intestine. *Johns Hopkins Medical Journal,* **135,** 17.

Rodgers, J. B. & O'Brien, R. J. (1975) The effect of acute ethanol treatment on lipid-re-esterifying enzymes of the rat small bowel. *American Journal of Digestive Diseases,* **20,** 354.

Roggin, G. M., Iber, F. L., Kater, R. M. H. et al (1969) Malabsorption in the chronic alcoholic. *Johns Hopkins Medical Journal,* **125,** 321.

Rubin, E., Rybak, B. J., Lindenbaum, J. et al (1972) Ultrastructural changes in the small intestine induced by ethanol. *Gastroenterology,* **63,** 801.

Schafer, D. F., Stephenson, D. V., Barak, A. J. et al (1974) Effects of ethanol on the transport of manganese by small intestine of the rat. *Journal of Nutrition,* **104,** 101.

Schneider, R. E. & Viteri, F. E. (1974) Studies on the luminal events of lipid absorption in protein-calorie malnourished (PCM) children; its relation with nutritional recovery and diarrhea. II. Alterations in the bile acids of the duodenal content. *American Journal of Clinical Nutrition,* **27,** 788.

Seitz, K., Korsten, M. A. & Lieber, C. S. (1978) Increased activity of intestinal microsomal enzymes after chronic ethanol feeding. *Gastroenterology,* **74,** 1092.

Small, M., Longarini, A. & Zamcheck, N. (1959) Disturbances of digestive physiology following acute drinking episodes in 'skid-row' alcoholics. *American Journal of Medicine,* **27,** 575.

Small, M. D., Gershoff, S. N., Broitman, S. A. et al (1960) Effect of alcohol and dietary deprivation on absorption of xylose from the rat small intestine. *American Journal of Digestive Diseases,* **5,** 801.

Smith, F. E. & Palmer, D. L. (1976) Alcoholism, infection and altered host defenses. A review of clinical and experimental observations. *Journal of Chronic Diseases,* **29,** 35.

Solomon, N., Solomon, T. E., Jacobson, E. G. et al (1974) Direct effects of alcohol on in vivo and in vitro exocrine pancreatic secretion and metabolism. *American Journal of Digestive Diseases,* **19,** 253.

Tandon, B. N., Banks, P. A., George, P. K. et al (1970) Recovery of exocrine pancreatic function in adult protein-calorie malnutrition. *Gastroenterology,* **58,** 358.

Tall, A. R., Green, P. H. R., Glickman, R. M. et al (1978) Metabolic rate of chylomicrons, phospholipids and apoproteins in the rat. *Circulation,* **58,** 11.

Tapper, E. J., Bushi, S., Ruppert, R. D. et al (1968) Effects of acute and chronic ethanol treatment on the absorption of iron in rats. *American Journal of Medical Science,* **255,** 46.

Theron, J. J., Wittmann, W., & Prinslov, J. G. (1971) The fine structure of the jejunum in kwashiorkor. *Experimental Molecular Pathology,* **14,** 184.

Thomson, A. D., Baker, H. & Leevy, C. M. (1970) Patterns of ^{35}S-thiamine hydrochloride absorption in the malnourished alcoholic patient. *Journal of Laboratory and Clinical Medicine,* **76,** 34.

Tomasulo, P. A., Kater, R. M. H. & Iber, F. L. (1968) Impairment of thiamine absorption in alcoholism. *American Journal of Clinical Nutrition,* **21,** 1341.

Verdy, M. & Caron, D. (1973) Ethanol et absorption du calcium chez l'humain. *Biologie et Gastroenterologie* (Paris), **6,** 157.

Viteri, F. E., Flores, J. M. & Alvarado, J. (1973) Intestinal malabsorption in malnourished children before and during recovery. Relation between severity of protein deficiency and the malabsorption process. *American Journal of Digestive Diseases,* **18,** 201.

Vlahcevic, Z. R., Juttijudata, P., Bell, C. C. et al (1972) Bile acid metabolism in patients with cirrhosis. II. Cholic and chenodeoxycholic acid metabolism. *Gastroenterology,* **62,** 1174.

Wilson, F. A. & Hoyumpa, A. M. Jr (1979) Ethanol and small intestinal transport. *Gastroenterology,* **76,** 386.

Yano, K., Rhoads, G. G. & Kagan, A. (1977) Coffee, alcohol and risk of coronary heart disease among Japanese men living in Hawaii. *New England Journal of Medicine,* **297,** 405.

16

Mucosal Histopathology of Malabsorption

ROBERT L. OWEN
LLOYD L. BRANDBORG

Correlation of intestinal mucosal structure with malabsorption and other pathophysiological conditions became possible only after development of peroral small intestinal suction biopsy techniques. Previously, rapid autolysis of the intestinal lining post mortem prevented study of the mucosa during the evolution of disease states. Suction biopsies are usually carried out with a multipurpose tube (Brandborg, Rubin and Quinton, 1959) or with biopsy devices (Crosby and Kugler, 1957). The use of these instruments has been described in detail (Perera, Weinstein and Rubin, 1975). The instrument used will depend upon availability and experience of the operator, but instruments which give more than one specimen are often preferable because of the patchy nature of many intestinal mucosal lesions. Unless specimens are removed from the biopsy instrument gently and oriented with care prior to fixation, subsequent interpretation will be difficult if not impossible. Because of contraction of the muscularis mucosae, specimens usually curl up into a porcupine-like ball with villi projecting out in all directions. A specimen is laid on a dry gloved finger and the opposed edges are spread apart with the shaft of a needle or probe. The specimen usually remains flattened due to adhesion to the operator's finger. This flattened specimen is then transferred onto plastic mesh or a small Millipore filter by adherence. The technician processing the disc-shaped biopsy must be instructed to embed it on edge so that subsequent sections are perpendicular to the luminal surface. Serial sectioning of mucosal biopsies is desirable to maximize opportunity for detection of patchy lesions. Biopsies are usually taken just beyond the duodenum near the ligament of Treitz. The end of the duodenal curve is a recognizable landmark which can be used for subsequent comparative biopsies. Detection of many important lesions, especially coeliac sprue and *Giardia* infection, is maximized at this location. Standardization of biopsy site is necessary because of a normal and physiological gradient in shape of villi along the intestine. In the duodenum, villi are broadened and may be fused or distorted by underlying Brunner's glands. In the usual biopsy site in the proximal jejunum, normal villi are usually finger- or tongue-shaped in patients from industrial western countries with a refined mixed diet. Patients eating a high-bulk vegetarian diet with small intestinal distension may have broadening and flattening of villi in the absence of pathological conditions (Owen and Brandborg, 1977).

Villi sectioned in an upright position are covered by tall columnar epithelial cells with basally located nuclei and an even luminal brush border of microvilli. Among columnar cells are mucus-filled goblet cells, and in spaces between epithelial cells are seen wandering lymphocytes and pseudopods of macrophages. Epithelial cells are generated by mitosis in adjacent crypts and are desquamated at the tips of villi. Furrows in the surfaces of villi produce serrations around the perimeter of villi, seen in sections (Figure 1). Beneath the villus surface, the lamina propria is physiologically inflamed, containing plasma cells, lymphocytes, macrophages, mast cells, and occasionally eosinophils.

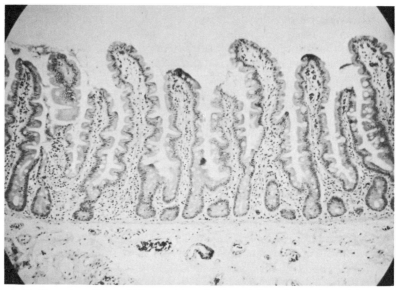

Figure 1. Normal small bowel biopsy with well-oriented finger-like villi. Nuclei are evenly situated at the bases of columnar cells and goblet cells over these villus surfaces. Villus height is two to three times as great as crypt depth. × 65. From Brandborg (1979), with kind permission of the author and the editor of *American Journal of Medicine*.

Any of a variety of processes which damage or shorten the life span of villus epithelial cells will produce a common appearance as damaged columnar cells more rapidly desquamate, producing villus shortening, and mitotic rate increases with lengthening of surrounding crypts. As the process continues, villi shorten, flatten and may join with adjacent villi, forming ridges or convolutions in the mucosal surface. Because of compensatory crypt hypertrophy, total mucosal thickness may remain the same but surface area is drastically reduced. This loss of surface area and the immaturity of epithelial cells rushed from the crypts to replace lost cells contribute to the clinical picture of malabsorption which accompanies this type of severe mucosal lesion. This lesion has been called total villus atrophy, but this term is misleading because mucosal thickness, cell renewal rate and metabolic activity are normal or increased rather than atrophic. This shift in mucosal architecture to a flattened surface with deep crypts resembles development of colon. During embryological development, the colon is also lined with villi which flatten as crypts assume their adult depth. A small intestinal biopsy with a severe mucosal lesion may, indeed, be mistaken for colonic tissue except for fewer numbers of goblets cells and presence of Paneth cells which are rarely found in colon.

Determination of the cause of jejunal villus flattening is made by correlation with the clinical history or by appropriate therapeutic trials. In North America and Europe, coeliac sprue is the most common cause of this appearance (Figure 2). In patients with a hereditary sensitivity, protein components of a variety of cereal grains produce a direct toxic destructive effect on villus epithelial cells, accompanied by increased cellular immune reactivity (see Chapter 10). Confirmation of the diagnosis is made by exclusion of wheat, barley, rye and oats from the diet and observation for clinical and histological improvement. Clinically controlled patients and their asymptomatic relatives may continue to show flattened villi in the

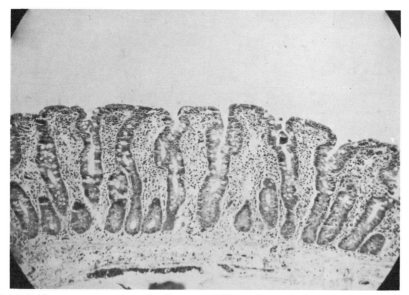

Figure 2. Flat mucosa in untreated coeliac sprue. Villi are short and widened by lymphoid cells in the lamina propria and infiltrating the epithelium. Crypts are increased in length. ×65. From Brandborg (1979), with kind permission of the author and the editor of *American Journal of Medicine.*

most proximal portion of the small intestine, suggesting proximal precipitation or inactivation of residual gluten with protection of the more distal intestine. The great reserve capacity for absorption of the small intestine permits adequate absorption without total resolution of the mucosal lesion. Patients with dermatitis herpetiformis, a skin disease characterized by pruritic vesicles and papules in a bilateral symmetrical distribution, frequently have villus flattening which also responds to a gluten-free diet (Weinstein et al, 1971). Patients with malabsorption with villus flattening who have been living in non-industrialized areas may have tropical sprue syndrome which responds to folic acid and broad spectrum antibiotics but not to gluten exclusion (Figure 3). Asymptomatic persons in developing countries, eating a high-bulk vegetable diet dictated by local custom and economic necessity, may show shortening and broadening of villi similar to that seen in white middle-class North American adults eating a vegetarian diet by choice (Owen and Brandborg, 1977). Symptomatic patients with tropical sprue have greater numbers of intraepithelial lymphocytes and round cell infiltration of the lamina propria (Perera, Weinstein and Rubin, 1975). Some patients with idiopathic chronic ulcerative enteritis have a mucosal lesion remote from the ulcers which is indistinguishable from the severe lesion seen in coeliac sprue (Mills, Brown and Watkinson, 1980).

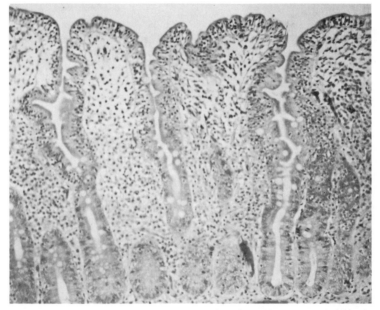

Figure 3. Tropical sprue syndrome. Villi are short, broad, and lymphocytes within the villus epithelium are markedly increased. Cells in the lamina propria appear widely spaced due to formalin fixation, compared to Bouin's fixation in Figures 1 and 2. × 140. From Brandborg (1979), with kind permission of the author and the editor of *American Journal of Medicine.*

Patients with acute gastroenteritis and accompanying malabsorption may have villus shortening in a patchy distribution which usually resolves spontaneously with time. Patients with chronic bacterial overgrowth in the small intestine due to impaired intestinal motility because of systemic disease, blind loops, partial obstruction or other impediments to intestinal transit may also develop malabsorption from a combination of intraluminal bacterial effects on bile salts and food items and on mucosal villus structure. Broad spectrum antibiotics or surgical correction of obstructive lesions improves symptoms. Histological normalization may be difficult to assess because of the patchy nature of such lesions.

Patients with severe dietary protein deficiency with kwashiorkor have a mucosal lesion which resembles untreated coeliac sprue or tropical sprue. This syndrome, which should be apparent from a dietary history, responds to high-quality protein but not to gluten exclusion or antibiotics.

The conditions of some patients with severe mucosal flattening and malabsorption which do not fall into any of the above categories and do not respond to gluten exclusion, antibiotics or dietary protein enhancement have been called unclassified or refractory sprue. The mucosal lesion in these patients may reflect a toxic or allergic response to dietary constituents (Baker and Rosenberg, 1978).

MALABSORPTION SYNDROMES WITH DIAGNOSTIC CHANGES

Whipple's disease is a systemic condition characterized by arthritis and diarrhoea, usually with an immunological deficiency which includes impairment of macrophage function. Villi are distorted in shape by macrophages filled with PAS-positive material (Figure 4) which, in plastic-embedded sections, is recognized as bacilli by light microscopy and by transmission electron microscopy. By endoscopy, highly infiltrated areas appear white and raised (Volpicelli et al, 1976). Although the bacillus type has not been identified, antibody staining techniques indicate that a particular organism is responsible for most cases of Whipple's disease (Keren, 1981). Lacteals may become obstructed and dilated by the engorged macrophages in the lamina propria. In patients with acquired immuno-deficiency syndrome (AIDS), a similar mucosal appearance has been observed with systemic *Mycobacterium avium-intracellulare*. In such cases the bacilli filling macrophages are larger (Figure 5), may be recovered by blood culture, and are also found in mesenteric and systemic lymph nodes. Antibiotics promote symptomatic and histological improvement with the Whipple's organism but have not been effective with *Mycobacterium avium-intracellulare*.

Primary intestinal lymphoma (Mediterranean lymphoma or heavy chain disease) is characterized by mucosal infiltration by lymphocytes replacing and displacing crypts with subsequent villus flattening. In this instance, villus shortening may indeed represent atrophy because of impaired crypt function (Figures 6 and 7). This appearance may resemble coeliac sprue in which patients initially responsive to gluten exclusion may also later develop lymphoma (Perera, Weinstein and Rubin, 1975).

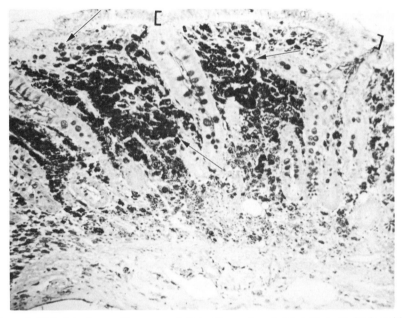

Figure 4. Whipple's disease. The mucosa is flat with very broad villi stuffed with PAS-positive macrophages (arrows) containing bacilli. The edges of a single broad villus are marked by brackets. ×70. From Brandborg (1979), with kind permission of the author and the editor of *American Journal of Medicine*.

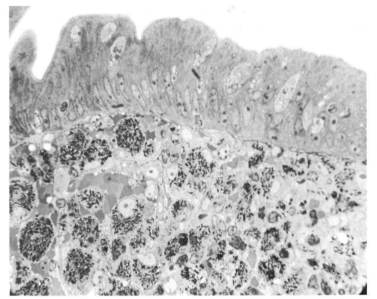

Figure 5. In a patient with Kaposi's sarcoma and acquired immunosuppression syndrome, macrophages containing *Mycobacterium avium-intracellulare* fill the lamina propria. ×350.

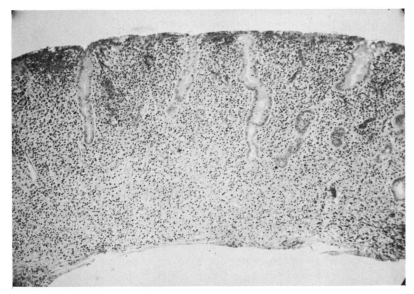

Figure 6. Diffuse infiltration of the intestinal mucosa by malignant lymphoma. Crypts are displaced and villi are completely flattened. ×65. From Brandborg (1979), with kind permission of the author and the editor of *American Journal of Medicine.*

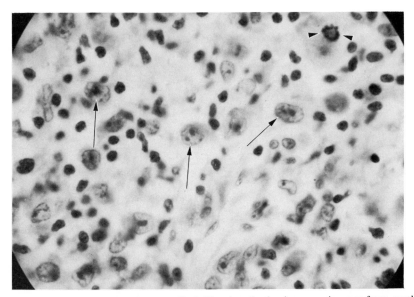

Figure 7. In malignant lymphoma, cells infiltrating the lamina propria vary from small, normal-appearing lymphoid cells to cells with large, frankly neoplastic nuclei (arrows). A cell in mitosis is present in the upper right corner (arrowheads). ×260. From Brandborg (1979), with kind permission of the author and the editor of *American Journal of Medicine.*

In eosinophilic gastroenteritis excessive numbers of eosinophilic leuco-cytes infiltrate the lamina propria (Cello, 1979 — see chapter 12). Any portion of the intestinal tract may be involved. A wide variety of intestinal symptoms can occur and no aetiology is yet apparent.

Rare systemic diseases may produce remarkably distinctive intestinal histological changes. In abetalipoproteinaemia, a defect in lipid transport due to failure to synthesize beta-lipoprotein, dietary lipid enters absorptive cells but cannot be transported to the lacteals. Large vacuoles filled with lipid distend and distort columnar cells over villi which are, themselves, normal in shape. Lipid is extracted by usual embedding techniques, so that vacuoles appear empty (Figure 8) (Gotto et al, 1971). In collagenous sprue, a broad band of collagen, demonstrated with trichrome stain, separates the epithelium from the lamina propria. Crypts are displaced and villi are absent (Figure 9) (Weinstein et al, 1970).

Intestinal parasitic infection

Protozoan and helminthic parasites produce malabsorption by a variety of mechanisms, including competition for food, damage to epithelial cells, and provocation of cellular immune reactions which damage columnar cells as innocent bystanders. *Giardia lamblia* is increasingly recognized as a source of intestinal symptoms, especially increased gas production and discomfort with or without diarrhoea. In most cases, villus shape is unchanged, although increased intraepithelial lymphocytes may be noted. Mucus from

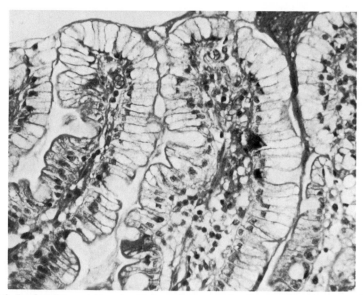

Figure 8. In abetalipoproteinaemia, triglyceride in vacuoles distends the columnar cells over villi. ×150. From Brandborg (1979), with kind permission of the author and the editor of *American Journal of Medicine.*

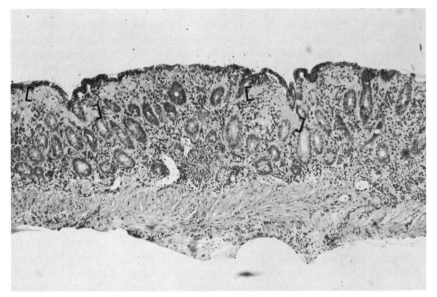

Figure 9. In collagenous sprue, a dense collagen band (brackets) lies just beneath the epithelium, replacing some crypts. ×65. From Brandborg (1979) with kind permission of the author and the editor of *American Journal of Medicine*.

the biopsy surface or fluid from the biopsy capsule placed between a slide and cover slip may permit immediate diagnosis when the characteristic tumbling motion of *Giardia* trophozoites is seen at high dry magnification. In sections, *Giardia* are recognized in the lumen and along the mucosal surface more easily when stained with Giemsa stain or trichrome stain than with haematoxylin and eosin (Figure 10) (Brandborg et al, 1967). Lymphocytes may be seen in the intestinal lumen in association with *Giardia* trophozoites (Brandborg et al, 1980). In patients with intestinal immunodeficiency, malabsorption and diarrhoea may be prominent with villus shortening which improves following treatment of giardiasis. In patients with normal immune systems and no apparent villus structural change, some secondary lactase deficiency appears to be present and symptoms of excess gas production are often relieved by avoidance of milk and milk products, pending resolution of infection by normal immunological clearance. *Giardia* normally remain within the lumen or adhere to microvillus surfaces of columnar cells. When mucosal integrity is damaged and large numbers of trophozoites are present in the lumen, *Giardia* may wander into the epithelium and lamina propria but do not proliferate. The primary pathophysiological importance of such *Giardia* invasion appears to be in initiating immunological clearance mechanisms (Owen, Allen and Stevens, 1981).

   Other protozoa, classified as coccidia, enter intestinal epithelial cells which are damaged by the organisms replicating within their cytoplasm. *Isospora belli* is found deep within and between columnar cells (Figure 11).

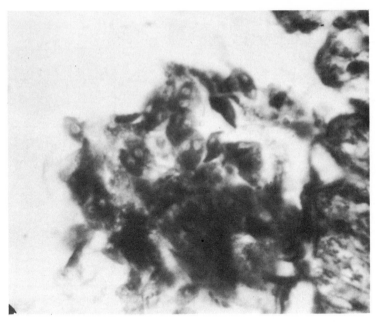

Figure 10. *Giardia* with paired nuclei in a mass of mucus and cellular debris lie in the intestinal lumen next to the villus epithelial surface to the right. ×70. Masson's trichrome stain. From Brandborg (1979), with kind permission of the author and the editor of *American Journal of Medicine*.

This organism is not often recognized but probably occurs with some frequency and is cleared by normal immune processes. There may be increased eosinophils in the lamina propria and villi may or may not be shortened (Brandborg, Goldberg and Breidenbach, 1970). In patients with immunodeficiency, chronic malabsorption and diarrhoea, careful search of villus epithelium may be worthwhile. In one patient with chronic malabsorption and *Isospora belli*, symptoms were alleviated by treatment with pyrimethamine and sulphadiazine (Trier et al, 1974).

Another member of the coccidia group, recognized with increasing frequency, is *Cryptosporidium*. This protozoon, commonly found in calves and pigs, produces a secretory diarrhoea and infects columnar cells just below the luminal surface membrane, effacing microvilli and producing villus shortening. In haematoxylin- and eosin-stained sections this organism can be recognized as 'dust particles' within the brush border (Figure 12a). When the diagnosis is in question, paraffin-embedded tissue may be re-embedded for transmission electron microscopy (Figure 12b) to verify the diagnosis. In patients with normal immune systems, infection resolves within two weeks (Reese et al, 1982). In immunosuppressed patients, no antibiotics have been effective, but infection has resolved when drug-induced immunosuppression has been terminated (Weinstein et al, 1981).

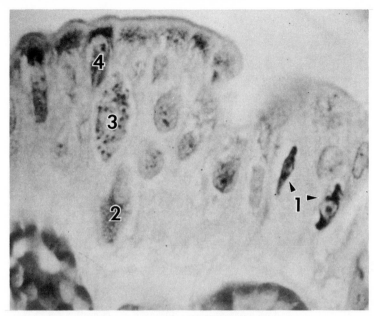

Figure 11. In *Isopora belli* infection, a variety of stages in the life cycle of the protozoon are found in nearby villus columnar, epithelial cells: 1 = merozoites, 2 = schizont, 3 = macrogametocyte, 4 = trophozoite (immature schizont). ×700. Colophonium Giemsa stain. From Brandborg et al (1970), with kind permission of the authors and the editor of *New England Journal of Medicine*.

The organisms are equally infective for man and for a variety of other mammals. Stools from patients induce marked villus shortening in experimental animals (Reese et al, 1982; Tzipori et al, 1982).

The nematode *Strongyloides stercoralis* may produce mild gastrointestinal symptoms, worms and larvae in the mucosa inducing an inflammatory reaction with villus flattening (O'Brien, 1975). In patients with characteristic cutaneous larva migrans, diagnosis is more likely to be made from stool examination. Because of autoinfection, patients infected in the Pacific in World War II continue to have active infection in the United States and Britain (Gill and Bell, 1979). Endemic domestic transmission during sexual contact also occurs.

Intestinal immunodeficiency syndromes

A variety of syndromes have been described with varying histological pictures related to specific cellular defects or exaggerated response to physiological and pathological intestinal infection (Boyd and Bachman, 1982). In hypogammaglobulinaemic sprue the mucosa resembles that in coeliac sprue except for absence of plasma cells and failure to respond to gluten exclusion. *Giardia* are frequently present. The incidence of *Giardia* infection may be no higher in such patients than in the normal population,

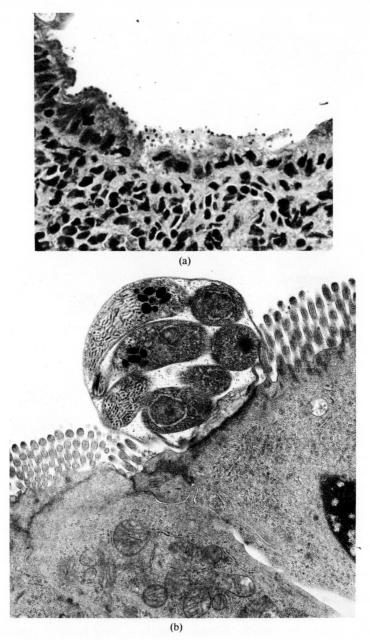

(a)

(b)

Figure 12. (a) *Cryptosporidium* infection in a twelve-year-old boy with congenital immuno-globulin deficiency. The dark round organisms lie among the microvilli along the surface of the epithelium over villi and in crypts. × 300. Haematoxylin and eosin stain. (b) *Cryptosporidium* from a patient with acquired immunodeficiency syndrome. The organism effaces microvilli and forms a dense attachment zone. This schizont is dividing into eight merozoites which upon release would infect adjacent cells. × 13 000.

but with failure to clear, prevalence may increase with time, especially in children in institutional settings and in adults with oral-anal sexual exposure. Villus architecture may improve following elimination of *Giardia* with antibiotics (Figures 13 and 14) (Ament and Rubin, 1972).

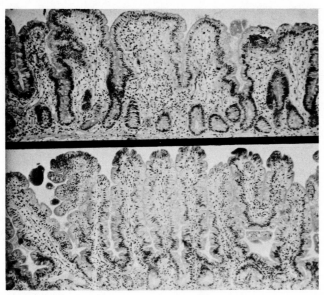

Figure 13. Intestinal biopsies from a patient with immunodeficiency disease complicated by *Giardia* infection. Above, villi are shortened and broadened with inflammatory infiltration of the lamina propria during active *Giardia* infection. Below, villus form has normalized following eradication of *Giardia* infection. ×65. (Illustration courtesy of Dr Marvin Ament.)

Benign lymphoid hyperplasia may be recognized as mucosal nodularity on x-ray studies. In intestinal biopsies, lymphoid nodules displace villi but villi between nodules are normal.

Rare jejunal biopsy abnormalities

In lymphangiectasia lymphatics which are normally not seen within villi are dilated. Lymphatics may be congenitally obstructed, distorting villus shape (Figure 15). Similar appearances may occur with secondary lymphatic obstruction.

When epithelial cell replacement is impaired by deficiency of vitamin B_{12} or folic acid, or following radiation or radiomimetic drugs, decreased mitosis within crypts will be noted with macrocytosis of individual intestinal columnar cells. Villus atrophy may develop, depending on the degree of inhibition of columnar cell replacement. Such abnormality may be patchy in distribution, possibly reflecting underlying differences in vascular perfusion which is greater along the mesenteric border and diminished

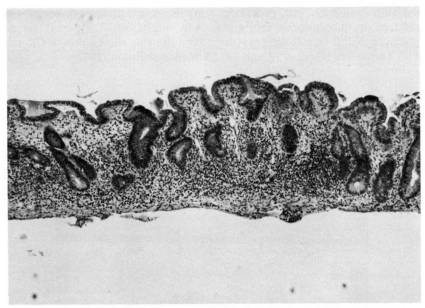

Figure 14. Hypogammaglobulinaemic sprue without *Giardia* infection. Villi are shortened and resemble coeliac sprue except for absence of plasma cells and failure to respond to gluten exclusion. ×70. From Brandborg (1979), with kind permission of the author and the editor of *American Journal of Medicine*.

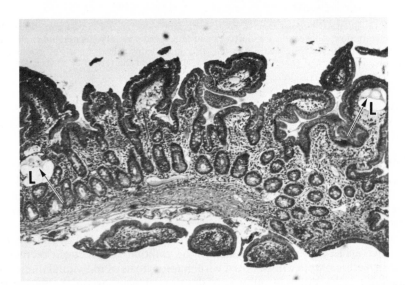

Figure 15. Lymphangiectasia. Lymphatics (L) are greatly dilated, especially at the left and far right of the biopsy. Foamy macrophages (arrows) are present in the lymphatics. ×60. From Brandborg (1979), with kind permission of the author and the editor of *American Journal of Medicine*.

along the opposite intestinal wall. Non-caseating granulomas of Crohn's disease, with or without giant cells, may be seen at any point throughout the intestinal tract, but Crohn's disease is relatively uncommon in the jejunum at the normal site of small bowel biopsy. Patients with gastrinoma (Zollinger-Ellison syndrome) produce greater amounts of gastric acid than can be neutralized by pancreatic secretions, distending the jejunum and producing small ulcers and inflammation of the mucosal surface. In amyloidosis, blood vessels in the lamina propria may contain material which reacts with congo red stain. In chronic granulomatis disease, vacuolated macrophages in the lamina propria may be filled with PAS-positive material without distortion of villus architecture. In acrodermatitis enteropathica, patients with vesicular dermatitis over projecting body points may have non-specific intestinal lesions which respond to zinc replacement. In lipid storage diseases, vacuolated ganglion cells may be observed in Meissner's plexus. In macroglobulinaemia, patients with intestinal involvement may have malabsorption with amorphous masses of hyalin located between cells in the lamina propria, especially in the ends of villi, producing a club-like shape.

REFERENCES

Ament, M. & Rubin, C. E. (1972) Relation of giardiasis to abnormal intestinal structure and function in gastrointestinal immunodeficiency syndromes. *Gastroenterology, 62*, 216-226.

Baker, A. L. & Rosenberg, I. H. (1978) Refractory sprue: recovery after removal of nongluten dietary proteins. *Annals of Internal Medicine, 89*, 505-508.

Boyd, W. P. Jr & Bachman, B. A. (1982) Gastrointestinal infections in the compromised host. *Medical Clinics of North America, 66*, 743-753.

Brandborg, L. L. (1979) Histologic diagnosis of diseases of malabsorption. *Americal Journal of Medicine, 67*, 999-1006.

Brandborg, L. L., Goldberg, S. B. & Breidenbach, W. C. (1970) Human coccidiosis: a possible cause of malabsorption. *New England Journal of Medicine, 283*, 1306-1313.

Brandborg, L. L., Rubin, C. & Quinton, W. (1959) Multipurpose instrument for suction biopsy of esophagus, stomach, small bowel, and colon. *Gastroenterology, 37*, 1-16.

Brandborg, L., L., Tankersley, C. B., Gottlieb, S. et al (1967) Histological demonstration of mucosal invasion by *Giardia lamblia* in man. *Gastroenterology, 52*, 143-150.

Brandborg, L. L., Owen, R. L., Fogel, R. et al (1980) Giardiasis and traveller's diarrhea. *Gastroenterology, 78*, 1602-1614.

Cello, J. P. (1979) Eosinophilic gastroenteritis — a complex disease entity. *American Journal of Medicine, 67*, 1097-1104.

Crosby, W. H. & Kugler, H. W. (1957) Intraluminal biopsy of the small intestine. *Americal Journal of Digestive Diseases, 2*, 236-241.

Gill, G. V. & Bell, D. R. (1979) *Strongyloides stercoralis* infection in former Far East prisoners of war. *British Medical Journal, ii*, 572-574.

Gotto, A. M., Levy, R. I., John, K. & Fredrickson, D. S. (1971) On the protein defect in abetalipoproteinemia. *New England Journal of Medicine, 284*, 813-818.

Keren, D. F. (1981) Whipple's disease: a review emphasizing immunology and microbiology. *CRC Critical Reviews In Clinical Laboratory Sciences, 14*, 75-100.

Mills, P. R., Brown, J. L. & Watkinson, G. (1980) Idiopathic chronic ulcerative enteritis. Report of five cases and review of the literature. *Quarterly Journal of Medicine, 49*, 133-149.

O'Brien, W. (1975) Intestinal malabsorption in acute infection with *Strongyloides stercoralis*. *Transactions of the Royal Society of Tropical Medicine and Hygiene, 69*, 69-77.

Owen, R. L. & Brandborg, L. L. (1977) Jejunal morphologic consequences of vegetarian diet in humans. *Gastroenterology, 72*, 1111 (abstract).

Owen, R. L., Allen, C. L. & Stevens, D. P. (1981) Phagocytosis of *Giardia muris* by macrophages in Peyer's patch epithelium in mice. *Infection and Immunity,* **33,** 591-601.

Perera, D. R., Weinstein, W. M. & Rubin, C. E. (1975) Small intestinal biopsy. *Human Pathology,* **6,** 157-217.

Reese, N. C., Current, W. L., Ernst, J. V. & Bailey, W. S. (1982) Cryptosporidiosis of man and calf: a case report and results of experimental infections in mice and rats. *Americal Journal of Tropical Medicine and Hygiene,* **31,** 226-229.

Trier, J. S., Moxey, P. C., Schimmel, E. M. & Robles, E. (1974) Chronic intestinal coccidiosis in man: intestinal morphology and response to treatment. *Gastroenterology,* **66,** 923-935.

Tzipori, S., Angus, K. W., Campbell, I. & Gray, E. W. (1982) Experimental infection of lambs with *Cryptosporidium* isolated from a human patient with diarrhea. *Gut,* **23,** 71-74.

Weinstein, L., Edelstein, S. M., Madara, J. L. et al (1981) Intestinal cryptosporidiosis complicated by disseminated cytomegalovirus infection. *Gastroenterology,* **81,** 584-591.

Weinstein, W. M., Saunders, D. R., Tytgat, G. N. & Rubin, C. E. (1970) Collagenous sprue — an unrecognized type of malabsorption. *New England Journal of Medicine,* **283,** 1297-1301.

Weinstein, W. M., Brow, J. R., Parker, F. & Rubin, C. E. (1971) The small intestinal mucosa in dermatitis herpetiformis. II. Relationship of the small intestinal lesion to gluten. *Gastroenterology,* **60,** 362-369.

Volpicelli, N. A., Salyer, W. R., Milligan, F. D. et al (1976) The endoscopic appearance of the duodenum in Whipple's disease. *Johns Hopkins Medical Journal,* **138,** 19-23.

17

The Use of Breath Tests in the Study of Malabsorption

CHARLES E. KING
PHILLIP P. TOSKES

Analysis of the breath as a means to monitor events taking place in the gastrointestinal tract is a technique which has been developed appreciably in the recent past. These breath tests offer tremendous advantages in terms of simplicity and aesthetic quality, especially when compared to the multitude of tube tests and non-respiratory secretory/excretory studies available for gastrointestinal diagnosis. Sensitivity and specificity of the tests has been moderately good to excellent, and has varied with the ability to focus the desired test parameter as a rate-limiting step in volatile metabolite (gas) generation. The purpose of this review will be to survey the current tests available for clinical evaluation of malabsorption, analysing the strengths and weaknesses of the tests and outlining potential changes necessary for improved clinical applicability.

PRINCIPLES OF DIAGNOSTIC GASTROINTESTINAL BREATH TESTS

Breath hydrogen (H_2) tests

Levitt has shown that the production of hydrogen gas in man occurs primarily as a result of contact between fermentable substrate and bacteria of the intestinal microflora. This is usually related to H_2 generation by the colon bacterial flora, although production is also seen in the small intestine when the usually sparse small bowel flora has been increased (bacterial overgrowth of the small intestine). Because this production by the intestinal microflora is reflected by approximately 14 per cent of the total H_2 produced as H_2 in the breath, respiratory H_2 excretion can be used as a monitor of H_2 production in the intestine (Levitt, 1969). Further evaluation has shown the utility of breath H_2 analysis as a marker for arrival of a fermentable substrate to the colonic flora, either as a test for small intestinal transit time or to demonstrate malabsorption of as little as 2 - 5 g of ingested substances by the small intestine, with secondary contact with the colonic flora (Levitt and Donaldson, 1970; Bond and Levitt, 1972, 1975). These

0300-5089/83/1202-591 $05.00©1983 W. B. Saunders Company Ltd

studies laid the groundwork for use of H_2 breath analysis as a clinical guide for abnormal contact of bowel bacteria with ingested nutrients, which is discussed in other sections of this review.

Isotopic CO_2 breath tests

Depending on the route of administration and substrate employed, administration of an isotopic (^{14}C or ^{13}C) labelled substrate can lead to the production of isotopic CO_2 as a result of metabolism: (a) in the gastrointestinal lumen, (b) in the host tissues following the absorption of orally administered substrate, and/or (c) in host tissues following intravenous administration of the substrate. Thus, when appropriately designed and interpreted, an isotopic CO_2 breath test can be used to detect abnormal intraluminal events (e.g., bacterial overgrowth, ileal malabsorption of bile salts), to detect the degree of intestinal absorption of the substrate (e.g., labelled triglyceride), and to quantify liver function and/or drug metabolism. The range of functions lending themselves to analysis by the breath test technique is thus wider with isotopic CO_2 tests than with H_2 breath tests, since the latter can measure only substrate which is not absorbed and/or has abnormal contact with intraluminal bacteria. This wider applicability of the CO_2 breath tests requires more rigorous design and validation in ascertaining that the cause of abnormal labelled CO_2 generation is the pathophysiological process which is being evaluated. In addition, since CO_2 generation and/or excretion may change as a result of acid-base reactions, metabolic activity of the subject, and pulmonary function, adequate control for these variables must be made for valid isotopic CO_2 test interpretation (Slanger, Kusubov and Winchell, 1970; King and Toskes, 1981).

METHODOLOGY AND LIMITATIONS

H_2 breath tests

The technique of H_2 breath analysis is relatively simple, primarily involving use of thermal conductivity gas chromatographic analysis of exhaled breath by means of a closed-rebreathing system (Bond and Levitt, 1972) or a simpler interval sampling technique (Metz et al, 1976a). Simple gas chromatographs dedicated to the measurement of H_2 alone and a system employing simple use of room air as the carrier gas have been developed, simplifying the technique for practical, inexpensive analysis in the routine diagnostic laboratory (Solomons, Viteri and Hamilton, 1977; Christman and Hamilton, 1982). An alternative electrochemical analysis system has also been recently described (Bartlett, Dobson and Eastham, 1980; Corbett et al, 1981). Breath can be collected as an end-tidal specimen using the Rahn-Otis sampler, coordinated aspiration from a nasal cannula, a Haldane-Priestley tube, or use of a two-bag system in which dead-space air is collected in a discard bag prior to filling of a second, analysis-specimen bag. These techniques, along with use of nasal prongs, were recently assessed for their reliability in H_2 breath tests, and all found to have comparable degrees of reliability (Gardiner et al, 1981a). For specimens which have appreciable dead-space air (i.e., in which the technique does not attempt to collect end-expiratory specimens) normalization of H_2 results to respiratory CO_2 (Niu, Schoeller and Klein, 1979) or to oxygen and nitrogen (Robb and Davidson, 1981) might improve reliability of results.

The major limitation of H_2 breath tests is the absence of H_2-producing bacteria in the microflora of up to 20 to 25 per cent of subjects (Gilat et al, 1978; Ravich, Bayless and Thomas, 1983). This limitation can usually be controlled by testing for H_2 production following oral administration of a large dose of the non-absorbable disaccharide lactulose as a second part of a normal or 'non-reactive' H_2 breath test. If there are H_2-producing bacteria in the subject's microflora, H_2 should appear in the breath when the lactulose passes into the colon. The relatively high incidence of subjects whose microflora is unable to generate H_2 could perhaps be limited by avoiding H_2 testing in subjects who have recently undergone mechanical bowel cleansing and/or antibiotic therapy, or who have severe diarrhoea (Gilat et al, 1978; Solomons et al, 1979). There is also a degree of pH-sensitivity in H_2 generation by bacteria (less H_2 production in an acidic environment) (Perman, Modler and Olson, 1981). This phenomenon is important because passage to the colon of fermentable carbohydrate often leads to the production of organic acids in addition to the potential H_2 production.

Minor limitations in the H_2 breath tests exist with respect to pulmonary H_2 excretion as a result of recent smoke inhalation or inhalation of organic solvent vapours (Tadesse and Eastwood, 1977). These factors are easily controlled for by disallowing cigarette smoking during the test, and performance of the test in ventilated rooms which have not been freshly painted and/or used for organic solvent storage. It has also been pointed out that breath H_2 concentrations during sleep and/or the night are higher than during waking hours, which requires some control over the time of testing and avoidance of prolonged periods of sleeping during the test (Solomons, Viteri and Rosenberg, 1978).

CO_2 breath tests

The most commonly used technique for isotopic CO_2 collection uses the bubbling of exhaled breath through an alkaline trapping solution, usually hyamine hydroxide. Usually 1 or 2 millimoles of ethanolic hyamine hydroxide are used to trap an equal quantity of CO_2 for analysis, with one to two drops of a pH indicator (e.g., phenolphthalein) to tell when complete neutralization of the alkaline trapping solution has occurred (Abt and von Schuching, 1966). Analysis from this solution for labelled CO_2 content is then made — by addition of a scintillant and performance of liquid scintillation counting for β activity during $^{14}CO_2$ tests, and by distillation of CO_2 between a dry ice-methanol trap and a liquid nitrogen trap, release of CO_2 from the alkaline solution by acidification, and mass spectrometric analysis for $^{13}CO_2$ tests (Schoeller et al, 1977). Isotopic ratio ($^{13}CO_2/^{12}CO_2$) analysis has also been carried out successfully on mixed specimens stored in 50 ml vacutainer vials (Schoeller and Klein, 1978). This simplified system actually reduces a tendency to fractionation of $^{13}CO_2$ and $^{12}CO_2$ during specimen handling, a problem which must be controlled to avoid non-specific changes in $^{13}CO_2/^{12}CO_2$ ratios (Schoeller et al, 1977).

For $^{14}CO_2$ tests, although it has been stated that photoluminescence and chemiluminescence may necessitate overnight adaptation of specimens before liquid scinitillation counting (Schwabe and Hepner, 1979), we have found that use of hyamine hydroxide (rather than the less expensive sodium hydroxide) along with the use of a quality scintillant affords reproducible, valid counting within two hours of specimen preparation (King and Toskes, 1982, unpublished observations). Thus, depending on availability of a liquid scintillation counter, results can be available within four hours of specimen collection.

We have analysed the applicability of an alternative $^{14}CO_2$ detection system developed at the University of Florida (Lorenz, Brookeman and Mauderli, 1978). This system, utilizing excitation of plastic filament rods coupled to photomultiplier tubes, has been found to be easily calibrated, sensitive, and reliable. The major advantage of this system is the direct readout of radioactive counts, affording interpretation of results during the test. Microprocessor automation of this system is currently being developed, which will afford technician-free sample collection, analysis, and system flushing. We have utilized this prototype system successfully for both repeated continuous flow testing in the experimental animal and for interval sampling for human clinical testing (Figure 1) (Toskes et al, 1978; King et al, 1979; King et al, 1980a).

Analysis for $^{13}CO_2$ concentration has been primarily performed using mass spectrometric analysis for $^{13}CO_2/^{12}CO_2$ ratios in breath specimens (Schoeller et al, 1977). It is also probable that alternative methods for

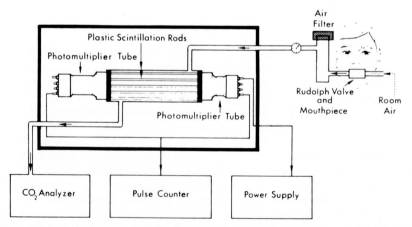

Figure 1. Schematic diagram of the $^{14}CO_2/CO_2$ analysis system. From King et al (1979), with kind permission of the authors and the editor of *Gastroenterology*.

determining breath $^{13}CO_2/^{12}CO_2$ ratios will be developed as use of stable
isotope CO_2 breath tests increases, such as shown recently with infrared
spectometric analysis of $^{13}CO_2$ (Hirano et al, 1979).

Use of interval sampling of breath during isotopic CO_2 breath tests has
simplified the technique, in contrast to earlier continuous sampling
techniques. Most laboratories using the interval sampling technique assume
that there is a constant production of 9 millimoles per kilogram hour of
endogenous CO_2 (the background against which labelled CO_2 generation is
measured) (Winchell et al, 1970). Because endogenous CO_2 production is
known to rise in the non-resting or febrile state (Slanger, Kusubov and
Winchell, 1970), isotopic CO_2 breath tests are performed only in the resting,
afebrile setting. We have recently demonstrated that there is an increase in
endogenous CO_2 production when greater than 100 kcal are administered as
part of the breath test (King and Toskes, 1981) (Figure 2). This is pertinent
because some breath tests utilize administration of a test meal as part of the
procedure. An increase in endogenous CO_2 production will lead to a

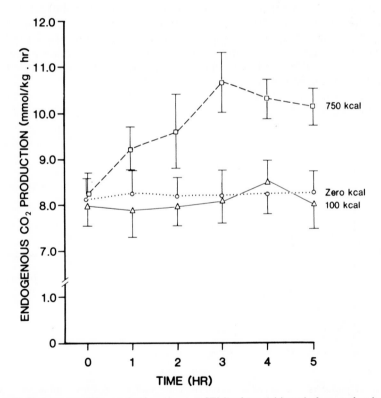

Figure 2. Endogenous CO_2 production (mean ± SEM) of ten subjects before, and at hourly
intervals following, administration of the three 'test meals' of zero, 100, and 750 kcal, the
latter as 200 kcal at time zero and 550 kcal at 2 h. Endogenous CO_2 production increased
significantly with administration of 200 kcal or more ($P<0.01$ at 2 h, $P<0.001$ after 2 h). From
King and Toskes (1981), with kind permission of the editor of *Journal of Nuclear Medicine*.

dilution of the labelled CO_2 concentration in the breath. If unaccounted for, changes in endogenous CO_2 production will lead to a less distinct separation of normal from abnormal labelled CO_2 generation, as depicted in Figure 3. The closer approximation of normal and abnormal values which would occur when changes in endogenous CO_2 production are not taken into account (assumed constancy of CO_2 production) would be accompanied by diminished sensitivity of the test in distinguishing normal from abnormal. During isotopic CO_2 tests which employ substantial caloric intake, analysis should include some measure of total CO_2 production (for example, measuring rate and volume of breath and total CO_2 content) during the collection of interval specimens for isotopic CO_2 measurement.

Stable isotopic $^{13}CO_2$ breath tests require, in addition, control for changes in labelled CO_2 production as a result of the ^{13}C-labelling of constituents of a carrier meal. In contrast to the rarity of ^{14}C in natural substances, $^{13}CO_2$ breath tests are performed against a substantial and variable (averaging 1.1 per cent) background (natural abundance) of ^{13}C. Since this natural abundance of ^{13}C varies, $^{13}CO_2$ generation and breath excretion varies according to ^{13}C content of any substances ingested and metabolized during the test (Schoeller et al, 1977). Schoeller and co-workers have demonstrated the need for controlling for $^{13}CO_2$ production as a result of meal constituents (by use of carrier meals having a ^{13}C abundance approximating that of fasting breath $^{13}CO_2$ and correction for meal-related changes in $^{13}CO_2$ abundance in the breath) (Schoeller et al, 1980).

Thus, isotopic ($^{14}CO_2$ and $^{13}CO_2$) CO_2 breath tests can be performed through simple determination of isotopic CO_2 content in the breath via

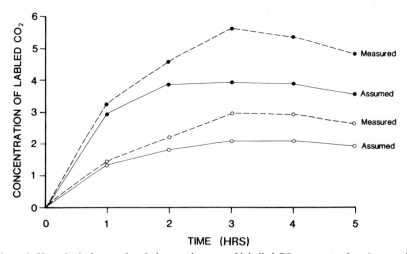

Figure 3. Hypothetical normal and abnormal curves of labelled CO_2 concentration, 'assumed' curves derived by dilution to the same degree as endogenous CO_2 is increased by a 750 kcal meal (Figure 2). Closer approximation of the 'assumed' curves than the 'measured' curves leads to more overlap of normal and abnormal ranges when endogenous CO_2 changes are not accounted for in data computation. From King and Toskes (1981), with kind permission of the editor of *Journal of Nuclear Medicine*.

interval sampling. As noted in Table 1, both types (radio- and stable-isotopic) require control and/or calculation of total CO_2 changes occurring as a result of metabolism changes (fever, exercise) or from ingestion of substantial calories. The stable isotopic ($^{13}CO_2$) tests require, in addition, control for labelled CO_2 production occurring as a result of ^{13}C content of substances ingested before or as part of the test.

Table 1. *Requirements of isotopic CO_2 breath tests*

General
Performance in afebrile, rested setting
Measurement of total CO_2 (in addition to labelled CO_2) if substantial (>100 kcal) calories
   administered

$^{14}CO_2$ *tests*
No excessive tissue retention

$^{13}CO_2$ *tests*
Avoid change in $^{13}CO_2$ breath excretion due to carrier meal ^{13}C content

SPECIFIC USES OF BREATH ANALYSIS

Intraluminal bacterial overgrowth

Small intestine bacterial overgrowth is the setting where altered killing or movement of bacteria in the small bowel leads to a marked increase of the usual sparse small bowel flora and which is accompanied by secondary nutrient malabsorption and/or diarrhoea (King and Toskes, 1979). Usual identification is by jejunal intubation and microbiological analysis of intestinal aspirates (looking for 10^6 or more organisms/ml, especially when containing the usually absent coliforms and anaerobes). Use of breath analysis to simplify identification of this setting has been evaluated with several different tests. A critical point in determining the utility of a breath test for bacterial overgrowth is how clearly one can distinguish between the normal, luxuriant (even in the setting of bacterial overgrowth) small bowel flora. As indicated in Table 1, desirable characteristics of a substrate for a bacterial overgrowth breath test affords improved distinction by means of one or more of several techniques: (a) maximizing contact of small bowel bacteria with the test probe, (b) minimizing contact of colonic bacteria with the test probe (e.g., using a test probe which is completely absorbed before the colon is reached), and (c) analysing time periods when the test probe is predominantly in the small intestine. Since no tissue production of H_2 occurs, an ideal H_2 breath test probe will require only avid bacterial catabolism and avid small bowel absorption, whereas an isotopic CO_2 probe requires, in addition, minimal host tissue metabolism.

Bile acid breath test

Following studies by Hofmann and co-workers regarding the deconjugation of bile salts, primarily by anaerobic bacteria, the ^{14}C-bile acid breath test was developed as a clinical aid in detecting bacterial contact with an orally administered labelled conjugated bile salt (cholyl-1-^{14}C-glycine) (Fromm and Hofmann, 1971; Sherr et al, 1971). Test procedure generally involves co-administration of a carrier meal to stimulate output of endogenous bile salts from the biliary tree. Breath analysis has been generally carried out hourly for six to eight hours. Patients with small intestine bacterial overgrowth and/or ileal malabsorption of bile salts have been shown by several other laboratories to have abnormal breath excretion of $^{14}CO_2$ (James, Agnew and Bouchier, 1973; Pedersen, Arnfred and Hess Thaysen, 1973; Scarpello and Sladen, 1977). In addition, a $^{13}CO_2$ bile acid breath test has been devised as a non-radioactive alternative (Solomons et al, 1977). By itself, it is difficult to use the bile acid breath test to distinguish whether abnormal labelled CO_2 excretion represents bacterial deconjugation in the small intestine or large intestine (i.e., bacterial overgrowth or ileal malabsorption of the test probe). Concomitant faecal ^{14}C testing can make the test more specific but strays from the aesthetic character of breath testing alone (Pedersen, Arnfred and Hess Thaysen, 1973; Scarpello and Sladen, 1977). We and others have noted that even normal subjects have a substantial (approximately fourfold) contribution of the colonic flora to catabolism of orally ingested labelled bile salt (James, Agnew and Bouchier, 1973; King et al, 1980a). With respect to detecting bacterial overgrowth of the small intestine this is a 'dirty' background which may diminish diagnostic sensitivity of the test. In fact, our evaluation of the bile acid breath test, as well as that of others, has shown that 30 to 35 per cent of patients with culture-proven overgrowth will have a normal test (Lauterburg, Newcomer and Hofmann, 1978; King et al, 1980a). A recent study had an even higher (60 per cent) false-negative rate (Watson et al, 1980). In our study of this test, even analysing more frequently during the first two hours of the test (a period during which one looks more specifically at small intestinal events) failed to avoid the 30 per cent false-negative rate of the bile acid breath test in detecting bacterial overgrowth. It is possible that the bile acid breath test, when combined with a sensitive test to rule out bacterial overgrowth, may have high sensitivity and specificity in detecting bile acid malabsorption, without resorting to faecal analysis.

One-gram xylose breath test

For the past four years we have employed the xylose (1 g, 10 μCi) breath test for the detection of bacterial overgrowth within the small intestine. Indeed, this breath test has become the primary test for the diagnosis of bacterial overgrowth at our medical centre. Our continuing experience has demonstrated this test to be as sensitive and specific as we originally suggested (King et al, 1979). This clinical breath test resulted from our work with the experimental rat blind loop syndrome, which demonstrated that the decreased urinary xylose excretion in this condition could be accounted for by the amount of $^{14}CO_2$ in the breath following the oral administration of ^{14}C-xylose, indicating catabolism of xylose to CO_2 by the overgrowth flora (Toskes et al, 1978).

Abnormally elevated breath $^{14}CO_2$ levels occur within the first 60 minutes in 85 per cent of the patients (in 53 per cent by the first determination at 30 minutes). In 15 per cent of patients who may have delayed gastric emptying (e.g., scleroderma, Crohn's disease) a diagnostic elevation in breath $^{14}CO_2$ may not be apparent until 180 minutes. Antibiotic therapy greatly reduces the breath $^{14}CO_2$ excretion towards normal. In patients with malabsorption not due to bacterial overgrowth, the ^{14}C-xylose breath test is not abnormal.

The sensitivity of the ^{14}C-xylose breath test has been compared to that of the cholyl-1-^{14}C-glycine breath test (King et al, 1980a) (Figures 4 and 5). In 12 patients with culture-proven overgrowth of the small intestine, the xylose

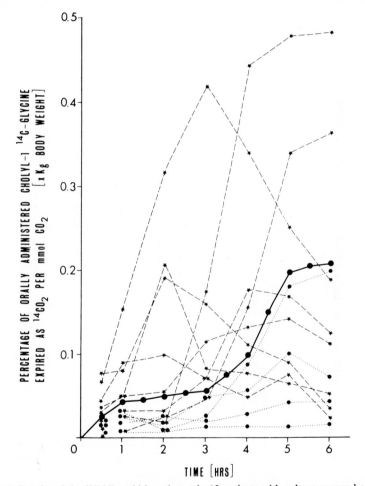

Figure 4. Results of the ^{14}C-bile acid breath test in 12 patients with culture-proven bacterial overgrowth. The upper limit of normal (95 per cent confidence range) breath $^{14}CO_2$ concentration is represented by the heavy line, showing a fourfold rise (colonic passage of substrate) after the third hour. Four of the twelve patients have no abnormal point (false-negative result). From King et al (1980a), with kind permission of the authors and the editor of *Digestive Diseases and Sciences*.

breath test was abnormal in all, but the bile acid breath test was abnormal in only eight of 12 patients. Thus, 33 per cent of these patients with bacterial overgrowth were not diagnosed by the bile and breath tests — a finding confirmed by other investigators (Lauterburg, Newcomer and Hofmann, 1978; Metz et al, 1976c). Two of the four patients in whom the bile acid breath test failed to detect bacterial overgrowth had marked malabsorption of cobalamin, xylose, and fat.

Very recently we evaluated the clinical utility of the xylose breath test after it had been made readily available to the clinicians at our medical

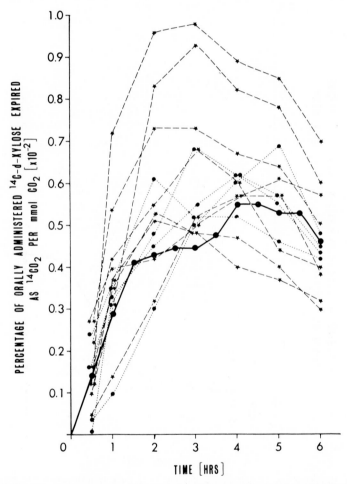

Figure 5. Results of the one-gram ^{14}C-xylose breath test in 12 patients with culture-proven bacterial overgrowth. Normal range (heavy line) shows minimal late rise secondary to colonic passage of substrate. In contrast to bile acid breath test, all twelve patients have abnormal xylose breath tests. From King et al (1980a), with kind permission of the authors and the editor of *Digestive Diseases and Sciences*.

centre (Tillman, King and Toskes, 1981). Over a 15-month period of assessment the xylose breath test was performed in 63 patients. In 38 patients strongly suspected of having malabsorption secondary to bacterial overgrowth, various clinicians ordered both the xylose breath test and an intestinal culture, thus subjecting the xylose breath test to their own 'test'. A number of patients received multiple breath tests and multiple cultures. The findings were remarkable: (a) the xylose breath test had a reproducibility of 92 per cent, the intestinal culture a reproducibility of only 38 per cent, and (b) although it was common to have a positive xylose breath test and a negative culture, multiple repeat cultures in the setting of a positive xylose breath test were likely to yield at least one positive culture. This study demonstrated the intestinal culture to have a high false-negative value, while false-negative values were rare with the xylose breath test.

In the same study four patients with clinically significant overgrowth and positive xylose breath tests had three intestinal cultures taken prospectively from the same intubation, with aspirates taken 10 cm apart beginning at the ligament of Treitz and going distally. In two the culture results were consistent. In the other two positive cultures were obtained in only one of the three sites. The intestinal culture being positive is dependent upon a random aspirate being from an area of pathological overgrowth, whereas a positive xylose breath test reflects total intraluminal catabolism of xylose by the flora. Thus, bacterial overgrowth is non-confluent in the small bowel and apt to be missed by an intestinal culture obtained from only one location.

Thus, the intestinal culture, which traditionally has been the gold standard for the diagnosis of bacterial overgrowth, must be reassessed in light of these findings. In our extensive referral practice for patients with bacterial overgrowth, we continue to see patients with malabsorption who have a positive xylose breath test, a negative intestinal culture, and reversal of their malabsorption following antimicrobial therapy — lending further support to our reliance upon the ^{14}C-xylose breath test as our primary means of detecting bacterial overgrowth.

Why does the xylose breath test given such fine results? Several reasons are apparent: (a) xylose is absorbed primarily in the proximal bowel and very little reaches the colonic bacteria, thus avoiding the problem of false-positive results, (b) xylose is catabolized by gram-negative aerobes whereas a positive bile acid breath test usually depends on the presence of anaerobes which may or may not be present in the overgrowth flora, and (c) the 1 g of xylose employed does not increase the endogenous CO_2 output, as may be seen with the bile acid breath test, and lead to false-negative results, particularly if a constant endogenous CO_2 production is assumed (King and Toskes, 1981). Thus, the ^{14}C xylose breath test is close to the ideal breath test for diagnosing bacterial overgrowth, as detailed in Table 2.

Glucose-H$_2$ breath test

Since glucose is so avidly absorbed in the small intestine, it can serve as an excellent probe for an abnormal small bowel flora while avoiding catabolism of the test substrate by the colonic flora. In addition, analysis of

Table 2. *Characteristics of the ideal substrate for a breath test to detect small intestine bacterial overgrowth*

1. Avid catabolism by bacteria
2. Avid absorption in the small intestine to minimize contact with luxuriant colonic flora
3. No production of gas as a result of host tissue metabolism
4. Unlimited safety
5. Substrate inexpensive and/or easily produced

H_2 as the marker of glucose catabolism makes it a specific test for bacterial overgrowth (since H_2 is not produced as a result of tissue metabolism of glucose). It has been demonstrated that a 50 g glucose-H_2 breath test will be abnormal in approximately two-thirds of subjects with bacterial overgrowth (Metz et al, 1976c). We are currently evaluating if a higher dose of glucose (80 g) can increase sensitivity of the test (by increasing contact of substrate with the small bowel flora) while avoiding non-specific colonic bacterial contact with the substrate.

Lactulose-H_2 breath test

One laboratory has used a 10 g lactulose-H_2 breath test in nine subjects with bacterial overgrowth, finding abnormal H_2 excretion in eight of them (Rhodes, Middleton and Jewell, 1979). All subjects had H_2 production due to colonic flora (at the time of arrival of the non-absorbed lactulose to the colonic flora). Rhodes et al claimed that there was no difficulty in distinguishing catabolism of the substrate in the small intestine from that in the colon. Because we have experienced difficulty in distinguishing the small bowel and colonic 'humps' in many subjects during evaluation of a high-dose (25 g) xylose and the bile acid breath tests (both of which had substantial passage of test probe to the colonic flora) (King et al, 1979; King et al, 1980b) we must reserve enthusiasm for the lactulose-H_2 breath test for bacterial overgrowth until studies confirming the ability to make this separation are made. This reservation regarding specificity of the lactulose-H_2 breath test is reflected in Table 3, which gives an overview of techniques for diagnosing bacterial overgrowth.

Potential future directions

Search for an optimum agent and dose for an H_2 breath test for bacterial overgrowth continues. Even an optimum test may not reach the sensitivity

Table 3. *Tests for small intestine bacterial overgrowth*

	Simplicity	Sensitivity	Specificity	Safety
Culture	Poor	Good	Excellent	Good
Breath tests:				
^{14}C-xylose	Excellent	>95%	Excellent	Good
^{14}C-bile acid	Excellent	Approx. 70%	Poor	Good
glucose-H_2	Excellent	Approx. 70%	Unknown	Excellent
lactulose-H_2	Excellent	Unknown	Poor—good	Excellent

of the one-gram ^{14}C-xylose breath test. This is because detection of catabolism of ^{14}C-labelled substances is more sensitive than that of H_2 generation, and to increase the H_2 'signal' so much substrate may be required that non-specific colonic bacterial fermentation may become a problem. The alternative approach to development of a non-radioactive breath test lies with the potential development of a [13]CO_2 breath test such as, but more specific than, the previously described ^{13}C-bile acid breath test (Solomons et al, 1977). Two potential candidates for this approach are ^{13}C-xylose and ^{13}C-taurine. We have shown in the experimental blind loop syndrome that taurine is potentially an excellent probe for bacterial overgrowth (King, Lorenz and Toskes, 1976), since no catabolism of the substance occurs in mammalian tissue (Sturman et al, 1975).

BREATH ANALYSIS AS AN ABSORPTIVE TEST

Analysis of absorption from the gastrointestinal tract is frequently a time-consuming procedure that may, in addition, require unaesthetic techniques such as intestinal perfusion or quantitative stool analysis. Even the 'aesthetic' absorptive studies (urinary xylose test and Schilling test) require patient cooperation and technician handling of urine specimens. Breath analysis has been used to analyse the intestinal absorption of several substances, aesthetically allowing rapid analysis of absorptive events. The absorptive breath tests have analysed either the part of the test meal that was not absorbed (e.g., H_2 breath test analysing malabsorption of carbohydrate, isotopic CO_2-bile acid breath test) or have evaluated that part of the meal which was absorbed and metabolized (e.g., isotopic CO_2 test for fat absorption).

Carbohydrate-H_2 Absorption Tests

Lactose malabsorption

Perhaps the most widely used breath test in gastroenterology is the hydrogen breath test employed to detect lactose malabsorption (Newcomer et al, 1975). In this group's evaluation of 25 subjects with decreased intestinal brush border lactase levels and 25 normal controls subjects with normal lactase levels, they noted that the 50 g H_2-lactose breath test was the most sensitive non-invasive test for lactose tolerance, this test having been compared to a ^{14}C-lactose breath test and to the blood lactose tolerance test. Several groups have since demonstrated the utility of the H_2-lactose breath test, including modifications using more physiological (and less symptom-producing) doses of lactose administered as either free lactose or lactose administered as milk (Metz et al, 1975; Bayless and Paige, 1979; MacLean and Fink, 1980; Solomons, Garcia-Ibanez and Viteri, 1980; Barr, Watkins and Perman, 1981). This test has been used in epidemiological field evaluations of lactose or milk intolerance in both the evaluation of the utility of lactase-treated milk as a nutritional source for lactase-deficient subjects and in the evaluation of paediatric subjects with diarrhoea of obscure aetiology. This test can be used to quantify the level of lactose ingestion that can be tolerated by individuals with partial lactase deficiency. This is important in nutritional management of subjects recovering from intestinal disease and/or protein-caloric malnutrition, which can lead to variable levels of lactose tolerance during the illness and recovery period.

Indeed, in respect to quantifying the amount of lactose tolerance, Bayless and Paige (1979) recently demonstrated that by using an H_2-lactose breath test it was possible to predict which patients with lactose malabsorption were unable to adequately digest the lactose in 240 ml (one glass) of milk. The blood lactose tolerance test was not able to distinguish those patients with lactose malabsorption who could or could not digest the 11 g of lactose in a glass of milk. Thus, this study appropriately emphasized that there is a great deal of variation in the amount of lactose tolerated among lactose malabsorbers, which can be predicted by the H_2-lactose breath test. Another recent study (Barr, Watkins and Perman, 1981) emphasized the H_2 lactose test as a better test of lactose tolerance than the so-called direct assessment by small bowel biopsy, since the breath test measures overall functional lactose tolerance in vivo, whereas the biopsy measures lactase activity at only one particular location.

Sucrose-isomaltose malabsorption

Excessive H_2 excretion in the breath has been consistently seen with a sucrose-H_2 breath test in subjects with congenital sucrase-isomaltase deficiency. Although this test has been shown to detect severe deficiency of sucrase, less consistency has been seen with acquired deficiency or where marginal enzyme levels are present (Metz et al, 1976b; Perman, Barr and Watkins, 1978; Douwes, Fernandes and Jongbloed, 1980). Part of the inconsistent results with acquired sucrase deficiency are related to the higher normal levels and less superficial placement (towards the lumen) of sucrase, as contrasted to lactase, in the brush border of the enterocyte. In terms of practical use of breath analysis, evaluation for possible disaccharidase deficiency as a cause for diarrhoea should probably start with a lactose-H_2 breath test, with a dose of 1.5-2.0 g/kg body weight up to a maximum of 50 g (although a 25 g maximum dose will probably give only slightly less sensitivity with a marked decrease in test-related side effects). If the results of the lactose-H_2 breath test are unclear, and if the absence of an H_2-producing flora is ruled out by performance of a lactulose-H_2 control (Metz, Blendis and Jenkins, 1976), performance of a sucrose-H_2 breath test would be reasonable to check for congenital sucrase-isomaltase deficiency.

Monosaccharide malabsorption

An attempt to use a 25 g xylose-H_2 breath test to aid in the evaluation of tropical malabsorption has been reported (Cook, 1980). Results of this test have been less than satisfactory, in part due to the generation of H_2 from the substrate in a substantial percentage of normal subjects. Because xylose is not absorbed as avidly as glucose in the small intestine, it is not an optimal test probe for this type of analysis (Levitt and Donaldson, 1970).

Although reports of H_2-glucose breath testing as a means of detecting primary monosaccharide malabsorption are scant in the literature, a graded dosing of glucose with breath H_2 monitoring would appear to be an excellent way of determining both the presence of congenital or acquired absorptive deficiency and also the degree of glucose that can be absorbed (as a nutritional guide). It is noted that one report of glucose-H_2 testing in a patient with primary monosaccharide malabsorption demonstrated negative results with glucose but positive production of H_2 with lactulose (Gardiner et al, 1981b). These results may relate to pH-sensitive generation of H_2 by the flora (Perman, Modler and Olsen, 1981), which at a given pH may be more notable with one substrate than another.

Fat Absorption Breath Tests

Breath analysis for $^{14}CO_2$ following the administration of ^{14}C-labelled triglyceride was one of the earliest proposed uses for both continuous (Schwabe et al, 1962) and interval sampling (Abt and von Schuching, 1966; Kaihara and Wagner, 1968) isotopic CO_2 breath testing. Despite this long availability and support from other laboratories regarding the utility of long-chain triglyceride CO_2 breath analysis (Bhatia et al, 1969; Burrows et al, 1974; Chen et al, 1974), this test was not used widely, probably because of concern over deposition of ^{14}C in slowly-metabolized fat pools and because of a degree of overlap of breath test results or normal and abnormal patients in some of the studies (Kaihara and Wagner, 1968; Burrows et al, 1974). The report from the Mayo Clinic (Newcomer et al, 1979) rejuvenated interest in this test, partly because potential relationship to non-radioactive $^{13}CO_2$ tests was by then more of a tangible entity and partly because their test results were so good. In this study the investigators compared three different labelled triglyceride breath tests (^{14}C-triolein, ^{14}C-tripalmitin and ^{14}C-trioctanoin) to serum carotene levels and qualitative and quantitative stool fat examinations. The labelled triolein breath test in their patient population had a sensitivity (100 per cent) that rivalled the less aesthetic 'gold standard' quantitative stool fat examination while attaining 96 per cent specificity. In their study, the qualitative stool fat examination attained an excellent sensitivity of 92 per cent and a specificity of 96 per cent, but required dietary preparation for several days; the serum carotene had a sensitivity of only a 64 per cent. Since ^{14}C-triolein gave better results than the other two breath tests (because of a 58 per cent and 69 per cent false-positive result with ^{14}C-tripalmitin and ^{14}C-trioctanoin, respectively), it seemed that problems with lack of sensitivity and specificity with the labelled triglyceride absorption CO_2 breath test were now solved. Unfortunately, our recent study of the ^{14}C-triolein breath test, using the same 20 g fat carrier meal and 5 μCi dose of ^{14}C-triolein, has shown such a high degree of overlap of patients with normal and abnormal 72 hour stool fat studies that the breath test, as performed, had no discriminatory value as a diagnostic tool (King, Snook and Toskes, 1982). In our study, no diagnostic parameter (peak $^{14}CO_2$ concentration, cumulative 6 hour or 8 hour $^{14}CO_2$, or any hourly rate) was found which would distinguish normal (defined by the 72 hour faecal fat excretion) from abnormal fat absorption. No selection of patients was made for entry. This factor is important because the high degree of sensitivity and specificity of the Mayo Clinic study may have been related to exclusion of patients with diabetes mellitus, thyroid disease, hyperlipidaemia and liver disease (Pedersen, 1980; Strange et al, 1980). Other recent reports of the ^{14}C-tripalmitin breath test (some including concomitant oral ^{14}C-palmitic acid studies as a means to distinguish problems of malabsorption from maldigestion) have given discouraging (Caspary, 1978; Levy-Gigi et al, 1978) or encouraging (Mills, Horton and Watkinson, 1979; Meeker et al, 1980) results. In addition, a very encouraging report regarding ^{13}C-labelled triolein and palmitic acid as a means to diagnose and differentiate fat malabsorption in children has recently been published (Watkins et al, 1982).

What then is the place of isotopic CO_2 breath testing in the evaluation of fat absorption? Although the full answer to this question is not at hand, a survey of the studies already performed reveals some guiding points. One is that many of the encouraging studies have used a high level of carrier fat, in the range of 0.75-1.0 g fat/kg body weight (Kaihara and Wagner, 1968; Bhatia et al, 1969; Watkins et al, 1982). Perhaps this greater stress on the absorptive capacity allows a better separation of normal from abnormal subjects. If high-calorie, high-fat carrier meals are to be used, accounting for changes in endogenous CO_2 production will undoubtedly be necessary for optimum reliability and sensitivity (King and Toskes, 1981). In addition to accounting for changes in endogenous CO_2 production (by measuring CO_2 production rates during the test, rather than assuming a constant CO_2 production of 9 mmol/kg.h) it may be necessary to also normalize for differences in fatty acid metabolism. For example, one could make intravenous fatty acid CO_2 testing a tandem or concomitant (if both ^{14}C and ^{13}C labels are used) part of the test. This use of fatty acid isotopic CO_2 testing would be more important than the current use of oral fatty acid CO_2 tests, which supply information which can be obtained from other mucosal tests. Finally, even in studies in which discrimination between normal and abnormal groups was difficult, the response of one individual's breath test result after therapy has been clearly different from the same subject's pretherapy test result (Chen et al, 1974; Goff, 1982; King, Snook and Toskes, 1982). Thus, the isotopic CO_2 fat absorption breath test has a future, but needs better validation, modification, and definition of where it fits into the evaluation of patients.

SAFETY OF ^{14}C BREATH TESTS

Because of the long physical half-life of ^{14}C there has been a fear, although probably unwarranted, stifling the use of ^{14}C-labelled breath tests. This occurred despite the calculations that the administration of 10 μCi ^{14}C-glycine would lead to a 400 day integrated radiation dose of 15 mrad (as contrasted to the 1200 mrad cosmic radiation dose) (Tolbert and Cozetto, 1964). In an attempt to allay anxiety about use of the ^{14}C-radioisotopes for human breath tests, we have performed dosimetry studies with ^{14}C-xylose and cholyl-1-^{14}C-glycine (substrates for the xylose and bile salt breath tests) (King et al, 1980b) and with ^{14}C-triolein (King et al, 1982). In all these studies maximum gonadal dosimetry ranged between 10 and 17 mrad. We thus feel very comfortable with use of these substrates in adult humans, since radiation exposure is less than that received with common procedures such as a plain gastrointestinal or chest x-ray, and certainly much less than that with barium contrast intestinal radiography or abdominal computed tomography.

SUMMARY

Breath analysis has evolved into a technique that can support nicely the evaluation of patients with diarrhoea and/or weight loss and in whom nutrient malabsorption is a possibility. The lactose and sucrose breath hydrogen tests offer direct (and probably the most sensitive) documentation of the malabsorption of carbohydrate and are currently widely used for clinical analysis. The ^{14}C-xylose breath test is the most sensitive and specific breath test for detecting bacterial overgrowth; it may be used in combination with the labelled bile acid breath test to make the latter a sensitive and specific test for ileal malabsorption of bile salts. The labelled fat breath test has promise in aiding the detection and/or cause of fat malabsorption, but requires modification for optimum sensitivity and utility in quantifying the level of fat absorption.

ACKNOWLEDGEMENT

The authors acknowledge the expert secretarial assistance of Frances T. Tucker.

REFERENCES

Abt, A. F. & von Schuching, S. L. (1966) Fat utilization test in disorders of fat metabolism. *Bulletin of the Johns Hopkins Hospital,* 119, 316-330.

Barr, R. G., Watkins, J. B. & Perman, J. A. (1981) Mucosal function and breath hydrogen excretion: comparative studies in the clinical evaluation of children with nonspecific abdominal complaints. *Pediatrics,* 68, 526-533.

Bartlett, K., Dobson, J. V. & Eastham, H. (1980) A new method for the detection of hydrogen in breath and its application to acquired and inborn sugar malabsorption. *Clinica Chimica Acta,* 108, 189-194.

Bayless, T. M. & Paige, D. M. (1979) Consequences of lactose malabsorption: breath hydrogen excretion after milk ingestion. *Gastroenterology,* 76, 1097.

Bhatia, S. K., Bell, T. K., Love, A. H. & Montgomery, D. A. D. (1969) An evaluation of a test using ^{14}C-labelled triglyceride in the diagnosis of steatorrhoea. *Irish Journal of Medical Science,* 2, 545-552.

Bond, J. H. & Levitt, M. D. (1972) Use of pulmonary hydrogen (H_2) measurements to quantitate carbohydrate absorption: study of partially gastrectomized patients. *Journal of Clinical Investigation,* 51, 1219-1225.

Bond, J. H. & Levitt, M. D. (1975) Investigation of small bowel transit time in man utilizing pulmonary hydrogen (H_2) measurements. *Journal of Laboratory and Clinical Medicine,* 85, 546-555.

Burrows, P. J., Fleming, J. S., Garnett, E. S. et al (1974) Clinical evaluation of the ^{14}C fat absorption test. *Gut,* 15, 147-150.

Caspary, W. F. (1978) Breath tests. *Clinics in Gastroenterology,* 7, 351-374.

Chen, I. W., Azmudeh, K., Connell, A. M. & Saenger, F. L. (1974) ^{14}C-tripalmitin breath test as a diagnostic aid for fat malabsorption due to pancreatic insufficiency. *Journal of Nuclear Medicine,* 15, 1125-1129.

Christman, N. T. & Hamilton, L. H. (1982) A new chromatographic instrument for measuring trace concentrations of breath hydrogen. *Journal of Chromatography,* **229,** 259-265.

Cook, G. C. (1980) Breath hydrogen after oral xylose in tropical malabsorption. *American Journal of Clinical Nutrition,* **33,** 555-560.

Corbett, C. L., Thomas, S., Read, N. W. et al (1981) Electrochemical detector for breath hydrogen determination: measurements of small bowel transit time in normal subjects and patients with the irritable bowel syndrome. *Gut,* **22,** 836-840.

Douwes, A. C., Fernandes, J. & Jongbloed, A. A. (1980) Diagnostic value of sucrose tolerance test in children evaluated by breath hydrogen measurement. *Acta Paediatrica Scandinavica,* **69,** 79-82.

Fromm, H. & Hofmann, A. F. (1971) Breath test for altered bile-acid metabolism. *Lancet,* **ii,** 621-625.

Gardiner, A. J., Tarlow, M. J., Sutherland, I. T. & Sammons, H. G. (1981a) Collection of breath for hydrogen estimation. *Archives of Disease in Childhood,* **56,** 125-127.

Gardiner, A. J., Tarlow, M. J., Symonds, J. et al (1981b) Failure of the hydrogen breath test to detect primary sugar malabsorption. *Archives of Disease in Childhood,* **56,** 368-372.

Gilat, T., Ben Hur, H., Gelman-Malachi, E. et al (1978) Alterations of the colonic flora and their effect on the hydrogen breath test. *Gut,* **19,** 602-605.

Goff, J. S. (1982) Two-stage triolein breath test differentiates pancreatic insufficiency from other causes of malabsorption. *Gastroenterology,* **83,** 44-46.

Hirano, S., Kanamatsu, T., Takagi, Y. & Abei, T. (1979) A simple infrared spectroscopic method for the measurement of expired $^{13}CO_2$. *Analytical Biochemistry,* **96,** 64-69.

James, O. F. W., Agnew, J. E. & Bouchier, I. A. D. (1973) Assessment of the ^{14}C-glycocholic acid breath test. *British Medical Journal,* **iii,** 191-195.

Kaihara, S. & Wagner, H. N. (1968) Measurement of intestinal fat absorption with carbon-14 labelled tracers. *Journal of Laboratory and Clinical Medicine,* **71,** 400-411.

King, C. E. & Toskes, P. P. (1979) Small intestine bacterial overgrowth. *Gastroenterology,* **76,** 1035-1055.

King, C. E. & Toskes, P. P. (1981) Alteration of CO_2 production during non-fasting isotopic CO_2 breath tests. *Journal of Nuclear Medicine,* **22,** 955-958.

King, C. E., Lorenz, E. & Toskes, P. P. (1976) The pathogenesis of decreased serum protein levels in the blind loop syndrome: evaluation including a newly developed ^{14}C-amino acid breath test. *Gastroenterology,* **70,** 43.

King, C. E., Snook, L. B. & Toskes, P. P. (1981) The ^{14}C-triolein breath test: is it ready for clinical use in its present form? *Gastroenterology,* **82,** 1100.

King, C. E., Toskes, P. P., Spivey, J. C. et al (1979) Detection of small intestine bacterial overgrowth by means of a ^{14}C-D-xylose breath test. *Gastroenterology,* **77,** 75-82.

King, C. E., Toskes, P. P., Guilarte, T. R. et al (1980a) Comparison of the one gram D-[^{14}C] xylose breath test to the [^{14}C] bile acid breath test in patients with small intestinal bacterial overgrowth. *Digestive Diseases and Sciences,* **25,** 53-58.

King, C. E., Toskes, P. P., Guilarte, T. R. et al (1980b) Safety of the ^{14}C-D-xyloze and ^{14}C-cholylglycine (bile acid) breath tests: elimination and tissue retention studies. *Clinical Research,* **28,** 483A.

King, C. E., Snook, L. B., Toskes, P. P. et al (1982) Safety of $^{14}CO_2$ breath tests: dosimetry evaluation of ^{14}C-triolein. *Gastroenterology,* **82,** 1100.

Lauterburg, B. H., Newcomer, A. D. & Hofmann, A. F. (1978) Clinical value of the bile acid breath test: evaluation of the Mayo Clinic experience. *Mayo Clinic Proceedings,* **53,** 227-233.

Levitt, M. D. (1969) Production and excretion of hydrogen gas in man. *New England Journal of Medicine,* **281,** 122-127.

Levitt, M. D. & Donaldson, R. M. (1970) Use of respiratory hydrogen (H_2) excretion to detect carbohydrate malabsorption. *Journal of Laboratory and Clinical Medicine,* **75,** 937-945.

Levy-Gigi, C., Mandelowitz, N., Peled, Y. & Gilat, T. (1978) Is the fat breath test effective in the diagnosis of fat malabsorption and pancreatic disease? *Digestion,* **18,** 77-85.

Lorenz, E., Brookeman, V. A. & Mauderli, W. (1978) Plastic scintillation filament detector system for $^{14}CO_2$ breath analysis tests. *Medical Physics,* **5,** 195-198.

MacLean, W. C. & Fink, B. B. (1980) Lactose malabsorption by premature infants: magnitude and clinical significance. *Journal of Pediatrics,* **97,** 383-388.

Meeker, H. E., Chen, I. W., Connell, A. M. & Saenger, E. L. (1980) Clinical experiences in ^{14}C-tripalmitin breath test for fat malabsorption. *American Journal of Gastroenterology,* **73,** 227-231.

Metz, G., Blendis, L. M. & Jenkins, D. J. A. (1976) H$_2$ breath test for lactase deficiency. *New England Journal of Medicine,* **294,** 730.

Metz, G., Jenkins, D. J. A., Peters, T. J. et al (1975) Breath hydrogen as a diagnostic method for hypolactasia. *Lancet,* **i,** 1155-1157.

Metz, G., Gassull, M. A., Leeds, A. R. et al (1976a) A simple method of measuring breath hydrogen in carbohydrate malabsorption by end-expiratory sampling. *Clinical Science and Molecular Medicine,* **50,** 237-240.

Metz, G., Jenkins, D. J. A., Newman, A. & Blendis, L. M. (1976b) Breath hydrogen in hyposucrasia. *Lancet,* **i,** 119-120.

Metz, G., Gassull, M. A., Drasar, B. S. et al (1976c) Breath hydrogen test for small-intestinal bacterial colonisation. *Lancet,* **i,** 668-669.

Mills, P. R., Horton, P. W. & Watkinson, G. (1979) Breath tests for the detection of fat malabsorption. *Scottish Medical Journal,* **24,** 324-325.

Newcomer, A. D., McGill, D. B., Thomas, P. J. & Hofmann, A. F. (1975) Prospective comparison of indirect methods for detecting lactase deficiency. *New England Journal of Medicine,* **293,** 1232-1236.

Newcomer, A. D., Hofmann, A. F., DiMagno, E. P. et al (1979) Triolein breath test: a sensitive and specific test for fat malabsorption. *Gastroenterology,* **76,** 6-13.

Niu, H., Schoeller, D. A. & Klein, P. D. (1979) Improved gas chromatographic quantitation of breath hydrogen by normalization to respiratory carbon dioxide. *Journal of Laboratory and Clinical Medicine,* **94,** 755-763.

Pedersen, N. T. (1980) Triolein breath test. *Gastroenterology,* **78,** 422-423.

Pedersen, L., Arnfred, T. & Hess Thaysen, E. (1973) Rapid screening of increased bile acid deconjugation and bile acid malabsorption by means of the glycine-1-[^{14}C] cholylglycine assay. *Scandinavian Journal of Gastroenterology,* **8,** 665-672.

Perman, J. A., Barr, R. G. & Watkins, J. B. (1978) Sucrose malabsorption in children: non-invasive diagnosis by interval breath hydrogen determination. *Journal of Pediatrics,* **93,** 17-22.

Perman, J. A., Modler, S. & Olson, A. C. (1981) Role of pH in production of hydrogen from carbohydrates by colonic bacterial flora. *Journal of Clinical Investigation,* **67,** 643-650.

Ravich, W. J., Bayless, T. M. & Thomas, M. (1983) Fructose: imcomplete intestinal absorption in man. *Gastroenterology,* **84,** 26-29.

Rhodes, J. M., Middleton, P. & Jewell, D. P. (1979) The lactulose hydrogen breath test as a diagnostic test for small-bowel bacterial overgrowth. *Scandinavian Journal of Gastroenterology,* **14,** 333-336.

Robb, T. A. & Davidson, G. P. (1981) Advances in breath hydrogen quantitation in paediatrics: sample collection and normalization to constant oxygen and nitrogen levels. *Clinica Chimica Acta,* **111,** 281-285.

Scarpello, J. H. B. & Sladen, G. E. (1977) Appraisal of the ^{14}C-glycocholate acid test with special reference to the measurement of faecal ^{14}C excretion. *Gut,* **18,** 742-748.

Schoeller, D. A. & Klein, P. D. (1978) A simplified technique for collecting breath CO$_2$ for isotope ratio mass spectrometry. *Biomedical Mass Spectrometry,* **5,** 29-31.

Schoeller, D. A., Schneider, J. F., Solomons, N. W. et al (1977) Clinical diagnosis with the stable isotope ^{13}C in CO$_2$ breath tests: methodology and fundamental considerations. *Journal of Laboratory and Clinical Medicine,* **90,** 412-421.

Schoeller, D. A., Klein, P. D., Watkins, J. B. et al (1980) ^{13}C abundances of nutrients and the effect of variations in ^{13}C isotopic abundances of test meals formulated for ^{13}CO$_2$ breath tests. *American Journal of Clinical Nutrition,* **33,** 2375-2385.

Schwabe, A. D. & Hepner, G. W. (1979) Breath tests for the detection of fat malabsorption. *Gastroenterology,* **72,** 216-218.

Schwabe, A. D., Cozzetto, F. J., Bennett, L. R. & Mellinkoff, S. M. (1962) Estimation of fat absorption by monitoring of expired radioactive cabon dioxide after feeding a radioactive fat. *Gastroenterology,* **42,** 285-291.

Sherr, H. P., Sasaki, Y., Newman, A. et al (1971) Detection of bacterial deconjugation of bile salts by a convenient breath analysis technic. *New England Journal of Medicine,* **285,** 656-661.

Slanger, B. H., Kusubov, N. & Winchell, H. S. (1970) Effect of exercise on human CO_2-HCO_3 kinetics. *Journal of Nuclear Medicine,* **11,** 716-718.

Solomons, N. W., Viteri, F. E. & Hamilton, L. H. (1977) Application of a simple gas chromatographic technique for measuring breath hydrogen. *Journal of Laboratory and Clinical Medicine,* **90,** 956-962.

Solomons, N. W., Viteri, F. & Rosenberg, I. H. (1978) Development of an interval sampling hydrogen (H_2) breath test for carbohydrate malabsorption in children: evidence for a circadian pattern of breath H_2 concentration. *Pediatric Research,* **12,** 816-823.

Solomons, N. W., Garcia-Ibanez, R. & Viteri, F. E. (1980) Hydrogen breath test of lactose absorption in adults: the application of physiological doses and whole cow's milk sources. *American Journal of Clinical Nutrition,* **33,** 545-554.

Solomons, N. W., Garcia, R., Schneider, R. et al (1979) H_2 breath tests during diarrhoea. *Acta Paediatrica Scandinavica,* **168,** 171-172.

Solomons, N. W., Schoeller, D. A., Wagonfeld, J. B. et al (1977) Application of a stable isotope (^{13}C)-labelled glycocholate breath test to diagnosis of bacterial overgrowth and ileal dysfunction. *Journal of Laboratory and Clinical Medicine,* **90,** 431-439.

Strange, R. C., Reid, J., Holton, D. et al (1980) The glyceryl (^{14}C) tripalmitate breath test: a reassessment. *Clinica Chimica Acta,* **103,** 317-323.

Sturman, J. A., Hepner, G. W., Hofmann, A. F. & Thomas, P. G. (1975) Metabolism of [^{35}S] taurine in man. *Journal of Nutrition,* **105,** 1206-1214.

Tadesse, K. & Eastwood, M. (1977) Breath-hydrogen test and smoking. *Lancet,* **ii,** 91.

Tolbert, B. M. & Cozetto, F. J. (1964) Respiration studies of substrate oxidation in man. *Proceedings of a symposium held at the Oak Ridge Institute of Nuclear Studies, October 21-25, 1963,* 107-133.

Toskes, P. P., King, C. E., Spivey, J. C. & Lorenz, E. (1978) Xylose catabolism in the experimental rat blind loop syndrome. Studies including use of a newly-developed D-[^{14}C]-xylose breath test. *Gastroenterology,* **74,** 691-697.

Tillman, R. T., King, C. E. & Toskes, P. P. (1981) Continued experience with the xylose breath test: evidence that the small bowel culture as the gold standard for bacterial overgrowth may be tarnished. *Gastroenterology,* **80,** 1304.

Watkins, J. B., Klein, P. D., Schoeller, D. A. et al (1982) Diagnosis and differentiation of fat malabsorption in children using ^{13}C-labelled lipids: trioctanoin, triolein, and palmitic acid breath tests. *Gastroenterology,* **82,** 911-917.

Watson, W. S., McKenzie, I., Holden, R. J. et al (1980) An evaluation of the ^{14}C-glycocholic acid breath test in the diagnosis of bacterial colonisation of the jejunum. *Scottish Medical Journal,* **25,** 27-32.

Winchell, H. S., Stahelin, H., Kusubov, N. et al (1970) Kinetics of CO_2-HCO_3 in normal adult males. *Journal of Nuclear Medicine,* **11,** 711-715.

Index

Note: Page numbers of article titles are in **bold** type